Diagnosis and Treatment of
Pituitary Tumors

Diagnosis and Treatment of
Pituitary Tumors

Proceedings of a Conference Sponsored jointly by the National
Institute of Child Health and Human Development and the National
Cancer Institute in Bethesda, Md., January 15–17, 1973

Editors: PETER O. KOHLER, M.D.
Professor of Medicine,
Baylor College of Medicine, Houston, Tex.

GRIFF T. ROSS, M.D, Ph.D.,
Clinical Director,
National Institute of Child Health and Development, Bethesda, Md.

 1973

Excerpta Medica Amsterdam
American Elsevier Publishing Co., Inc. New York

International Congress Series No. 303

ISBN Excerpta Medica 90 219 0245 1
ISBN American Elsevier 0 444 15098 6
Library of Congress Catalog Card Number 73-88894

Publisher: Excerpta Medica
335 Jan van Galenstraat
Amsterdam
P. O. Box 1126

Sole Distributors for the USA and Canada:
American Elsevier Publishing Company, Inc.
52 Vanderbilt Avenue
New York, N. Y. 10017

Printed in The Netherlands by Drukkerij Dijkstra Niemeyer bv, Groningen

Preface

The management of patients with actual or suspected pituitary tumors has frequently been frustrating to clinicians. The extent of the work-up varies from institution to institution. The criteria for initiation of therapy may be strictly ophthalmologic or radiographic. Furthermore, many modalities for therapy have been used. None of these has seemed completely and uniformly successful, and the choice of a treatment modality frequently appears to be governed by local expertise alone. There have been no large series comparing the newer surgical and X-ray treatment techniques.

To collect the existing data regarding pituitary tumors, a committee of NIH physicians was formed to plan a symposium at which experts in the area of diagnosis and treatment could present their accumulated experiences. The members were:

G. DiCHIRO   *Head, Section on Neuroradiology*
                  National Institute of Neurological Diseases & Stroke

B. HATHAWAY   *Chief, Dept. of Diagnostic Radiology, Clinical Center*

M. LIPSETT   *Associate Scientific Director (RB), OSD*
                  National Institute of Child Health and Human Development

P. KOHLER   *Head, Endocrinology Service*
                  National Institute of Child Health and Human Development

A. RABSON   *Deputy Chief of Laboratory of Pathology*
                  National Cancer Institute

C. KUPFER   *Director, National Eye Institute*

G. ROSS   *Clinical Director*
                  National Institute of Child Health and Human Development

K. LAMOUREUX   *Radiation Branch*
                  National Cancer Institute

J. VAN BUREN   *Chief, Surgical Neurology Branch*
                  National Institute of Neurological Diseases and Stroke

In planning this symposium, the Organizing Committee had three basic objectives:

1. To summarize the present status of the art and science of diagnosing and treating human pituitary tumors.
2. To critically evaluate the results obtained among patients treated by experts using each of the several methods and to compare these results.
3. To define areas requiring further investigation.

N. I. Berlin, Director, Division of Cancer Biology and Diagnosis, National Cancer Institute, and C. U. Lowe, Scientific Director (OSD), National Institute of Child Health and Human Development, agreed with the committee's impression that these were laudable objectives and provided financial support for the meeting. Local arrangements for the conduct of the meeting were made by Mrs. M. Lebowitz, Office of Associate Director for Program Services, National Institute of Child Health and Human Development.

The following text consists of the data presented at the conference and the discussions. The manuscripts are in the style of the authors. A section on patient management has been included to allow proponents of various diagnostic techniques and therapeutic approaches to express their views. The final summary is a brief critique on the accomplishments on the conference with a comment on the need for further studies.

October 8, 1973   PETER O. KOHLER
Bethesda, Md.   GRIFF T. ROSS

Participants

Dr. Erik Olof Backlund
Department of Neurosurgery
Karolinska Sjukhuset
104 01 Stockholm 60
Sweden

Dr. H. L. Baker Jr
Consultant in Radiology
Mayo Clinic
Associate Professor in Radiology
Mayo Medical School
Rochester, Minnesota 55901

Dr. Ulrich Batzdorf
Associate Professor
Dept. of Surgery/Neurosurgery
UCLA School of Medicine
760 Westwood Plaza
Los Angeles, California 90024

Dr. John R. Bentson
Assistant Professor
Department of Radiology
UCLA School of Medicine
760 Westwood Plaza
Los Angeles, California 90024

Dr. John J. Canary
Professor of Medicine
Georgetown University Hospital
Washington, D.C. 20007

Dr. Claude Y. Chong
Radiotherapist
Donner Laboratory
Lawrence Berkeley Laboratory
University of California
Berkeley, California 94720

Dr. William H. Daughaday
Professor of Medicine
Director, Metabolism Division
Washington University School of
    Medicine
660 South Euclid Avenue
St. Louis, Missouri 63110

Dr. Michael D. F. Deck
Associate Professor of Radiology
Division of Neuroradiology
New York Hospital-Cornell Medical
    Center
525 East 68th Street
New York, New York 10021

Dr. Giovanni DiChiro
Head, Neuroradiology Section
National Institute of Neurological
    Diseases and Stroke
Bethesda, Maryland 20014

Dr. Kenneth M. Earle
Chief, Neuropathology Branch
Armed Forces Institute of Pathology
Washington, D. C. 20305

Dr. Charles A. Fager
Chairman, Department of Neurosurgery
Lahey Clinic Foundation
605 Commonwealth Avenue
Boston, Massachusetts 02215

Dr. Andrew G. Frantz
Associate Professor
Department of Medicine
Presbyterian Hospital
630 West 168th Street
New York, New York 10032

Dr. Russell Fraser
Professor, Royal Postgraduate Medical
School
University of London
Ducane Road
London W12, OHS England

Dr. Henry G. Friesen
Professor and Chairman
Department of Physiology
University of Manitoba
Winnipeg, Manitoba
R3EOW3,
Canada

Dr. Philip Gorden
Senior Investigator
National Institute of Arthritis, Me-
tabolism and Digestive Diseases
Bethesda, Maryland 20014

Dr. Gerard Guiot
Professor
Department of Neurosurgery
Hospital Foch
40, Rue Worth 92
Suresnes,
France

Dr. J. Jules Hardy
Professor of Neurosurgery
Faculty of Medicine
University of Montreal
Department of Neurosurgery
Notre Dame Hospital
1560 Sherbrooke Street E.
Montreal 133, P. Q.,
Canada

Dr. Robert W. Hollenhorst
Consultant in Ophthalmology
Mayo Clinic
Professor of Ophthalmology
Mayo Graduate School of Medicine
University of Minnesota
Rochester, Minnesota 55901

Dr. Melvin Horwith
Associate Professor of Medicine
Cornell University Medical School
1300 York Avenue
New York, New York 10021

Dr. William E. Hoyt
Professor of Neurology, Neurosurgery
and Ophthalmology
University of California Medical Center
San Francisco, California 94143

Dr. Benjamin Kaufman
Professor of Radiology
Department of Radiology
Case Western Reserve University
Cleveland, Ohio 44106

Dr. Raymond N. Kjellberg
Associate Clinical Professor of Surgery
Harvard Medical School
Visiting Neurosurgeon
Department of Neurology
Massachusetts General Hospital
Boston, Massachusetts 02114

Dr. Bernard Kliman
Associate Professor of Medicine
Harvard Medical School
Associate in Medicine
Department of Endocrinology
Massachusetts General Hospital
Boston, Massachusetts 02114

Dr. Simon Kramer
Professor and Chairman
Department of Radiation Therapy
Jefferson Medical College
Philadelphia, Pennsylvania 19107

Dr. Dorothy T. Krieger
Associate Professor of Medicine
Mt. Sinai School of Medicine
1 East 100th Street
New York, New York 10029

Dr. Howard E. Kulin
Associate Professor of Pediatrics
Head, Division of Pediatric Endo-
crinology
Hershey School of Medicine
Hershey, Pennsylvania 17033

Dr. Ann M. Lawrence
Professor of Medicine
Pritzker School of Medicine
University of Chicago Hospital
850 East 59th Street
Chicago, Illinois 60637

Dr. John H. Lawrence
  Regent, University of California
  And Director (Emeritus)
  Donner Laboratories
  Berkeley, California 94720

Dr. Harold E. Lebovitz
  Professor of Medicine
  Duke University Medical Center
  Durham, North Carolina 27710

Dr. Seymour Levin
  Assistant Professor of Medicine
  UCLA School of Medicine
  Chief, Metabolic Unit
  Wadsworth Veterans Administration
  Hospital
  Los Angeles, California 90073

Dr. John A. Linfoot
  Physician in Charge
  Donner Pavillion
  Cowell Memorial Hospital
  University of California
  and Research Associate
  Donner Laboratories
  at Berkeley
  Berkeley, California 94720

Dr. Collin S. MacCarty
  Chairman and Consultant
  Department of Neurosurgery
  Mayo Clinic
  Professor of Neurosurgery
  Mayo Medical School
  Rochester, Minnesota 55901

Dr. Robert S. Mecklenburg
  Staff Fellow
  Division of Endocrinology
  Department of Medicine
  University of Washington Hospital
  Seattle, Washington 98105

Dr. Gordon L. Noel
  Staff Fellow
  Department of Endocrinology and
    Metabolism
  Walter Reed Army Institute of Research
  Washington, D. C. 20012

Dr. William D. Odell
  Chairman, Department of Medicine
  Harbor General Hospital
  Professor of Physiology
  UCLA School of Medicine
  Torrance, California 90509

Dr. Ayub K. Ommaya
  Deputy Chief, Surgical Neurology
    Branch
  Head, Applied Research
  National Institute of Neurological
    Diseases and Stroke
  Bethesda, Maryland 20014

Dr. David N. Orth
  Director of Cancer Center
  Professor of Medicine, Endocrinology
  Department of Medicine
  Vanderbilt University
  Nashville, Tennessee 37203

Dr. Olof Pearson
  Professor of Medicine
  Case Western Reserve University
  2065 Adelbert Road
  Cleveland, Ohio 44106

Dr. Robert W. Rand
  Professor of Neurological Surgery
  UCLA School of Medicine
  760 Westwood Plaza
  Los Angeles, California 90024

Dr. Raymond Randall
  Head of a Section and
    Consultant, Division of Endocrinology
  Mayo Clinic
  Professor of Medicine
  Mayo Medical School
  Rochester, Minnesota 55901

Dr. Alan Robinson
  Assistant Professor of Medicine
  Division of Endocrinology and
    Metabolism
  Department of Medicine
  University of Pittsburgh
  Pittsburgh, Pennsylvania 15213

Dr. Jesse Roth
Chief, Diabetes Section
Clinical Endocrinology Branch
National Institute of Arthritis,
Metabolism and Digestive Diseases
Bethesda, Maryland 20014

Dr. Glenn E. Sheline
Professor and Vice-Chairman
Department of Radiology
University of California Medical Center
San Francisco, California 94143

Dr. Richard J. Sherins
Senior Investigator
Reproduction Research Branch
National Institute of Child Health and
Human Development
Bethesda, Maryland 20014

Dr. Barry Sherman
Assistant Professor of Internal Medicine
University of Iowa Hospital and Clinics
Iowa City, Iowa 52240

Dr. George Udvarhelyi
Professor of Neurosurgery
Johns Hopkins University
Baltimore, Maryland 21205

Dr. John M. Van Buren
Acting Clinical Director, IR
National Institute of Neurological
Diseases and Stroke
Bethesda, Maryland 20014

Dr. Nicholas T. Zervas
Associate Professor of Surgery
Harvard Medical School
Beth Israel Hospital
Boston, Massachusetts 02215

Contents

V. Radiation Treatment of Pituitary Tumors

A. Conventional radiation therapy

B. Heavy particle radiation therapy

VI. Miscellaneous Ablative Procedures for Pituitary Adenomas

VII. Medical Treatment of Pituitary Tumors

I. Pathology, pathogenesis, and endocrine evaluation

Pathology of adenomas of the pituitary gland*

KENNETH M. EARLE and SAMUEL H. DILLARD, Jr

Neuropathology Branch, Armed Forces Institute of Pathology, Washington, D.C., U.S.A.

When the clinical history, X-ray and operative findings, and histologic pattern are compatible with an adenoma of the pituitary, the diagnosis can be confirmed with ordinary histologic techniques with a high degree of accuracy. The diagnosis may be difficult when the biopsy is: (a) from the coverings of the tumor, (b) complicated by hemorrhages or necrosis, (c) altered by surgical compression, freezing or coagulation, (d) small or from a tumor that has been irradiated, frozen or previously biopsied.

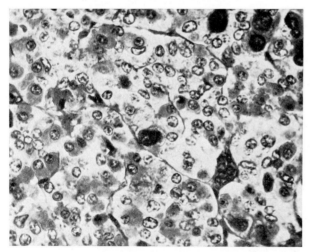

Fig. 1. Normal pituitary showing three types of cell: the large dark cells are basophilic; the middle size cells with lighter cytoplasm are eosinophilic; the small cells with few or no granules in the cytoplasm are chromophobe. H&E stain, ×275, AFIP Neg. 72-8386.

Even when the biopsy is adequate and unaltered, the differential diagnosis between chromophobe adenoma and acidophilic adenoma may be difficult. Secretory granules undergo autolysis so rapidly[1, 2, 3, 4, 7] that good fixation and differential staining is necessary in order to observe these granules by light microscopy (Fig. 1). The cytoplasm of a chromophobe cell will often

---

* The opinions or assertions contained herein are the private views of the authors and are not to be construed as official or as reflecting the views of the Department of the Army or the Department of Defense.

stain a bright red color with hematoxylin and eosin even though the PAS-orange G, iron-PAS, and aldehyde thionine fail to confirm the presence of secretory granules. [6, 9, 10, 19] This discrepancy has led to the diagnosis of 'acidophilic adenomas' without acromegaly or gigantism and, conversely, to 'chromophobe adenomas' occurring in acromegalics.

In the past, when a biopsy of a pituitary adenoma in an acromegalic revealed the features of a chromophobe adenoma, we reasoned that the tumor had been originally an acidophilic adenoma and that pressure effects had caused the eosinophilic cells to degranulate.[5] We are now persuaded that some *chromophobe* adenomas, without definite secretory granules by light microscopy, secrete hormones and may cause acromegaly. Electron micrographs of well fixed biopsies of chromophobe adenomas have shown a few secretory granules in most of the cells of any chromophobe adenoma, even though the cells appeared to be strictly chromophobes by light microscopy.[8, 15–18] The statement has been made recently that there are no such cells as chromophobes, since nearly all chromophobe cells show at least a few secretory granules by electron microscopy of well fixed specimens.[8]

Asymptomatic adenomas of all types have been reported to occur in approximately 25 % of all pituitary glands. Kernohan and Sayre[5] report adenomas in 225 of 1000 normal pituitary glands, of which 52.8 % were chromophobic, 7.5 % eosinophilic and 27.2 % basophilic. Some degree of adenomatous hyperplasia can be found in almost every pituitary gland.

Chromophobe adenomas

Chromophobe adenomas are by far the most common type of pituitary adenoma (if you accept the definition of light microscopy). They tend to occur in adults, to grow slowly and to enlarge the sella turcica in a downward and lateral direction before they emerge through the dural roof to press upon the optic chiasm and protrude into the third ventricle.[5, 12, 13] Rarely, they will grow outside the sella and cause a large suprasellar mass without any enlargement of the sella turcica. In other cases, massive erosion of the floor of the skull has been seen. The combination of expansion above and into the sella is the most common biological behavior. Some of these tumors enlarge laterally into the region of the limen insulae; rarely, they become so large laterally that they may appear to the surgeon to be a

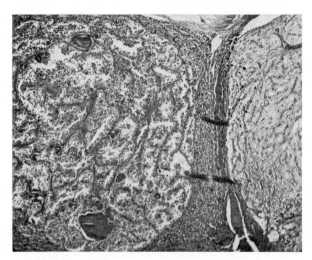

Fig. 2 Chromophobe adenoma, incidental finding at autopsy. Note lobular pattern and focal mineralization. H&E stain, ×40, AFIP Neg. 72-8397.

tumor of the temporal lobe. In some cases the tumor protrudes into the frontal lobe. Grossly, it appears to be a multilobulated, more or less encapsulated tumor composed of moderately firm or soft grayish tissue with many small vascular channels. Areas of recent and old hemorrhage are common and cystic changes may result and may grossly resemble a cranio-pharyngioma. As stated previously, small chromophobe adenomas are common incidental findings at autopsy (Fig. 2).

The most common histologic pattern in hematoxylin and eosin (H&E) preparations con-sists of masses of uniformly small cells with round to oval nuclei, irregular chromatin, and either absent nucleoli or one or more small nucleoli. The cytoplasm is scanty and frequently the cell boundaries are poorly defined. In H&E stains, the cytoplasm stains red and the nuclei stain blue, but no definite intracytoplasmic granules are visible. The stroma consists of many thin-walled capillaries that separate the tumor cells into irregular globoid masses. The endothelium of the vessels appears to be swollen in many areas. This is the so-called 'endocrine pattern' that we expect to see in well preserved tumors. Areas of necrosis, prob-ably due to infarction, are common in slowly growing as well as in rapidly growing types. Spontaneous hemorrhage (so-called 'pituitary apoplexy') occurs in about 1 % of cases and may be the first sign.

With the trauma of surgical biopsy and other secondary changes, the characteristic pattern is frequently not present and we are presented with a few masses of relatively small, poorly stained cells slightly larger than mononuclear cells of the blood with no definite stroma or

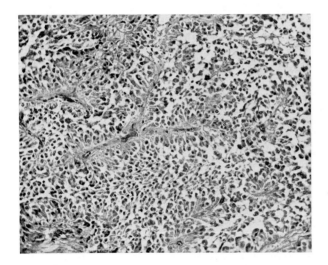

Fig. 3 Chromophobe adenoma. Perivascular pseudorosette pattern resembling ependymoma. H&E stain, × 100, AFIP Neg. 72-8059.

pattern. Such biopsies are inadequate but we usually record that they are 'compatible with but not diagnostic of' a chromophobe adenoma.

Other histologic patterns include (*a*) a perivascular pseudorosette pattern resembling ependymomas (Figs. 3 and 4), (*b*) a pattern of small cells with halos around the nucleus resembling oligodendrogliomas (Figs. 5 and 6), and (*c*) compact masses of cells with a ten-dency to whorl and with considerable intercellular collagen resembling a meningioma. Such patterns have been described as papillary, diffuse, and sinusoidal types. In some cases there is a bimodal cell type consisting of larger cells mixed with smaller ones. In other cases the cells forming a perivascular pattern are small and dark with scanty cytoplasm. This variant is termed 'fetal adenoma' which is a misnomer since it does not resemble the developing pituitary gland. The differential diagnosis between chromophobe adenoma, ependymoma, oligodendroglioma, and meningioma would not ordinarily be difficult with large biopsies or with optimum fixation, but it is a constantly recurring problem with the ordinary biopsies that we receive in the laboratory.

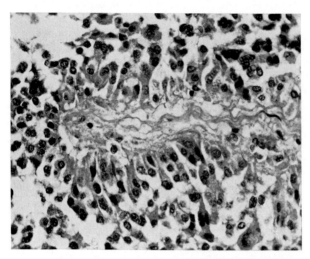

Fig. 4   Chromophobe adenoma. Higher power view of Fig. 3 showing perivascular pseudorosette pattern resembling ependymoma. H&E stain, ×275, AFIP Neg. 72-8064.

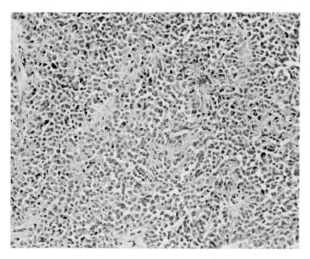

Fig. 5   Chromophobe adenoma. Masses of cells with scanty cytoplasm resembling oligodendroglioma. AFIP Neg. 72-8060.

Rarely, in small biopsies, a granuloma or other chronic inflammatory process may be difficult to differentiate from a chromophobe adenoma. Biopsies of chromophobe adenomas frequently contain portions of the posterior hypophysis that may be mistaken for a glioma. Portions of the pars intermedia containing glandular structures may resemble an adenocarcinoma.

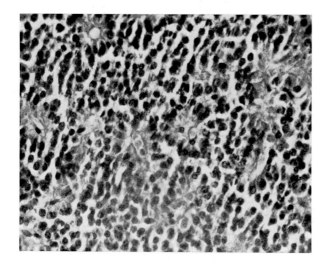

Fig. 6 Chromophobe adenoma. Masses of small cells with scanty cytoplasm and a tendency toward perivascular arrangement. H&E stain, ×275, AFIP Neg. 72-8392.

The type of adenoma that imitates the perivascular pseudorosette pattern of an ependymoma is called the sinusoidal or papillary type. These types are often mixed. The cells have elongated cytoplasms that radiate around small blood vessels in a pseudorosette pattern. In some planes of section, the anatomy of the blood vessel may not be completely visible and the pattern resembles the Homer–Wright type of rosette that is seen in medulloblastomas and retinoblastomas. The histologic type does not seem to influence the prognosis of a chromophobe adenoma. Rapid growth, invasion, mitoses, and pleomorphism are more reliable criteria of malignancy than the histologic pattern.

In summary, the diagnosis of a chromophobe adenoma is not difficult if a well fixed, undistorted biopsy of reasonable size can be obtained. Biopsies of the coverings of the neoplasm, changes produced by hemorrhage, necrosis, previous biopsy, radiation or infection can conspire to make the diagnosis difficult or impossible. Various patterns may be encountered, including patterns resembling ependymoma, oligodendroglioma or meningioma. Special stains and better material may be required in order to resolve the differential diagnosis.

Malignant adenomas and carcinoma of the pituitary

The terms 'malignant adenoma' or 'primary carcinoma' of the pituitary are very rarely justified. In fact, the distinction between an ordinary chromophobe adenoma and a 'malignant adenoma' or 'carcinoma' is somewhat arbitrary. We are reluctant to classify pituitary adenomas as 'malignant' or 'carcinomatous' on the basis of nuclear pleomorphism alone. In our experience, nuclear pleomorphism with infrequent mitoses is common in many of the slowly growing adenomas. Invasion of adjacent structures may be found in slowly growing adenomas as well as in rapidly growing ones. Adenomas that recur may subsequently tend to grow more rapidly than the original history would suggest and such cases are considered to have transformed into a malignant neoplasm (Fig. 7). Some invasive chromophobe adenomas appear to be carcinomatous at first operation by virtue of widespread invasion of the floor of the skull and anaplastic histologic features.

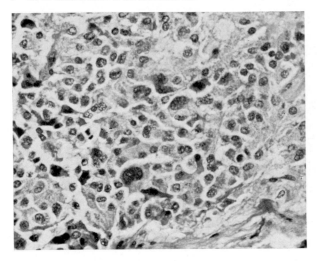

Fig. 7 Chromophobe adenoma, recurrent after surgery. Note marked nuclear pleomorphism. H&E stain, ×275, AFIP Neg. 72-8062.

In summary, the terms malignant adenoma or primary carcinoma of the pituitary are not often applicable, especially at the time of initial biopsy, but a few chromophobe adenomas invade the floor of the skull, grow rapidly, and show the usual anaplastic features of malignancy. Variations in the size, mode of spread and invasiveness of chromophobe adenomas are common but are not always correlated with the histologic evidence of malignancy.

Eosinophilic adenomas

Biopsies of actively secreting eosinophilic adenomas are rarely received by the pathologist even in cases of gigantism or acromegaly, for two important reasons. Until recently such adenomas were not biopsied in the majority of cases, therapy being given on the basis of clinical data and X-ray findings only. Secondly, when they were biopsied, they were usually 'burned out' (degranulated) by their own compression, or by X-ray or other means of therapy. In the past, relatively few biopsies of eosinophilic adenomas (Fig. 8), in which many secretory granules could be demonstrated by H&E or by special stains, have been submitted to us by neurosurgeons who felt that surgical removal was the treatment of choice or that histologic confirmation was desirable prior to therapy. X-ray therapy alone had been used in most of our cases.

In cases in which a biopsy is taken months or years after other forms of therapy, it is common to find no definite secretory granules by light microscopy. These are presumably the degranulated types of eosinophilic adenomas that appear to be chromophobe adenomas. We have seen some unhappy reactions when a pathologist reports one of these cases as chromophobe adenoma in an obviously acromegalic patient. Grossly, eosinophilic adenomas usually expand at the expense of the sella turcica, and seldom extend far above the sella as chromophobe adenomas are prone to do. Small eosinophilic adenomas tend to be located in one or the other lateral lobes of the pituitary.

In summary, in the past, eosinophilic adenomas were infrequently biopsied by craniotomy prior to X-ray therapy. When the biopsy was taken after therapy, the secretory granules may have disappeared and the remaining cells may show only the features of chromophobes. Electron microscopic evidence of secretory granules in chromophobe cells suggests that

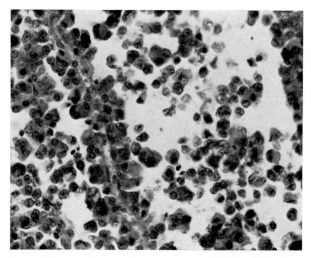

Fig. 8 Surgical biopsy of an actively secreting eosinophilic adenoma. Many secretory granules can be seen in the cytoplasm of the cells. H&E stain, ×275, AFIP Neg. 72-8394.

some cases of acromegaly may be produced by adenomas that show the characteristics of chromophobe cells by light microscopy. In the future, with the increasing use of the intranasal approach and microsurgery, we can expect to receive more biopsies from actively secreting eosinophilic adenomas than we have in the past.

Basophilic adenomas

These adenomas are usually small and do not enlarge the sella turcica. They are usually found incidentally at autopsy. Histologically they consist of masses of large cells containing intracytoplasmic basophilic granules. The nuclei are moderately pleomorphic and often

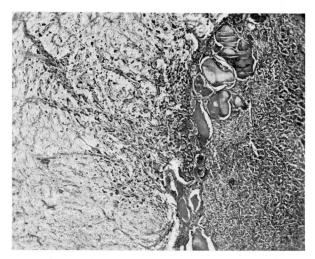

Fig. 9 Basophilic invasion of the posterior lobe (left side of picture) in an elderly person. H&E stain, ×40, AFIP Neg. 72-8398.

obscured by the granules. True adenomas show signs of compression of adjacent parenchyma but no erosion of bone. If there is no evidence of compression of adjacent structure by irregular enlarged masses of basophiles, they are considered to be 'adenomatous hyperplasia' and not true adenomas.[13] Both basophilic adenomas and adenomatous hyperplasia are common incidental findings at autopsy. In elderly people, so-called basophilic invasion of the posterior lobe (Fig. 9) is very frequently an incidental finding at autopsy.

By using special stains and rapid fixation of good material, the basophilic cell can be differentiated into several sub-types[9] but this differentiation serves no useful purpose in most surgical cases and autopsy material is notoriously poor for the staining of secretory granules that is necessary to make the differential diagnosis. The sub-types have been designated as beta 1, beta 2, delta 1, delta 2 cells or as MSH and ACTH-O-cyte, TSH-O-cyte, LH-O-cyte and FSH-O-cyte.[9, 10]

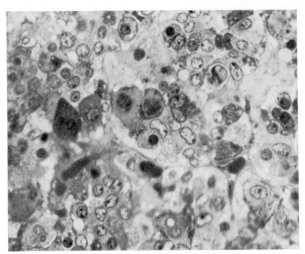

Fig. 10   Crooke's hyaline change. The two large cells in the center of the photograph show the hyaline material in a perinuclear location. H&E stain, ×275, AFIP Neg. 72-8387.

In cases of Cushing's syndrome we look for Crooke's hyaline change (Fig. 10) which is an intracytoplasmic accumulation of basophilic hyaline material displacing secretory granules.[9, 13, 14] The hyaline material usually accumulates in the perinuclear zone first and gradually increases to replace all the granules in some cells. Presumably this hyaline material is induced in some way by high levels of circulatory exogenous or endogenous corticosteroids, but it is not common practice to try to distinguish between MSH, ACTH, TSH, LH and FSH secreting cells in surgical biopsy material as a routine procedure. Ultrastructurally Crooke's change is composed of fine filaments[17] that do not give a positive reaction for ACTH by immunologic staining procedures.

Statistical studies from the files of the Armed Forces Institute of Pathology

The Automatic Data Processing Service of the Armed Forces Institute of Pathology, in collaboration with the authors, reviewed the records of 941 cases in which the diagnosis of an adenoma of the pituitary had been made by surgical biopsy, at autopsy, or both. All were chromophobe adenomas except 18, which were eosinophilic adenomas. The authors confirmed the diagnosis on the symptomatic cases by review of the slides.

The Armed Forces Institute of Pathology receives cases from all the Armed Services of the USA, from the Veterans Administration Hospitals, and from civilian hospitals upon request and within the limits of their resources. The source of referral is reflected by the preponderance of males in this study.

Some of the tables contain fewer cases than the total because the pertinent information was absent in some of the records.

Table I   *Type of case*

Type of case	Total	Percent
Total	941	100.0
Incidental	487	51.8
Symptomatic	454	48.2

The term 'incidental' means that the adenoma was an unexpected finding at autopsy and no symptoms were recorded. The number of 'incidental' adenomas is deceivingly small because incidental adenomas of the pituitary are so common that many pathologists do not record them routinely as a significant diagnosis. Those that were diagnosed in this series were probably larger than usual.

Table II   *Symptomatic adenomas: sex*

Sex	Total	Percent
Total	448	100.0
Male	333	74.3
Female	115	25.7

The marked preponderance of males in this series reflects the fact that most of these cases were referred from military or veterans' hospitals. Other studies show only a slight preponderance in males.

Table III   *Symptomatic adenomas: race*

Race	Total	Percent
Total	418	100.0*
White	353	84.4
Negro	57	13.6
American Indian	1	0.2
Other	7	1.7

* Percentages do not add to 100.0 due to rounding. No clear preponderance by race emerged from this study.

Table IV   *Symptomatic adenomas: age at time of diagnosis*

Age (years)	Total	Percent
Total	443	100.0
0– 9.9	—	—
10–19.9	19	4.3
20–29.9	59	13.3
30–39.9	100	22.6
40–49.9	91	20.5
50–59.9	86	19.4
60–69.9	69	15.6
70–79.9	18	4.1
80 and over	1	0.2
Oldest 81 yrs		
Youngest 13 yrs		
Range 68 yrs		
Mean 44.9 yrs		
Median 43.0 yrs		

These figures agree with other studies showing that the peak incidence is between 30 and 50 years.

Table V   *Symptomatic adenomas: size*

Size (cm)	Total	Percent
Total	103	100.0*
Less than 1	4	3.9
1–1.9	18	17.5
2–2.9	11	10.7
3–3.9	21	20.4
4–4.9	19	18.4
5–5.9	11	10.7
6–6.9	6	5.8
7–7.9	6	5.8
8–8.9	2	1.9
9–9.9	2	1.9
10 and over	3	2.9

Largest size	$11.5 \times 9.5 \times 6.8$ cm (weight 325 g)
Smallest size	0.50 cm
Range	11.0 cm
Mean	4.875 cm
Median	3.500 cm

* Percentages do not add to 100.0 due to rounding.
This table shows that most of the symptomatic adenomas are more than 1 cm in diameter and that some grow to a very large size. Compare this table with Table XIII showing the size of the incidental adenomas in this series. The largest incidental (presumably asymptomatic) adenoma was 12 cm in diameter.

Table VI   *Duration of preoperative signs and/or symptoms*

Duration (months)	Total	Percent
Total	306	100.0*
0– 11.9	126	41.2
12– 23.9	51	16.7
24– 35.9	38	12.4
36– 47.9	20	6.5
48– 59.9	13	4.2
60– 71.9	13	4.2
72– 83.9	11	3.6
84– 95.9	7	2.3
96–107.9	6	2.0
108–119.9	5	1.6
120 and over	16	5.2

Longest duration	300.0 months
Shortest duration	0.03 months
Range	299.97 months
Mean	31.3 months
Median	14.0 months

* Percentages do not add to 100.0 due to rounding.
This table indicates that the diagnosis will be made in most cases within 1 or 2 years after the onset of symptoms, but a significant number will wait several years before diagnosis.

Table VII *Males with impotence*

Impotence	Total	Percent
Total	322	100.0
Impotence	17	5.3
No impotence recorded	305	94.7

Impotence in our series was recorded only 17 times in males in those cases where the history indicated that the question had been raised. This may be an underestimation of the frequency of decreased libido or impotence.

Table VIII *Women with amenorrhea*

Amenorrhea	Total	Percent
Total	113	100.0
Amenorrhea	48	42.5
No amenorrhea recorded	65	57.5

Amenorrhea was recorded in less than half of the cases in which the history indicated that the question had been asked.

Table IX *X-ray findings (incidence)*

X-ray findings	Total	Percent
Total	245	—
Ballooning of sella turcica	218	89.0
Erosion of sella turcica	104	42.4
Involvement of surrounding structure	7	2.8

Ballooning of the sella was clearly the most common finding in those cases in which the X-ray reports were available.

Table X *Type of treatment*

Treatment	Total	Percent
Total	406	100.0
Radiation	31	7.6
Surgery only	235	57.9
Surgery and radiation	74	18.2
No treatment	66	16.3

The preponderance of surgery as the major type of treatment is probably due to the fact that only 18 cases in this series were eosinophilic adenomas and all the rest were chromophobe adenomas. Most of the cases of eosinophilic adenoma were treated with radiation alone.

Table XI   *Duration from diagnosis to last known status*

Duration (years)	Total	Percent
Total	262*	100.0**
Under 1	30	11.5
1–1.9	16	6.1
2–2.9	13	5.0
3–3.9	18	6.9
4–4.9	19	7.3
5–5.9	24	9.2
6–6.9	17	6.5
7–7.9	10	3.8
8–8.9	17	6.5
9–9.9	12	4.6
10 and over	86	32.8

Longest duration	38.33 yrs
Shortest duration	0.08 yrs
Range	38.25 yrs
Mean	8.57 yrs
Median	6.50 yrs

* Sixty-one cases with post-op of less than 1 month's duration were excluded from this table.
** Percentages do not add to 100.0 due to rounding.
See Table XII for the condition when last known. These 2 tables indicate the relatively good prognosis of pituitary adenomas, most of which were treated by surgery.

Table XII   *Last known status*

Status	Total	Percent
Total patients	432	100.0*
Alive, status of tumor unknown	97	22.5
Alive and well	42	9.7
Alive with recurrence	3	0.7
Dead, status of tumor unknown	6	1.4
Dead, no tumor or metastasis	2	0.5
Dead with recurrence or metastasis	5	1.2
Dead with tumor	277	64.1

* Percentages do not add to 100.0 due to rounding.
Although follow-up was obtained in only slightly more than half the cases, the relatively good prognosis is obvious.

Table XIII   *Size of tumor: incidental cases*

Size (cm)	Number	Percent
Total	26	100.0*
1–1.9	3	11.5
2–2.9	5	19.2
3–3.9	8	30.8
4–4.9	2	7.7
5–5.9	4	15.4
6–6.9	2	7.7
7–7.9	—	—

(*Table XIII cont.*)

8–8.9	1	3.8
9–9.9	—	—
10 and over	1	3.8

Largest	12.0	cm**
Smallest	1.0	cm
Range	11.0	cm
Mean	3.881	cm
Median	3.0	cm

---

* Percentages do not add to 100.0 due to rounding.
** Only one dimension (no weight) recorded.

The surprising finding in this series of adenomas found incidentally was the large size of a few of the presumably asymptomatic cases. Only the incidental adenomas over 1 cm in size were recorded in this series.

Summary

The anatomic pathology of chromophobe, eosinophilic and basophilic adenomas is reviewed. Growth is considered in relation to histologic features. Statistical studies of 454 symptomatic and 487 incidental adenomas of the pituitary are reported. The problems encountered in the differential diagnosis of an adenoma of the pituitary are reviewed.

Acknowledgments

The authors are indebted to Dr. William F. McCormick and Dr. Sidney S. Schochet for the loan of histologic preparations during work on this manuscript.

References

(1) BERGLAND, R. M. and TORACK, R. M. (1969): An ultrastructural study of follicular cells in the human anterior pituitary. *Amer. J. Path.*, *57*, 273.

(2) EZRIN, C. and MURRAY, S. (1963): The cells of the human adenohypophysis in pregnancy, thyroid disease, and adrenal cortical disorders. In: *Cytologie de l'Adénohypophyse*, pp. 183–201. Editors: J. Benoit and C. Da Lage. Centre National de la Recherche Scientifique, Paris.

(3) HALMI, N. S., MCCORMICK, W. F. and DECKER, D. A. (1971): The natural history of hyalinization of ACTH-MSH cells in man. *Arch. Path.*, *91*, 318.

(4) HALMI, N. S. and MCCORMICK, W. F. (1969): The delta cell of the human hypophysis in childhood. *J. clin. Endocr.*, *29*, 1036.

(5) KERNOHAN, J. W. and SAYRE, G. P. (1956): Tumors of the pituitary gland and infundibulum. In: *Atlas of Tumor Pathology*, *1st Series*. Fascicle 36, Armed Forces Institute of Pathology, Washington, D.C.

(6) KRAUS, E. J. (1926): The hypophysis. In: *Handbuch der speziellen pathologischen Anatomie und Histologie, Vol. 8*. Editors: F. Henke and O. Lubarsch. Springer, Berlin.

(7) MCCORMICK, W. F. and HALMI, N. S. (1970): The hypophysis with coma dépassé (respiratory brain). *Amer. J. clin. Path.*, *54*, 374.

(8) MCCORMICK, W. F. and HALMI, N. S. (1971): Absence of chromophobe adenomas from a large series of pituitary tumors. *Arch. Path.*, *92*, 231.

(9) NETTER, F. H. and FORSHAM, P. H. (1965): In: *The Ciba Collection of Medical Illustrations, Vol. 4*, pp. 10–11. Ciba Pharmaceutical Co., New York, N.Y.

(10) PAIZ, C. and HENNIGAR, G. R. (1970): Electron microscopy and histochemical correlation of human anterior pituitary cells. *Amer. J. Path.*, *59*, 43.

(11)   ROMEIS, B. (1940): Hypophyse. In: *Handbuch der microscopischen Anatomie des Menschen*, *Vol. 8/3*. Editor: W. von Möllendorff. Springer, Berlin.

(12)   RUBINSTEIN, L. J. (1972): Tumors of the central nervous system. In: *Atlas of Tumor Pathology*, *2nd Series*. Fascicle 6, Armed Forces Institute of Pathology, Washington, D.C.

(13)   RUSSELL, D. S. (1966): Pituitary gland (hypophysis). In: *Pathology, Vol. 20, 5th ed.*, pp. 1052–1073 Editor: W. A. D. Anderson. C. V. Mosby Co., St. Louis, Mo.

(14)   RUSSFIELD, A. B. (1968): Adenohypophysis. In: *Endocrine Pathology*. Editor: J. M. B. Bloodworth, Jr. Williams and Wilkins Co., Baltimore, Md.

(15)   SCHECHTER, J. (1972): Ultrastructural changes in the capillary bed of human pituitary tumors. *Amer. J. Path.*, *67*, 109.

(16)   SCHELIN, U. (1962): Chromophobe and acidophil adenomas of the human pituitary gland. a light and electron microscopic study. *Acta path. microbiol. scand.*, *Suppl. 158*, 5.

(17)   SCHOCHET, S. S., HALMI, N. S. and MCCORMICK, W. F. (1972): PAS-positive hyalin change in ACTH-MSH cells of man. *Arch. Path.*, *93*, 457.

(18)   SCHOCHET, S. S., MCCORMICK, W. F. and HALMI, N. S. (1972): Adenomas with intracytoplasmic aggregates. *Arch. Path.*, *94*, 16.

(19)   PHIFER, R. F., SPICER, S. S. and ORTH, D. N. (1970): Specific demonstration of the human hypophyseal cells which produce adrenocorticotropic hormone. *J. clin. Endocr.*, *31*, 347.

Table I (*b*)   *Most common early symptoms of pituitary tumor in 64 patients*

	No.
Headache	12
Amenorrhea	11
Decreased visual acuity	10
Decreased potentia	8
Decreased libido	7
Acromegaly	5

Table I (*c*)   *Most common presenting symptoms: 64 patients*

	No.
Decreased visual acuity	24
Decreased visual field	13
Headaches	9
Double vision	5
Fatigue	3
Incidental radiographic diagnosis	2

Endocrine related symptoms were analyzed in greater detail by 2 different approaches:

1. Evidence of pituitary target organ failure: if patients were grouped according to the presence of at least 1 or more symptoms of target organ failure, the incidence of such symptoms was as shown in Table II(*a*). Some patients provided a history of deficiency states of pituitary target organs, due to prior ablative surgery or extensive disease, which preceded other manifestations of an intrasellar tumor. These data are represented in Table II(*b*).

Table II (*a*)   *Evidence of pituitary target organ failure: one or more symptoms in 64 patients*

	No. of patients
Gonadal insufficiency	62
Thyroid insufficiency	53
Adrenal insufficiency	36

Table II (*b*)   *Pituitary target organ ablation or extensive disease*

	No. of patients
Oophorectomy	5
Disease of testes	3
Adrenalectomy	2
Thyroidectomy	0

2. Clinical syndromes of abnormal pituitary function: for purposes of this classification a scoring system* was applied jointly to symptoms and to findings on physical examination

---

* Available from the authors on request.

Patients exceeding a predetermined score were then grouped into different syndrome categories. These data are presented in Table III.

Table III   *Abnormal physical findings in 64 patients with pituitary tumor*

	%
Visual field defects	
Bilateral, all degrees	83
Unilateral, all degrees	5
Visual acuity impairment, distant vision	
Bilateral, all degrees	64
Unilateral, all degrees	23
Visual acuity impairment, near vision	
Bilateral, all degrees	45
Unilateral, all degrees	14
Optic atrophy	
Bilateral, all degrees	50
Unilateral, all degrees	16
Loss of hair, including thin brows	45
Skin dry, coarse and cool	30
Cranial nerve palsies (N. III, IV, VI), unilateral and bilateral combined	30
Testicular or uterine atrophy	28

3. Eight patients had, at some time in their history, developed symptoms thought to be due to acute hemorrhage into the pituitary tumor, or pituitary apoplexy. Seven of these patients had chromophobe adenomas and 1 had an eosinophilic tumor.

Physical examination

The most commonly encountered abnormal findings on physical examination are listed in Table III.

Endocrine symptoms

The method employed for obtaining the data for this tabulation is detailed above. Table IV provides the incidence of various types of endocrine abnormalities encountered in the group of patients under investigation.

Table IV   *Endocrine syndromes encountered in 64 patients operated on for pituitary tumor*

	Patients	Chromo-phobe	Mixed	Eosino-phile
Hypopituitarism:				
scored by history and findings	41	37	4	—
	(26)*	(23)	(3)	
Acromegaly: by findings	11	6	3	2
Nelson's syndrome	2	2		
Amenorrhea: by history	16			
assoc. with hypopituitarism	6	5	1	
assoc. with acromegaly	5	3	1	1
Galactorrhea: by history and/or findings	8	5	2	1
assoc. with amenorrhea	7			
ADH insufficiency: by history	9	9		

* The figures in parentheses are obtained when the minimum score required to establish the presence of hypopituitarism is raised by 1 point.

Diagnostic studies

The studies carried out on this group of patients reflect the procedures available and in general use at the time of the patient's hospitalization, and therefore do not necessarily represent the studies which would be performed today. In order to gain an impression of the usefulness of the studies in a group of patients known to have pituitary adenomas, the percentage of *abnormal* results was calculated for those studies carried out on at least 30 of the patients under investigation. The data are summarized in Table V. The table also shows that this group of patients included many with sizeable pituitary tumors. Some laboratory determinations showed good correlation with the pathological state of the patient, but were carried out in a smaller number of patients. These included plasma cortisol levels and adrenal stimulation tests, serum growth hormone determinations and glucose tolerance tests, the ratio of urine to serum osmolarity and the response to water loading.

Table V *Laboratory studies performed on 30 or more patients with pituitary tumors*

	No. of patients tested	% of abnormal results in all patients tested	No. of tested patients with large suprasellar tumor extension	No. of patients with large suprasellar extension showing abnormal lab. results
17-Ketosteroids, urinary	54	64.8	27	18
Follicle stimulating hormone, urine	45	57.8	17	14
Radioactive iodine uptake, 24 hours	39	56.4	16	14
Radioactive iodine uptake, 6 hours	36	50.0	14	10
17-Hydroxysteroids, urinary	51	39.2	9	7
17-Ketogenic steroids, urinary	30	30.0	5	4
Urine specific gravity	38	21.1	6	6
Protein bound iodine, serum	57	15.8	4	4
Sodium, serum	38	7.9	—	—
Protein, cerebrospinal fluid	36	66.7	16	16

Table VI *Radiological studies: 64 patients with pituitary tumor*

Sella on plain skull X-rays	Normal	Sella eroded and minimally enlarged	Sella eroded and significantly enlarged	Sella severely eroded		Study not performed
	(0)	(8)	(35)	(21)		(0)
Tumor size by pneumoencephalography	Normal	Sella enlarged; no suprasellar mass	Intrasellar mass; small suprasellar extension	Suprasellar extension exceeds intrasellar; no third ventricle distortion	Suprasellar extension with third ventricle distortion	
	(0)	(2)	(14)	(1)	(32)	(15)
Carotid angiography	Normal	Intrasellar mass	Intrasellar and suprasellar mass			
	(3)	(10)	(18)			(33)

Radiological studies carried out on this group of patients are summarized in Table VI. The classification of radiological abnormalities was described in a previous publication.[15]

Electroencephalography was routinely carried out on many of the patients in this study but this does not indicate that the patients necessarily had clinical seizure activity. The results of this study are summarized in Table VII. Diffuse EEG changes were seen most frequently in patients with tumors assessed by air encephalography as the largest, but other patients with tumors of similar size had normal electroencephalograms.

Table VII   *Preoperative electroencephalograms performed on 46 patients*

	No.	Patients with preop. seizures	Patients who had previous surgery
Normal study	20	—	1
Frontotemporal 5–7 cps slow wave activity	7	2	—
Focal frontal changes	5	—	3
Diffuse changes	14	2*	1*

* Patient common to both groups.

Surgical pathology

Cysts of various size were found at the time of surgery in 15 patients, including 13 associated with chromophobe adenomata and 1 each with a mixed and an eosinophilic tumor. Four of these cysts occurred in patients who had previously undergone irradiation therapy. Two of these 4 patients had also undergone prior surgery elsewhere. An additional cyst was encountered in a patient who underwent a second UCLA operation for a recurrent tumor. Fifty-four patients were considered to have chromophobe adenomata; 7 tumors were diagnosed as mixed and 3 patients harbored eosinophilic adenomata. No malignant adenomata were encountered in this series. The correlation of tumor type and endocrine abnormality is represented in Table IV.

Table VIII   *Comparison of tumor size evaluation: pneumoencephalography versus surgeon's estimate*

Pneumo-encephalo-graphy	Size categories	Normal	Sella enlarged; no suprasellar mass	Intrasellar mass with small suprasellar extension	Suprasellar extension exceeding intrasellar; no third ventricle distortion	Suprasellar extension with third ventricle distortion
Surgeon's estimate of suprasellar tumor extension	Moderate or present, degree not specified	0	1	4	2	13
	Large elevation, 1.5 cm or greater	0		2		17
	No elevation of diaphragma sellae		1	6		10
	No information			2		8

Estimates of tumor height in relation to the diaphragma sellae were given by the surgeon in many instances, and Table VIII correlates these observations with the more objective evaluation of tumor size by pneumoencephalography. The surgeon commonly also made observations on the appearance of the optic nerves and chiasm, and these observations were correlated with the patient's visual status. A high degree of correlation was evident between pallor or thinning of the optic nerves and impaired near vision, presence of visual field defects and optic atrophy. Correlation was least accurate with respect to distant vision. In general, even though pallor or thinning was described in only 1 optic nerve, visual impairment was present bilaterally. Alterations in appearance of the optic chiasm correlated less well with visual changes.

Discussion

In a consideration of pituitary adenomata, functional activity, size and relationship to the neighboring visual and other neural structures are of most fundamental significance. It is still almost universally accepted that tumors which produce significant visual field impairment and tumors with large suprasellar extension as well as tumors which fail to respond to radiation therapy require surgery by one approach or another. Thus, small hormone-secreting adenomas tend to be treated by radiotherapy,[4] and pituitary tumor series collected by surgical clinics[1,5,10,16] tend to be selective in the direction of larger tumors. It is therefore not surprising that our series of patients includes a significant percentage of large tumors (Table VI) and relatively few acromegalic patients.

Unfortunately, very few other series attempt to quantitate pituitary tumor size.[10,15] By pneumoencephalographic criteria, 33, or 67 %, of the 49 patients undergoing this study had 'large' tumors, i.e. tumors with large suprasellar extensions with or without distortion of the third ventricle. Large size of the tumors also correlates with the high incidence of headache and visual disturbances. The incidence of headache in our patients, 77%, is similar to that in other series.[2,12,13,16] Visual symptoms have been emphasized by many previous authors.[1,2,5,7,9,11–16] The findings on ophthalmological examination correspond closely to the incidence of visual symptoms and also agree with similar analyses of other authors.[1,11]

The frequency of manifestation of hypopituitarism in our group of patients, 64 %, also is in keeping with the proportion of large tumors in our study. This high incidence has been reported in other surgical series.[1,9,10,14,16] Of particular interest is the fact that symptoms suggestive of hypogonadism are among the earliest to develop, although they do not often constitute the reason for which the patient will consult a physician for the first time.[10,11] Amenorrhea is a particularly important early symptom, and is seen both in the absence or presence of other evidence for hypopituitarism and in association with acromegaly. All patients in the present study who had galactorrhea were females, although the condition has also been described in male patients with pituitary tumors.[8]

Recent advances in laboratory medicine have introduced many new and sophisticated tests for endocrine function. Among these have been the indirect tests for adrenal reserve (metyrapone) and the direct assay techniques for growth hormone, cortisol and prolactin. Basal urinary 17-hydroxysteroid levels were below normal in almost 40 % of patients tested, a figure comparable to that obtained from more accurate plasma 17-hydroxysteroid determinations by Nieman et al.[11] but exceeding the number of patients with low urinary levels of these steroids in their series. These authors did not include any patients with impaired ADH function. Nine of our patients with chromophobe adenomata, 8 of which indented the third ventricle, had symptoms suggestive of mild diabetes insipidus. However, none was associated with an abnormal urine/serum osmolarity ratio.[6]

The sequence in which elaboration of various pituitary trophic hormones is lost as the tumor enlarges is suggested in Table II(a). While our preliminary findings agree with some of the older work, recent studies have suggested that impairment of ACTH secretion is slightly more common than that of TSH secretion, while growth hormone production is reduced before that of any of the trophic hormones.[11]

In a retrospective study it is not always clear whether replacement medication was absolutely indicated. The most commonly encountered interference with pituitary end-organ relationships is probably due to the administration of thyroid preparations. The tabulation (Table II(b)) is therefore confined to the small number of patients who had evidence of loss of target organ function before their pituitary adenoma became symptomatic.

Table IV indicates that certain tests, such as the protein bound iodine, routinely ordered in a 'battery' of tests, are apparently of little value. Obviously the sensitivity of the analytical technique of each test is of great importance in such a comparative evaluation. By contrast to the variable correlation between pathology and alterations in metabolism, the fact that all patients had abnormal sellae and air encephalograms (Table VI) emphasizes the value of these studies. It is hoped that future surveys will relate the numerous variables, particularly the endocrine parameters, to a quantitative estimate of tumor size.

Although endocrine deficiency states may cause electroencephalographic changes,[3] the obvious importance of an irritative focus in the medial temporal lobe resulting from compression by a laterally expanding pituitary adenoma is well known to produce EEG abnormalities.[10] Detailed analysis of EEG abnormalities in our series (Table VII) is beyond the scope of this report. The cerebrospinal fluid protein was elevated in 67 % of our patients, including 16 with 'large' tumors, a frequency far exceeding that reported by Nieman et al.[11] but in agreement with other data.[10]

The comparison of the surgeon's estimate of tumor size with the quantification of the pneumoencephalographic data reveals that such size estimates at the time of tumor exposure are often inaccurate. Observations on the state of the optic nerves, however, correlate well with the visual examination. It is worth noting that tumor cysts were encountered in 22 % of our patients. It is possible that some tumor cysts form as a consequence of irradiation. Since anamnestic data obtained from patients suspected of having pituitary tumors are often very inadequate, the physical examination incomplete with respect to significant details and the surgeon's report of his operative findings too often deficient in vital facts, we have attempted to systematize data collection for future analysis. A series of forms has been devised which orient the physician toward a more complete and organized evaluation of the pituitary tumor patient.* These forms have been a valuable teaching aid, and may partly replace the more laborious long-hand records. The information is so entered on these forms that it lends itself readily to key punching of computer cards.

The value of computer analysis for the comprehensive evaluation of such complex problems as pituitary adenomas is apparent. It is hoped that a broadly based study would allow sufficient data to be collected to permit development of definite criteria for therapy by irradiation or by one of the various surgical modalities available today. In addition, this type of analysis should enhance our understanding of the changes which take place in patients harboring such tumors, allow a more discriminating selection of laboratory tests to evaluate the endocrine status and facilitate the collection of follow-up data on these patients. Since recurrence of an adenoma sometimes many years after therapy is a well recognized problem,[15] such information is of critical importance.

Acknowledgments

The authors wish to thank Robert W. Rand, M.D., Paul H. Crandall, M.D., and Maxwell M. Andler, M.D. for kind permission to include their patients in the present study. They also wish to

---

* Sample forms may be obtained on request from the authors.

acknowledge the advice of Gunnar Heuser, M.D. and Josiah Brown, M.D. regarding the endocrinological aspects of this study; Prof. Peter T. Kirstein, University of London, Institute of Computer Science, Alan B. Forsythe, Ph. D. and Mr Onelio Clark UCLA Health Science Computer Facility, and Joan Westlake, Ph. D. for their patience and help in dealing with the numerous computer problems associated with this project.

References

(1) BAKAY, L. (1950): The results of 300 pituitary adenoma operations (Prof. Herbert Olivecrona's series). *J. Neurosurg.*, *7*, 240.

(2) BAKER, G. S. (1960): Treatment of pituitary adenomas. *Arch. Surg.*, *81*, 842.

(3) BOSELLI, F. and JEFFERSON, A. A. (1957): Electroencephalogram with chromophobe adenomata and Rathke pouch cysts: modification by associated metabolic disorder. *Electroenceph. clin. Neurophysiol.*, *9*, 275.

(4) CORREA, J. N. and LAMPE, I. (1962): The radiation treatment of pituitary tumors. *J. Neurosurg.*, *19*, 626.

(5) CUSHING, H. (1912): In: *The Pituitary Body and its Disorders*. Editor: J. B. Phil. Lippincott Co., Philadelphia, Pa.

(6) DASHE, A. M., CRAMM, R. E., CRIST, C. A., HABENER, J. F. and SOLOMON, D. H. (1963): A water deprivation test for the differential diagnosis of polyuria. *J. Amer. med. Ass.*, *185*, 71.

(7) DOTT, N. M. and BAILEY, P. (1925): A consideration of the hypophysial adenomata. *Brit. J. Surg.*, *13*, 314.

(8) FINN, J. E. and MOUNT, L. A. (1971): Galactorrhea in males with tumors in the region of the pituitary gland. *J. Neurosurg.*, *35*, 723.

(9) HIRSCH, O. (1952): Symptoms and treatment of pituitary tumors. *Arch. Otolaryng.*, *55*, 268.

(10) JEFFERSON, A. A. (1957): Some clinical features of the pituitary chromophobe adenomata and of the Rathke pouch cysts. *Ann. roy. Coll. Surg. Engl.*, *21*, 358.

(11) NIEMAN, E. A., LANDON, J. and WYNN, V. (1967): Endocrine function in patients with untreated chromophobe adenomas. *Quart. J. Med.*, *36*, 357.

(12) NURNBERGER, J. I. and KOREY, S. R. (1953): *Pituitary Chromophobe Adenomas*. Springer Publishing Co., New York, N.Y.

(13) RAND, C. W. (1957): Notes on pituitary tumors. *Clin. Neurosurg.*, *3*, 1.

(14) RAY, B. S. and PATTERSON Jr, R. H. (1971): Surgical experience with chromophobe adenomas of the pituitary gland. *J. Neurosurg.*, *34*, 726.

(15) STERN, W. E. and BATZDORF, U. (1970): Intracranial removal of pituitary adenomas. An evaluation of varying degrees of excision from partial to total. *J. Neurosurg.*, *33*, 564.

(16) YOUNGHUSBAND, O. Z., HORRAX, G., HURXTHAL, L. M., HARE, H. F. and POPPEN, J. L. (1952): Chromophobe pituitary tumors. I. Diagnosis. *J. clin. Endocr.*, *12*, 611.

The role of the hypothalamus in the pathogenesis of pituitary tumors*

WILLIAM H. DAUGHADAY, PHILIP E. CRYER** and LAURENCE S. JACOBS***

Metabolism Division, Department of Medicine, Washington University School of Medicine, St. Louis, Mo., U.S.A.

Since the application of the radioimmunoassay concept to the measurement of growth hormone (GH) in human serum in 1962[1] nearly 60 patients with acromegaly have been studied in this laboratory. The 50 patients who underwent, at a minimum, an oral glucose tolerance test with measurement of growth hormone levels, form the basis of the concept of regulated though excessive growth hormone secretion in acromegaly as elaborated in the following paragraphs.

The development of a radioimmunoassay system for the measurement of human serum prolactin,[2] a decade after the GH assay, has permitted study of the prolactin secretory patterns in women with high circulating levels of prolactin, some of whom exhibit galactorrhea.

Regulation of growth hormone secretion in acromegaly

Oral glucose tolerance tests. Serum GH responses to the ingestion of 100 g of glucose in 50 patients with acromegaly are summarized in Table I. Baseline values in these 50 patients ranged from 5 to 1800 ng/ml, with a median value of 50 ng/ml.

No change in serum GH concentrations followed glucose ingestion in 31 patients. However, suppression of the serum GH level, a qualitatively normal response,[3] occurred in 12 acromegalic patients. The suppressive response of serum GH to the ingestion of glucose was consistent in a given patient when restudied. For example, the serum GH levels in patient A. Sa. fell from 160 to 80 ng/ml and 120 to 65 ng/ml following glucose ingestion on 2 separate occasions.

---

 * Supported by Research Grant AM05105 and Training Grant AM05027 from the National Institute of Arthritis, Metabolic and Digestive Diseases, National Institutes of Health, Bethesda, Maryland. Clinical studies were done on the Clinical Research Center, supported by RR00036, Division of Research Resources, General Clinical Research Centers Branch, National Institutes of Health, Bethesda, Maryland.
 ** Teaching and Research Scholar of the American College of Physicians.
*** Research Career Development Awardee of the National Institute of Arthritis, Metabolic and Digestive Diseases (IK04 AM70521), National Institutes of Health, Bethesda, Maryland.

Table I   *Serum GH response to oral glucose, intravenous arginine and insulin-induced hypoglycemia in acromegalic patients*

	No. of patients	Serum growth hormone responses		
		No change	Decrease*	Increase**
Oral glucose tolerance tests	50	31 (62 %)	12 (24 %)	7 (14 %)
Arginine infusion	33	18 (55 %)	—	15 (45 %)
Insulin-induced hypoglycemia	20	8 (40 %)	—	12 (60 %)

 * Decrease to $< 50 \%$ of baseline.
** Increase to $> 150 \%$ of baseline.

Failure of the serum GH concentration to suppress into the normal range following oral glucose has been considered a criterion for the diagnosis of acromegaly.[3, 4] In this series of 50 acromegalic patients, 2 suppressed to less than 5 ng/ml. From baseline values of 13 and 10 ng/ml, these patients suppressed to 3 ng/ml following glucose ingestion. Of the remaining 48 patients, none suppressed to less than 15 ng/ml.

Paradoxical stimulation of GH secretion following glucose ingestion occurred in 7 of 50 acromegalic patients. In 5 patients the glucose-induced increment in serum GH ranged from 2- to 5-fold. This pattern was also consistent when a given patient was studied repetitively. For example, in patient M.G. the GH level rose from 25 to 130 ng/ml, 20 to 72 ng/ml and 12 to 100 ng/ml during 3 separate glucose tolerance tests. Paradoxical GH secretion in response to ingested glucose is not unique to acromegaly. It has been described in patients with tumors encroaching upon the hypothalamus[5] and in patients with a variety of disorders without recognized structural lesions of the hypothalamus or pituitary.[6]

Arginine and insulin provocative tests.   As listed in Table I, serum GH concentrations rose following the infusion of 30 g of arginine hydrochloride in 15 of 33 acromegalic patients and during insulin-induced hypoglycemia in 12 of 20 patients. These responses, like those to glucose, were consistent in a given patient. For example, in patient N.P. the GH levels rose from 27 to 124 ng/ml and 50 to 118 ng/ml following arginine infusion on 2 occasions, and in patient V.Y. the GH levels rose from 200 to 345 ng/ml, 41 to 224 ng/ml, 64 to 456 ng/ml and 60 to 123 ng/ml during insulin-induced hypoglycemia on 4 occasions.

Thus, changes in GH secretion following glucose ingestion, arginine infusion or insulin-induced hypoglycemia occurred in 31 of 50 acromegalic patients. Of the 14 patients in whom all 3 tests were performed, GH responses to at least one maneuver occurred in 12. These findings are comparable to those of Lawrence and co-workers[7] who found GH responses to hyperglycemia, hypoglycemia, arginine or exercise in 20 of 24 acromegalic patients.

The GH secretory response to hypoglycemia is mediated through the hypothalamus. Hypothalamic lesioning[8] and intrahypothalamic glucose infusion[9] inhibit the GH response to hypoglycemia in monkeys. In man, pituitary stalk section blocks the GH response to hypoglycemia, even when the capacity of the pituitary to secrete GH is preserved as evidenced by the presence of measurable circulating GH in the baseline state.[10] It is often assumed that the GH secretory response to arginine is mediated through the hypothalamus, but evidence comparable to that cited for glucose effects on GH secretion is lacking.

Twenty-four-hour growth hormone profiles.   Hourly serum GH levels throughout a 24-hour period, drawn through an indwelling intravenous line, have been obtained in 24 acromegalic patients. As shown in Figure 1, mean serum GH concentrations over a 24-hour period ranged from 6 to 532 ng/ml. The median of the mean values was 60 ng/ml.

A striking feature of the 24-hour GH profiles was the marked variation in serum GH concentration in a given patient, as noted previously.[11] The observed values ranged up to 24-fold (5–119 ng/ml) during a 24-hour period in patient N.P. Of the 24 acromegalic patients studied, the coefficient of variation* of the serum GH concentration during a 24-hour period exceeded 25 % in 18 patients and 50 % in 7 patients.

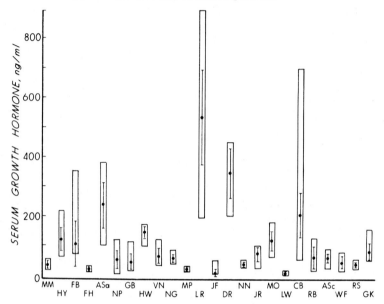

Fig. 1 24-hour serum GH values in 24 acromegalic patients. The points and brackets indicate the mean ± one standard deviation; the rectangles indicate the observed range.

We have previously noted an apparent relationship between serum GH peaks and meals and physical activity during a 24-hour period in selected acromegalic patients.[11] These patients exhibited postprandial GH peaks and had higher serum GH levels during the day. However, a sharply defined serum GH peak following the onset of sleep, a characteristic feature of GH secretion in normal subjects,[12] was not seen. This has also been the experience of others.[13] However, we have recently studied a patient who had higher levels at night than during the day on 2 occasions (Fig. 2). These rather broad nocturnal peaks may be analogous to the sleep-related spike in GH secretion observed in non-acromegalic normal subjects.

Thyrotropin releasing hormone (TRH) and L-dihydroxyphenylalanine (L-DOPA). Synthetic TRH has been administered intravenously, and L-DOPA orally, to a small number of acromegalic patients. Examples are illustrated in Figure 3. GH secretory responses to TRH in acromegalic patients have been reported by others;[14] TRH does not stimulate GH secretion in normal subjects.[15]

Adrenergic control of GH secretion. There is considerable evidence that alpha-adrenergic mechanisms trigger GH secretion.[16–18] Studies in non-human primates suggest that this

---

* Standard deviation over the mean, expressed as a percentage.

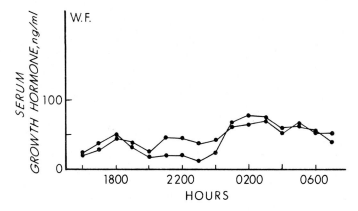

Fig. 2 Serum GH profiles obtained from acromegalic patient W.F. on 2 separate studies.

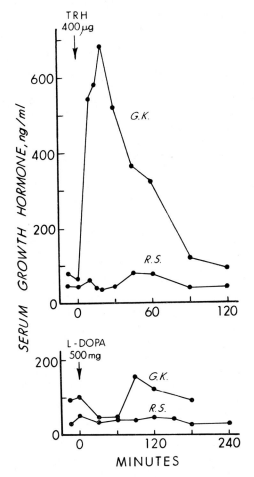

Fig. 3 Serum GH levels following intravenous thyrotropin releasing hormone and oral L-DOPA in acromegalic patients G.K. and R.S.

effect is exerted at the level of the hypothalamus rather than at the pituitary level.[19] Whether adrenergic stimuli are major determinants or only modulating influences on GH secretion in normal subjects remains to be determined. However, the possibility that deranged adrenergic mechanisms may play a role in the pathologic physiology of acromegaly[20] is currently under investigation in our laboratory.

Comment. From these observations it is clear that the secretion of GH from the pituitaries of the majority of acromegalic patients is not autonomous. In most acromegalics, qualitatively appropriate GH secretory responses occur following provocative manipulations, e.g. glucose ingestion, arginine infusion or insulin-induced hypoglycemia, and during the more subtle stimuli, e.g. meals, activity and others, exerted during a 24-hour observation period. Indeed, in one acromegalic patient a sleep-related increase in GH secretion, the hallmark of normal GH secretion in non-acromegalic subjects, may have occurred. Thus, despite quantitatively excessive GH secretion, regulatory influences on GH secretion persist in most acromegalic patients.

In view of the intimate functional relationship between the hypothalamus and pituitary GH secretion, and the fact that the glucose-mediated (and perhaps other) GH secretory stimuli described above are mediated via the hypothalamus, we have hypothesized that a defect in hypothalamic regulation of GH secretion may underlie the development of acromegaly in some patients.[11]

Diminished hypothalamic sensitivity to normal suppression of growth hormone releasing factor production is a potential mechanism for the putative regulatory defect in these acromegalic patients. Evidence that feedback suppression of GH secretion is operative in acromegalic patients has been adduced. The administration of estrogens, which block the effects of GH, has been shown to facilitate the GH secretory response to hypoglycemia in acromegalic patients.[21] In addition, GH secretory responses to provocative stimuli in acromegalic patients with normal baseline serum GH levels after pituitary irradiation have been reported to be obliterated by the infusion of GH, to produce serum GH levels comparable to those preceding therapy.[22] Furthermore, Hagen, Lawrence and Kirsteins have detected bioassayable GH releasing activity in acromegalic plasma,[23] an observation also reported by Strachma, Frohman and Dhariwal.[24] Hagen and co-workers have observed increased GH releasing activity in acromegalic plasma after hypophysectomy and decreased activity during effective medical therapy.[25]

Thus, the concept of diminished hypothalamic sensitivity to (or elevated threshold for) normal suppression of GH releasing factor secretion, with resultant excessive production of releasing factor and GH, is consistent with available data. However, there are certain limitations to this simplified view. It is unlikely, for example, that fixed hypersecretion of GH releasing factor underlies the excessive GH secretion in these patients since, with serial GH determinations, some patients may at times have serum GH values in the normal range. Furthermore, it is unlikely that the defect is a failure of GH alone to feedback normally on hypothalamic GH releasing factor secretion, since we have observed definite increments in serum GH in response to arginine in a patient whose baseline GH levels were normal following cryogenic hypophysectomy.[11] Similarly, patients with normal serum GH levels following irradiation have been observed by others to respond to provocative secretory stimuli.[22]

Regulation of prolactin secretion in patients with pituitary tumors

Excessive prolactin secretion is frequently encountered in patients with pituitary tumors.[2,26-30] While some patients with excessive prolactin secretion experience galactorrhea, often no manifestations are recognized clinically. Infrequently, excessive prolactin secretion is en-

ACROMEGALY WITH GALACTORRHEA

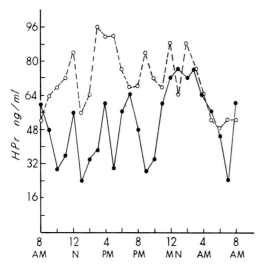

Fig. 4 Serum prolactin levels during a 24-hour observation period in 2 patients with acromegaly.

countered in patients with acromegaly. In 2 such cases we have observed the same instability of prolactin secretion observed for growth hormone (Fig. 4).

We have now completed 24-hour profile studies in 5 patients with prolactin-secreting pituitary tumors. In 4 of these 5 a high degree of variance of the serum prolactin concentration was encountered (Fig. 5). In no case was the normal circadian nocturnal rise in serum prolactin recognized. It is of interest that in the physiologic hyperprolactinemia of late pregnancy a similar variance of serum prolactin levels was observed (Fig. 5).

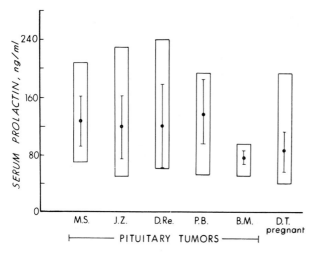

Fig. 5 24-hour serum prolactin levels in 5 patients with hyperprolactinemia and pituitary tumors and one normal subject with the physiologic hyperprolactinemia of late pregnancy. The points and brackets indicate the mean ± one standard deviation; the rectangles indicate the observed range.

Prolactin secretion by pituitary tumors may be inhibited by the administration of L-DOPA.[31, 32] We have given 0.5 g of L-DOPA orally to 10 such patients (Fig. 6). Unequivocal suppression of serum prolactin levels followed L-DOPA in 4 patients, less definite falls were observed in 3, and in 3 patients no significant change in serum prolactin occurred. In one patient, responsiveness to L-DOPA appeared after external irradiation to the pituitary. In 3 patients with prolactin-secreting pituitary tumors no rise in serum prolactin followed the injection of 50 mg of chlorpromazine.

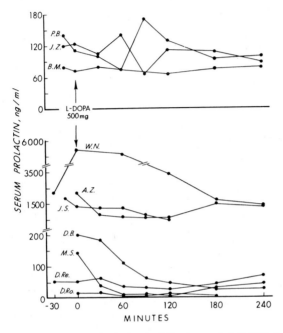

Fig. 6   Serum prolactin levels following oral L-DOPA in 10 patients with hyperprolactinemia and pituitary tumors.

This experience with prolactin-secreting tumors appears to be analogous to that we have had with growth hormone-secreting tumors. A high degree of cyclic variation in secretion occurs and secretion is modified by agents acting through the hypothalamus.

Summary

Reproducible changes in serum GH concentrations in the majority of acromegalic patients following oral glucose, intravenous arginine and insulin-induced hypoglycemia, and marked variation during the more subtle stimuli of a 24-hour observation period, indicate that GH secretion, though quantitatively excessive, remains responsive to regulatory influences in these patients. Since at least some of these secretory stimuli are mediated through the hypothalamus, we have suggested that the primary defect in some acromegalic patients lies at the level of the hypothalamus rather than the pituitary. Reports of bioassayable GH releasing activity in the plasma of acromegalic patients are consistent with the hypothesis that excessive GH releasing factor production from the hypothalamus underlies GH hypersecretion in these acromegalic patients.

Marked variation in the serum prolactin concentrations occurs during serial observation of patients with prolactin-secreting pituitary tumors. In some of these patients, the serum prolactin levels are suppressed following L-DOPA ingestion. Thus, there is considerable similarity between the patterns of GH and prolactin secretion in disorders characterized by pituitary tumors and excessive secretion of GH or of prolactin.

References

(1) UTIGER, R. D., PARKER, M. L. and DAUGHADAY, W. H. (1962): Studies of human growth hormone. I. A radioimmunoassay for human growth hormone. *J. clin. Invest., 41*, 254.

(2) JACOBS, L. S., MARIZ, I. K. and DAUGHADAY, W. H. (1972): A mixed heterologous radio-immunoassay for human prolactin. *J. clin. Endocr., 34*, 484.

(3) EARLL, J. M., SPARKS, L. L. and FORSHAM, P. H. (1967): Glucose suppression of serum growth hormone in the diagnosis of acromegaly. *J. Amer. med. Ass., 201*, 628.

(4) ROTH, J., GLICK, S. M., CUATRECASAS, P. and HOLLANDER, C. S. (1967): Acromegaly and other disorders of growth hormone secretion. *Ann. intern. Med., 66*, 760.

(5) BECK, P., PARKER, M. L. and DAUGHADAY, W. H. (1966): Paradoxical hypersecretion of growth hormone in response to glucose. *J. clin. Endocr., 28*, 463.

(6) CATT, J. K. (1970): Growth hormone. *Lancet, 1*, 933.

(7) LAWRENCE, A. M., GOLDFINE, I. D. and KIRSTEINS, L. (1970): Growth hormone dynamics in acromegaly. *J. clin. Endocr., 31*, 239.

(8) ABRAMS, R. L., PARKER, M. L., BLANCO, S., REICHLIN, S. and DAUGHADAY, W. H. (1966): Hypothalamic regulation of growth hormone secretion. *Endocrinology, 78*, 605.

(9) REICHLIN, S. (1966): Functions of the median eminence gland. *New Engl. J. Med., 275*, 600.

(10) ANTONY, G. J., VAN WYK, J., FRENCH, F. S., WEAVER, R. P., DUGGER, G. S., TIMMONS, R. L. and NEWSOME, J. F. (1969): Influence of pituitary stalk section on growth hormone, insulin and TSH secretion in women with metastatic breast cancer. *J. clin. Endocr., 29*, 1238.

(11) CRYER, P. E. and DAUGHADAY, W. H. (1969): Regulation of growth hormone secretion in acromegaly. *J. clin. Endocr., 29*, 386.

(12) TAKAHASHI, Y., KIPNIS, D. M. and DAUGHADAY, W. H. (1968): Growth hormone secretion during sleep. *J. clin. Invest., 47*, 2079.

(13) CARLSON, H. E., GILLIN, J. C., GORDEN, P. and SNYDER, F. (1972): Absence of sleep-related growth hormone peaks in aged normal subjects and in acromegaly. *J. clin. Endocr., 34*, 1102.

(14) IRIE, M. and TSUSHIMA, T. (1972): Increase of serum growth hormone concentration following thyrotropin-releasing hormone injection in patients with acromegaly or gigantism. *J. clin. Endocr., 35*, 97.

(15) ANDERSON, M. S., BOWERS, C. Y., KASTIN, A. J. et al. (1971): Synthetic thyrotropin-releasing hormone. A potent stimulation of thyrotropin secretion in man. *New Engl. J. Med., 285*, 1279.

(16) BLACKARD, W. G. and HEIDINGS SELDER, S. A. (1968): Adrenergic receptor control mechanism for growth hormone secretion. *J. clin. Invest., 47*, 1407.

(17) BLACKARD, W. G. and HUBBELL, G. J. (1970): Stimulatory effect of exogenous catecholamines on plasma HGH concentrations in presence of beta-adrenergic blockade. *Metabolism, 19*, 547.

(18) IMURA, H., KATO, Y., IKEDA, M., MORIMOTO, M. and YAWATA, M. (1971): Effect of adrenergic blocking or stimulating agents on plasma growth hormone, immunoreactive insulin and blood free fatty acids in man. *J. clin. Invest., 50*, 1069.

(19) TOIVOLA, P. T. K., GALE, C. C., GOODNER, C. J. and WERRBACH, J. H. (1972): Central alpha-adrenergic regulation of growth hormone and insulin. *Hormones, 3*, 193.

(20) SHERMAN, L. and KOLODNY, H. D. (1971): The hypothalamus, brain catecholamines and drug therapy for gigantism and acromegaly. *Lancet, 1*, 682.

(21) LIPMAN, R., TAYLOR, A., SCHENK, A. and MINTZ, D. H. (1972): Acromegaly: a disorder of growth hormone feedback (abstract). *Clin. Res., 20*, 432.

(22) LAWRENCE, A. M., HAGEN, T. C. and KIRSTEINS, L. (1971): Regulation of growth hormone secretion in normals and in acromegaly (abstract). In: *Second International Symposium on Growth Hormone. Excerpta Medica International Congress Series No. 236, Abstract 140*, p. 63.

(23) HAGEN, T. C., LAWRENCE, A. M. and KIRSTEINS, L. (1971): In vitro release of monkey pituitary growth hormone by acromegalic plasma. *J. clin. Endocr., 33*, 448.

(24) STRACHMA, M. E., FROHMAN, L. A. and DHARIWAL, A. P. S. (1971): Effect of purified hypothala-
      mic extract and acromegalic plasma on growth hormone synthesis and release in vitro (abstract).
      Endocrinology, *88*, A-81.
(25) HAGEN, T. C., LAWRENCE, A. M. and KIRSTEINS, L. (1972): Growth hormone releasing factor in
      acromegalic plasma. Reduction during successful medical management (abstract). *J. clin.
      Invest.*, *51*, 35a.
(26) PEAKE, G. T., MCKEEL, D. W., JARETT, L. and DAUGHADAY, W. H. (1969): Ultrastructural,
      histologic and hormonal characterization of a prolactin-rich human pituitary tumor. *J. clin.
      Endocr.*, *29*, 1383.
(27) FORSYTH, I. A., BESSER, G. M., EDWARDS, C. R. W., FRANCIS, L. and MYRES, R. P. (1971):
      Plasma prolactin activity in inappropriate lactation. *Brit. med. J.*, *3*, 225.
(28) TURKINGTON, R. W. (1972): Secretion of prolactin by patients with pituitary and hypothalamic
      tumors. *J. clin. Endocr.*, *34*, 159.
(29) FRIESEN, H., WEBSTER, B. R., HWANG, P., GUYDA, H., MUNRO, R. E. and READ, L. (1972):
      Prolactin synthesis and secretion in a patient with the Forbes-Albright syndrome. *J. clin.
      Endocr.*, *34*, 192.
(30) NASR, H., MOZAFFARIAN, G., PENSKY, J. and PEARSON, O. H. (1972): Prolactin secreting
      pituitary tumors in women. *J. clin. Endocr.*, *35*, 505.
(31) MALARKEY, W. B., JACOBS, L. S. and DAUGHADAY, W. H. (1971): Levodopa suppression of
      prolactin in nonpuerperal galactorrhea. *New Engl. J. Med.*, *285*, 1160.
(32) TURKINGTON, R. W. (1972): Inhibition of prolactin secretion and successful therapy of the
      Forbes-Albright syndrome with L-Dopa. *J. clin. Endocr.*, *34*, 306.

The assessment of the endocrine effects and the effectiveness of ablative pituitary treatment by ^{90}Y and ^{198}Au implantation

RUSSELL FRASER, F. DOYLE, G. F. JOPLIN, C. W. BURKE, P. HARSOULIS, M. TUNBRIDGE, R. ARNOTT and D. CHILD

Royal Postgraduate Medical School, Hammersmith Hospital, London, United Kingdom

This review of our experience comes when our Unit is just completing its second decade of experience with pituitary ablations by implantation of radioactive material into the sella turcica.[1] Apart from pituitary ablations done for breast cancer or diabetic retinopathy, we have available for review after 1 year's follow-up over 200 partial or suppressive pituitary ablations by ^{90}Y or ^{198}Au implants[2-6] for Cushing's disease, acromegaly or 'functionless' pituitary tumours. I hope to cull from this experience any evidence about the best available procedures for the postoperative assessments of such or similar pituitary ablative treatments.

The problem

We have two different situations needing these assessments. (1) Sometimes, as in treating breast cancer or diabetic retinopathy, the objective has been total ablation; here, cortisol replacement must be planned from the operation day and our postoperative tests will be concerned with the completeness and the likely persistence of the ablation. (2) More often, however, the primary disease is a pituitary tumour or overactivity, and here we must assess postoperatively both the adequacy of the elimination of the primary disease, and also the extent of any incidental destruction of other pituitary function. The latter gauges both the 'cost' of the treatment and the need for replacement therapy. After attempted total ablation, clearly, we must test especially those functions most resistant to ablation, while after partial or suppressive ablation to treat pituitary hyperactivity or tumours we must test the functions most sensitive to pituitary damage or ischaemia. In either case we must also appraise the relief of symptoms and signs of the original disease.

Grading anterior pituitary function and its timing

For posterior pituitary function, any clinically important abnormality makes itself obvious as diabetes insipidus. But several anterior pituitary hormones need assessment, of which most, excluding only GH and prolactin, can be validly measured either directly or from the peripheral target gland's activity. Feasibility can best determine which of these to select for

Table I   *Grading anterior pituitary function*

I. Each hormone	Gonadotrophins		Prol	GH	ACTH	TSH
1. Hyperactive (or premature)						
2. Normal	LH	FSH				
3. Reserve low						
4. Basally *a.* Low *b.* Very low						
5. Peripheral gland failure						

II. Summated hypopituitarism (if any)
    A. Isolated deficiency ←——————————→
    B. Partial hypopit. ←————————————————→
    C. Panhypopit. ←————————————————————————→

assessment, e.g. cortisol is perhaps more easily measured than ACTH, but LH more easily than oestradiol. We find that 4 of the 5 hormones listed in Table I may need appraising; prolactin also will probably be helpful in certain circumstances still awaiting precise definition. As is noted, the secretory status of each can usefully be placed in one of 4 or 5 grades.

We must also look at the summated status. It is of course a familiar fact that isolated deficiencies of any pituitary hormone can occur. But after non-specific damage such as operative hypophysectomy or implant, we find most commonly that an isolated loss affects the gonadotrophins, as for example we found in assessing the functional status of our ^{90}Y or ^{198}Au implanted 'functionless' pituitary tumours. Indeed among our implanted subjects, the only serious exception is the isolated ACTH deficiency not infrequently seen following pituitary implant for Cushing's disease – possibly reflecting the large number of these based on an ACTH-producing tumour.[2, 7] When assessing for completeness of ablation, e.g. with diabetic and breast cancer patients, we find that thyroid function is the strictest criterion; with diabetic subjects it is also a good guide that insulin needs should fall more than 30 % if ablation is complete.

When should such postoperative testing be done? We routinely assess at 3 and 12 months and thereafter only as indicated. Earlier tests would be convenient but they may not adequately reflect the persisting status and may be complicated by postoperative cortisol replacement. Gonadotrophins may be measured at 10–14 days after pituitary implants or operations aiming at complete ablation (Fig. 1); this could perhaps pick out incomplete operations but not validate the completeness.

Testing hypopituitarism

Tests available to check for hypopituitarism (to assess the need for replacement treatment or the completeness of the pituitary ablation) include:

1. Gonadotrophin testing

Radioimmunoassays can only supplement the clinical assessment of gonad function from prostate and uterine size. We find the serum LH levels more sensitive than FSH to minor damage and also more responsive in stimulation tests. Of course with some pituitary tumours, especially in females, gonad function may be defective even though the basal levels of LH are normal. We are at present assessing the usefulness of LH-RH[8] and clomiphene tests[9, 10]

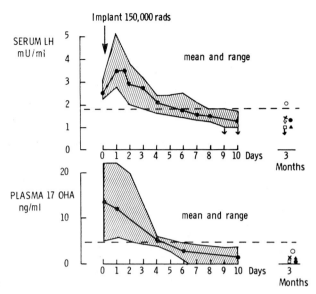

Fig. 1   Early changes in serum LH and in plasma 17-OH androgens following pituitary implant for total ablation in 6 diabetic men. (1 LH unit charted = 2 I.U.) (71/2583-2).

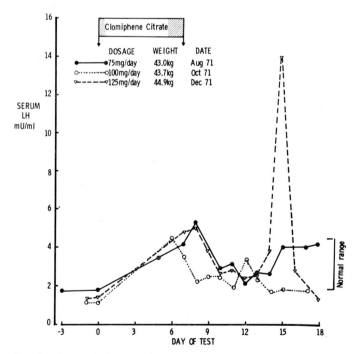

Fig. 2a   Serum LH levels after the administration of clomiphene citrate in recovering anorexia nervosa; a series of tests while the patient recovers responsiveness. (1 LH unit charted = 2 I.U.) (72/171-5).

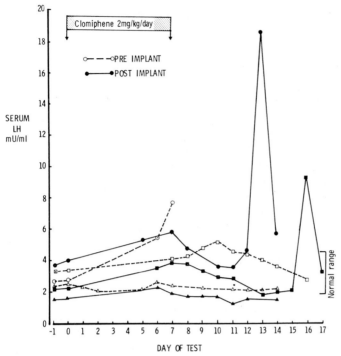

Fig. 2b   Clomiphene test results in 3 patients with 'functionless' pituitary tumours and amenorrhoea and after pituitary implant. Note recovery of LH surge in 2 patients. (1 LH unit charted = 2 I.U.) (72/171-1).

of gonadotrophin responsiveness in these and other cases. We must of course remember that functional disturbances, as for example in anorexia nervosa, can not only impair this responsiveness but also lower basal levels (Fig. 2a).[10] Recovery of responses to clomiphene may also be found with functionless pituitary tumours, after suppressive or small ^{90}Y implants (Fig. 2b). Further appraisal is needed to assess the place of LH-RH in such testing; it is a quicker test but does not involve the hypothalamus.

2. Assessing GH and ACTH

Where there is no question of hyperactivity of these functions, we rely on two main tests: after stopping for 24 hours any cortisol replacement of under 5 months' duration, an insulin tolerance test (ITT) for GH and cortisol responsiveness, followed by observing whether a cortisol deficiency syndrome supervenes within 5–7 days. The latter avoids full dependence on the ITT in assessing the need for replacement therapy. Figure 3a illustrates the usefulness of the ITT in revealing GH deficiency along with normal ACTH responsiveness in a subject with a tumour in the lining of the 3rd ventricle. With pituitary damage also, GH seems to be more susceptible to loss than ACTH (Fig. 3b).[22]

Other tests may be as good as the ITT, for example a glucagon test or an arginine test, but evidence of their consistent performance in subjects with normal pituitaries must be well established to warrant their advocacy in preference. Over hundreds of these ITTs,[12] our standard precautions have avoided any untoward complications. Figure 4 shows the peak growth hormone (GH) and cortisol levels attained in a series of such tests, performed both pre-implant and at 3–18 months post-implant, in a group of our subjects with 'functionless'

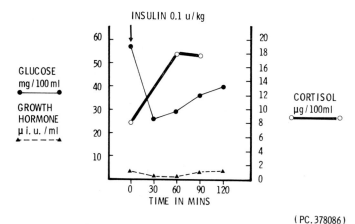

(PC. 378086)

Fig. 3a   I.v. ITT (0.1 U/kg) in 14-year-old boy later found to have hypothalamic tumour involving 3rd ventricle lining. Note normal cortisol response and no GH response. (72/1429).

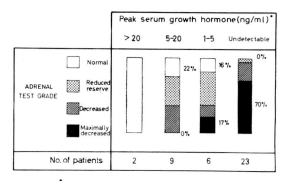

* Peak serum level during an insulin tolerance test   27-7-68

Fig. 3b   Peak serum GH and cortisol responses in diabetic subjects 3 months after implanting for diabetic retinopathy. Note more extensive GH than cortisol suppression. (68/4089).

pituitary tumours.[4] This offers good evidence that this 'suppressive' dosage of ^{90}Y implant, giving peripherally 20 Krads, usually at least preserves the GH and the ACTH functions which were residual at the time of the implant.

3. Tests of TSH and thyroid function

After pituitary implants aiming at total ablation, our patients are discharged on prednisone but without thyroxine replacement until they return for their 3 months' assessment. Then a standard ^{131}I test, combined with serum cholesterol and thyroxine or PBI, has proved very efficient in picking out those incompletely ablated and needing reimplantation. For this purpose the TSH assay is not yet sensitive enough at subnormal levels. With these patients the preceding tests of LH, GH and ACTH are useful but less stringent supplements.

After partial ablation treatments, such as implants for acromegaly, Cushing's disease or 'functionless' pituitary tumours, thyroid failure is rarely recognisable at the first or 3- to 12-month assessment, unless the pre-implant pituitary disease was extensive. However, we have been examining the usefulness of thyrotrophin-releasing hormone (TRH) tests[1, 13] for

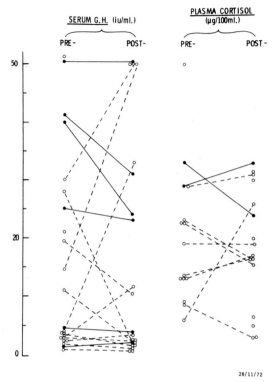

Fig. 4 Peak serum GH and cortisol responses in subjects implanted for 'functionless' pituitary
tumours. Note minimal changes from pre- to post-implant. (72/3138-1).

assessing the apparently euthyroid subjects with pituitary disease, to see whether those with
impending thyroid failure can be segregated by this test performed either pre- or post-
implant.

The standard TRH test measures serum TSH at 0, 20 and 60 min after a single maximal
i.v. injection of TRH, for which we use 200 μg. This produces a fairly but not completely
reproducible response.

We are not yet sure whether this is a sufficiently prolonged stimulus to gauge reduced
pituitary reserve and segregate the low responses from the very low ones, which may be the
distinction this clinical problem needs. We have been assessing a more prolonged test on
this problem. This test first measures the same standard response and then also gives a more
extended stimulus. Occasional cases are not as responsive on this prolonged test, but its
prognostic value is still under appraisal.

What can the standard TRH test add to the assessment of euthyroid subjects with pituitary
disease? Figure 5 shows our findings in two groups of these subjects – those with either
'functionless' pituitary tumours or acromegaly, all euthyroid when tested pre-implant. Among
the 'functionless' pituitary tumours, most had on this test low or normal responses; subsequently none of these have developed hypothyroidism as the test suggested. On the other
hand, half of the euthyroid acromegalics showed no response to the TRH; yet none of these
unresponsive acromegalics have subsequently developed hypothyroidism even after their
pituitary implant, although 2 who had fair or normal responses to TRH have developed
this thyroid failure. Further follow-up is needed to appraise this test, but it does seem that
in acromegaly it is not a valid prognosticator of impending TSH failure. The response to

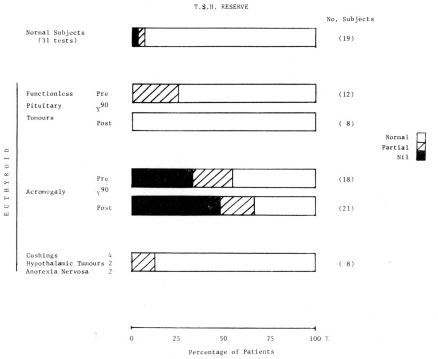

Fig. 5   Standard TRH tests (200 μg i.v.) in euthyroid subjects with 'functionless' pituitary tumours or acromegaly, compared with normals. Note nearly all normal increments in TSH seen with 'functionless' pituitary tumours and large proportion of acromegalics with no response. (72/1127-10).

TRH is evidently atypical in acromegaly for reasons which have not yet been defined. The LH-RH test may offer more hopeful prospects here but full appraisal is still awaited for both tests.

Occasionally, thyrotrophin-producing pituitary tumours are now being discovered,[14-16] for whose follow-up TSH measurements will be important, as is GH for acromegaly. However, sometimes the TSH levels become unmeasurable without the associated hyperthyroidism remitting fully.[16]

Assessing the curbing of the disease

Before implanting we normally do an aeroencephalogram (AEG) whenever the X-rays have shown a tumour.[2,4] We do not routinely do an AEG at follow-up unless (*a*) the initial tumour extended well up into the cranium, or (*b*) the visual field problem had recurred, or until (*c*) a reimplant is planned.

1. Cushing's disease

To assess remission in this disease, not only should we see recession of the syndrome but also we need evidence of recession of the hypercortisolism. For this last purpose, we find specific cortisol assays now available utilising binding proteins are the most helpful measurements, either checking that the midnight plasma cortisol is normally suppressed, or using

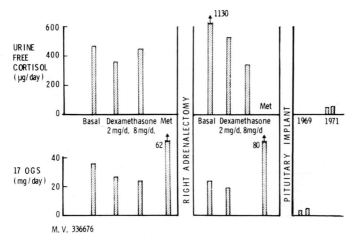

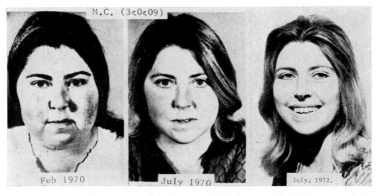

Fig. 6   Serial urinary steroid measurements in a subject with Cushing's disease with nodular adrenal hyperplasia. Note satisfactory remission after pituitary implant. (72/2839-11).

Fig. 7   Subject M.G. treated by pituitary implant for Cushing's disease. (72/2109-2).

the 24-hour urinary free or unconjugated cortisol.[17-19] While measuring the ACTH level is of great help in assessing the preoperative basis of a discovered Cushing's syndrome, functional tests of the pituitary basis for hyperadrenalism, by the metyrapone and dexamethasone tests, are perhaps more important for assessing the pituitary dependence of these cases. When the Cushing's syndrome has not remitted at 3 months after treatment of the pituitary, we find the metyrapone the most reliable test for reassessing the patient. Even in cases of Cushing's disease with nodular adrenal hyperplasia, these tests seem to have their usual significance, as illustrated in Figure 6.

For our follow-up assessments at 1 and 5 years among 55 cases of Cushing's disease treated by pituitary implant, we have divided our cases by the sella X-rays.[2, 3] Cases with clearly enlarged sellae pre-implant have clearly a much more serious prognosis, even though we have usually given them 2 implants and often an associated total adrenalectomy. On the other hand, among the other cases without enlarged sellae, 80 % are fully remitted at 1 year and 60 % at 5 years (Fig. 7). Less than half of these patients need replacement therapy.

2. Acromegaly

Serum GH levels offer an obvious gauge of the therapeutic response in this condition, provided the normal lability of this level is minimised by using an indwelling sampler and the mean level of the 2nd hour of an oral GTT.[6, 20] It is important to corroborate this with assessments of the acromegalic features, for which purpose the soft tissues seen in the skin and facies (Fig. 8) and measurement of skin thickness are preferable to heel thickness;[21] long-term remission may be seen in the bones. Both these clinical signs and the assay levels offer an index of the primary disease activity.[3, 6]

Tables II and III give an analysis of the serum GH and other responses among our first

Table II *Acromegaly: serum GH response at 1 year (after single low-dose ⁹⁰Y implant) (median and range)*

Pre-implant serum GH		No.	Post-implant serum GH*	
			ng/ml	% pre-implant
	I. *By implant dosage:*			
72 (14–1900)	50 Krad	(45)	20 (1–494)	28 %
60 (2–387)	Less	(27)	27 (1–213)	45 %
	50 Krad group			
	II. *By clinical response subgroups:*			
70 (13–185)	Satisfactory	(15)	7 (1–29)	10 %
69 (16–1900)	Partial	(20)	22 (5–494)	32 %
102 (14–346)	Nil	(10)	70 (2–590)	71 %

* GH value used = median of samples 1–2½ hours of 50 g oral GTT.

Table III ⁹⁰Y *implants for acromegaly: complications in first 125 implants (109 patients)*

	First implants		Second implants		Total
	50 Krad	Other	50 Krad	> 50 Krad	
Operative					
(a) CSF leak (+ infections or needing plug)	1 (2 %)	8 (12 %)	1 (11 %)	1 (14 %)	11 (9 %)
(b) Visual loss or paresis (> 2 months)	2 (5 %)	1 (2 %)	2 (22 %)	—	5 (4 %)
Hypopituitarism					
(a) (Ant.) needing replacement	15 (33 %)	16 (25 %)	5 (45 %)	6 (85 %)	42 (33 %)
(b) Diabetes insipidus (> 2 months)	2 (5 %)	1 (2 %)	—	1 (14 %)	3 (2 %)
Mortality within 1 year	1	2	—	—	3 (2 %)
No. free of any of the above	21 (47 %)	38 (60 %)	3	1	63 (51 %)
(No. of implants)	(45)	(64)	(9)	(7)	(125)

* 1 meningitis + 2 cardiac.

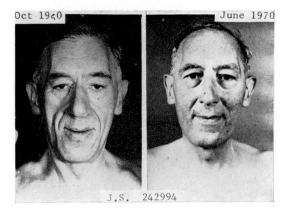

Fig. 8   Subject J.S. treated by pituitary implant for acromegaly. (71/2024-7).

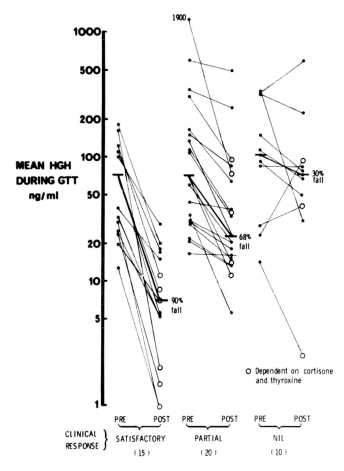

Fig. 9   Serum GH results pre- and 1 year post-implant for acromegaly, grouped by clinical response (72/486-3).

72 subjects given low dose implants. Figure 9 shows that unsatisfactory results often emerged when the pre-implant level was over 100 ng/ml, and such subjects now get higher dose implants. Figure 9 also indicates that the clinical remission is a good guide to the GH response, and that a good percentage drop in serum GH is needed as well as a drop to near normal levels. Our current objective is to drop the serum GH both by at least 50 % and to below 50 I.U./ml. This sharp regression to near normal levels has been attained in two-thirds of our subjects without inducing hypopituitarism needing replacement therapy. Thus this therapy seems very suited to the subjects with a mild form of the disease and to those without greatly expanded tumours.

3.   'Functionless' pituitary tumours

We find this term useful for those subjects whose tumour has not obviously added hyper-secretory features to the syndrome. These tumours were previously unfortunately called chromophobe tumours, which may at times be very hypersecretory.[5] Most of these tumours are not strictly chromophobe.

Here the activity of the disease can only be indexed by tumour size or some reflection of it. Sellar reconstitution, when it can be seen, is a useful sign of tumour shrinkage;[22] or it may be indexed from the visual fields,[23] or the AEG, as already noted.

Sometimes improvement in pituitary function gives the needed evidence of regression, as we have seen from the changes in pituitary function found after ⁹⁰Y implants to these patients. As Figure 4 shows we only rarely see improvement in GH or ACTH reserve after this treatment, but gonad function may recover fully when it was the only function disturbed preoperatively (Fig. 2b). Thus, partial pituitary ablation with ⁹⁰Y is a good treatment for 'functionless' pituitary tumours which have not extended too far beyond the sella, and one which rarely induces hypopituitarism needing replacement therapy when this was not needed pre-implant.

Summary

After pituitary disease has been treated by any partially or totally ablative procedure, post-operative assessments of endocrine function should be done at 3 and 12 months. These can both seek evidence of hypopituitarism needing replacement therapy, and also help to assess the curbing of the primary disease.

Gonadotrophin assessments are the most sensitive to minor hypopituitarism and thyroid function assessments the most valid indicators of the completeness of pituitary ablation.

Review of our 1-year follow-up results of over 200 partially ablative pituitary implants done for Cushing's disease, acromegaly or 'functionless' pituitary tumours has indicated the relative usefulness of some of the available tests; also that this treatment can usually curb these diseases without inducing hypopituitarism needing replacement therapy.

References

(1)   FRASER, T. R. and WRIGHT, A. D. (1968): Treatment of acromegaly and Cushing's disease by ⁹⁰Y implant for partial ablation of the pituitary. In: *Clinical Endocrinology, Vol. 2*, pp. 78–92. Grune and Stratton, New York, N.Y.

(2)   BURKE, C. W., DOYLE, F. H., JOPLIN, G. F., ARNOT, R. N., MACERLEAN, D. P. and FRASER, T. R. (1973): Cushing's disease: treatment by pituitary implantation of radioactive gold or yttrium. In press.

(3)   FRASER, T. R., DOYLE, F. H., JOPLIN, G. F., BURKE, C. W. and ARNET, R. (1972): The treat-ment of pituitary Cushing's syndrome by pituitary implant of ⁹⁰Y or ¹⁹⁰Au. In: *Cushing's*

Syndrome: Diagnosis and Treatment, pp. 119–125. Editors: C. Binder and P. Hall. William Heinemann Medical Books Ltd., London.

(4)   FRASER, T. R., DOYLE, F. H., JACKSON, R. and JOPLIN, G. F. (1973): Influence of pituitary implantation on endocrine function and visual defects in patients with functionless pituitary tumours. In press.

(5)   LEWIS, P. D. and VAN NOORDEN, S. (1972): Pituitary abnormalities in acromegaly. *Arch. Path.*, *94*, 119.

(6)   WRIGHT, A. D., HARTOG, M., PALTER, H., TEVAARWERK, G., DOYLE, F. H., ARNOT, R., JOPLIN, G. F. and FRASER, T. R. (1970): The use of yttrium-90 implantation in the treatment of acromegaly. *Proc. roy. Soc. Med.*, *63*, 221.

(7)   O'NEAL, L. W. (1964): Pathologic anatomy in Cushing's syndrome. *Ann. Surg.*, *160*, 860.

(8)   BESSER, G. M., McNEILLY, A. S., ANDERSON, D. C., MARSHALL, J. C., HARSOULIS, P., HALL, R., ORMSTON, B. J., ALEXANDER, L. and COLLINS, W. P. (1972): Hormonal responses to synthetic luteinizing hormone and follicle stimulating hormone-releasing hormone in man. *Brit. med. J.*, *3*, 267.

(9)   ANDERSON, D. C., MARSHALL, J. C., YOUNG, J. L. and FRASER, T. R. (1972): Stimulation tests of pituitary-Leydig cell function in normal male subjects and hypogonad men. *Clin. Endocr.*, *1*, 127.

(10) MARSHALL, J. C. and FRASER, T. R. (1971): Amenorrhoea in anorexia nervosa: Assessment and treatment with clomiphene citrate. *Brit. med. J.*, *4*, 590.

(11) WRIGHT, A. D., KOHNER, E. M., OAKLEY, N. W., HARTOG, M., JOPLIN, G. F. and FRASER, T. R. (1969): Serum growth hormone levels and the response of diabetic retinopathy to pituitary ablation. *Brit. med. J.*, *2*, 346.

(12) FRASER, T. R. and SMITH, P. H. (1941): The diagnosis of panhypopituitarism (anterior) by 2 tests. *Quart. J. Med.*, *10*, 297.

(13) FRASER, T. R. (1972): Effects of TRH on TSH release in patients with pituitary-hypothalamic disease. *Frontiers of Hormone Research*, *1*, 76.

(14) HAMILTON, C. R., ADAMS, L. C. and MALOOF, F. (1970): Hyperthyroidism due to thyrotropin-producing pituitary chromophobe adenoma. *New Engl. J. Med.*, *283*, 1077.

(15) EMERSON, C. H. and UTIGER, R. D. (1972): Hyperthyroidism and excessive thyrotropin secretion. *New Engl. J. Med.*, *287*, 328.

(16) O'DONNELL, J., HADDEN, D. R., WEAVER, J. A. and MONTGOMMERY, J. (1973): Thyrotoxicosis recurring after surgical removal of a thyrotrophin-secreting pituitary tumour. *Proc. roy. Soc. Med.*, *66*, 441.

(17) BUTLER, P. W. P. and BESSER, G. M. (1968): Pituitary-adrenal function in severe depressive illness. *Lancet*, *1*, 1234.

(18) BURKE, C. W. and BEARDWELL, C. G. (1973): Cushing's syndrome: an evaluation of the clinical usefulness of the urinary free cortisol and other urinary steroid measurements in diagnosis. *Quart. J. Med.*, *42*, 175.

(19) GALVAO-TELES, A., BURKE, C. W. and FRASER, T. R. (1973): Cortisol status in obesity. In press.

(20) FRASER, T. R. and WRIGHT, A. D. (1968): Standard procedures for assessing hypersecretion or secretory capacity of human growth hormone, using the radioimmunoassay. *Postgrad. med. J.*, *44*, 53.

(21) KHO, K. M., WRIGHT, A. D. and DOYLE, F. H. (1970): Heel pad thickness in acromegaly. *Brit. J. Radiol.*, *43*, 119.

(22) McLACHLAN, M. S. F., WRIGHT, A. D., DOYLE, F. H. and FRASER, T. R. (1971): Sellar reconstruction and serum levels of growth hormone in acromegaly before and after pituitary implant. *Clin. Radiol.*, *22*, 502.

(23) FRASER, T. R. (1970): Human pituitary disease. *Brit. med. J.*, *4*, 449.

Discussion

DR. HORWITH: Dr. Earle, in acromegalics does eosinophilic tissue tend to be spread diffusely or is it discretely located within the pituitary?

DR. EARLE: I have the impression from autopsy specimens consisting of the entire pituitary, that it is more inclined to be lateralized in one lobe or the other and to be more or less discrete.

DR. A. LAWRENCE: What do other areas of the anterior pituitary look like in acromegalics who have one discrete area of adenomatous hyperplasia? This, of course, pertains to these intriguing notions that perhaps some disorder in the hypothalamus acts to cause hyperplasia first and then in some we see bona fide adenomas develop.

DR. HARDY: In my experience in acromegalic patients without an enlarged sella, there is always a well localized, circumscribed nodule in the lateral wing of the gland. I do not think it is diffuse hyperplasia, but an adenoma. If it is smaller than 10 mm in diameter, we call it a microadenoma.

DR. RANDALL: I think it would be worth while to talk a bit more about microadenomas.
     There is a paper on this subject which is one of the most ignored and overlooked papers in the pituitary literature. It is entitled 'Subclinical Adenoma of the Pituitary Gland', was written by Russel P. Costellow, and appeared in the *American Journal of Pathology, Volume 12*, page 205, March 1936.
     Dr. Costello examined the pituitaries of 1000 consecutive autopsied patients, who did not have any endocrine disease. There were 224 glands, 22.4%, which contained 265 microadenomas. Of these, 140 or 52.8% were chromophobes, 20 or 7.5% were eosinophilic, 72 or 27.2% were basophilic, and 33 or 12.4% were mixed tumors. These tumors varied from small aggregates of cells up to fairly significantly sized adenomas which almost completely filled the pituitary. 66% of these patients were men and 34% were women. This corresponds quite closely to the number of men and women in the series of 1000 patients.
     These tumors have always intrigued me. These may be the forerunners of pituitary tumors which we are talking about today. These small adenomas may grow up to be the tumors which become clinically significant.

DR. LEBOVITZ: If one examines the embryology of the anterior pituitary gland, it seems possible that pituitary tumor tissue may be present in ectopic locations outside the sella such as in the ependymal area. We have seen acromegalic patients in whom extensive surgical procedures have been purported to clean out the sellar fossa, yet growth hormone levels remain high. Do you have any information on this?

DR. EARLE: We occasionally find little remnants of anterior pituitary in the sellas of people who were thought to have been totally cleaned out surgically. However, there may be parts of the brain other than the pituitary that produce hormones.

DR. LEVIN: In partial answer to Dr. Lebovitz' question, the embryology text of Patten in 1947 suggests that ectopic pituitary tissue should be considered a rule rather than an exception although he doesn't give any percentages. McGrath (*Brit. J. Surg.*, 1969) found that there are slips of anterior pituitary tissue lying in the tract left by Rathke's pouch. I ask, then, whether the partial responses that we see in some of our acromegalic patients in whom sellar approaches have been used may be related to the fact that tissue is present outside the sella. Dr. Patten stated that the three most common sites are in the floor of the sella, in the bony tissue behind the sphenoid sinus, and in the mucoperiosteum just above the posterior pharynx. Presence of tissue in these sites should be considered especially in patients who do not seem to respond to pituitary ablation.

DR. HARDY: I think this is an interesting observation from the embryological point of view, but it is not borne out by my surgical experience. I have explored more than 200 sellas in the course of normal pituitary ablation and I have never seen this sort of ectopic tissue in the sphenoid sinus or elsewhere.

DR. LEVIN: The absence of visible extrasellar pituitary tissue at transsphenoidal microdissection does not necessarily mean that no tissue is present. A dissection into the posterior wall of the sphenoid sinus might reveal such tissue.

DR. VAN BUREN: Some years ago in reviewing our hypophysectomy series, we had undertaken serial section studies of the pharyngeal hypophysis which we found at the junction of the vomer with the sphenoid bone. If you serially section this area, you will find the glandular tissue in just about all patients.

The dimensions for the pharyngeal hypophysis were established a number of years ago by Melciona and Moore. In our series of hypophysectomy patients, we did not find any pharyngeal hypophysis which exceeded the sizes of the normal. We did, however, find that there were occasional acidophilic cells and basophilic cells in the pharyngeal hypophysis. Thus, the tissue did not appear to hypertrophy after hypophysectomy but it did appear to have a potential secretory function.

DR. DAUGHADAY: The current literature indicates a very clear potential for secretion by pharyngeal pituitary tissue namely in the demonstration by immunofluorescence of the presence of small amounts of hormone. However, I am unaware of any clinical or experimental evidence to really establish that significant amounts of this hormone ever get into the circulation. Further, I am not aware of any primary tumors that have been definitely associated with pharyngeal pituitary.

We have also seen a patient with elevated serum growth hormone levels in whom the surgeon visualized no residual pituitary tissue. This patient was panhypopituitary by all our function tests, but still had active acromegaly after two surgical approaches to the pituitary. Cerebrospinal fluid growth hormone was elevated. To determine the source of growth hormone, we have differentially catheterized this patient. Peripheral blood growth hormone levels were 20 ng/ml at all sampling sites except the internal jugular vein where the growth hormone was close to 60 ng/ml. We feel that growth hormone is coming from the head in this patient.

DR. KOHLER: How many non-functioning adenomas are cystic? Do you think cyst formation is frequently caused by therapy?

DR. EARLE: Most of our material was obtained after treatment. It is my impression that cystic changes were present in the order of 10 to 15 % of our cases if you include cysts equal to or greater than 5 mm in size. In addition, microscopically we see a number of microcysts a little less than 1 mm in diameter.

DR. SHERINS: What is the sex ratio for human pituitary tumors in an unselected series?

DR. FRASER: I might attempt to answer that, since our patients have been referred without particular relevance to gynecological biased sources.

I think that both among patients with Cushing's disease and among patients with functionless tumors, we have a preponderance of females, perhaps in a 6 to 4 ratio. I don't think the same is true of acromegaly.

DR. SHERMAN: Dr. Earle, what was the incidence of pituitary apoplexy in your series?

DR. EARLE: I think it is no more than 1 or 2 %.

DR. PEARSON: Does electron microscopy have any value in assessing pituitary cells?

DR. EARLE: Yes. I think EM has certainly shown that there is probably no such thing as a chromophobe cell. All of the cells contain a few secretory granules. Now with immuno-tagging experiments and electron microscopy, it is becoming increasingly possible to identify the different hormones.

DR. ORTH: We seem to be hung up on the term 'chromophobe'. I think a 'chromophobe tumor' is a perfectly valid term. The question is whether the staining properties have any relationship to the content of hormones in the cell. In regard to this, I was fortunate to collaborate in a study with the late Dr. Robert Phifer and Dr. Samuel Spicer, using the immunoperoxidase bridge technique on normal pituitary cells using antisera specific for ACTH and for beta-MSH. The reference stain used in these studies was alcian blue-PAS-orange G. In general, in the normal pituitary cells, there was good correlation between those cells which stained a blue or blue-purple color and those cells which immunostained for ACTH and beta-MSH.

However, there are situations in which this correlation does not appear to hold. In the pituitaries of two patients who had been chronically treated with prednisone, for example, it was interesting that there were very few cells that gave this purple-blue stain. In the normal pituitary there were occasional cells which stained red or intensely red, and which stained weakly or not at all with the antiserum. In these patients treated with prednisone however, similar red staining cells stained intensely with both ACTH and beta-MSH antisera. This suggests that the stain for granules may not correlate very well with the cellular content of hormone even when secretory granules are present.

In addition, there was a patient who had so-called Schmidt's syndrome, primary hypo-adrenocorticism and hypothyroidism. In this patient there were microadenoma areas which were chromophobe. These cells also stained very well with antisera to ACTH and beta-MSH.

I should like to point out that, in all of the pituitaries Dr. Phifer examined, every cell that stained with the ACTH antiserum also stained with the beta-MSH antiserum, and every cell that stained for beta-MSH also stained for ACTH. This includes, incidentally, the areas of basophilic infiltration in the posterior lobe. Thus, it would appear that the same cells secrete both these hormones in the normal human pituitary.

DR. MECKLENBURG: Dr. Fraser, do you have any data on the frequency of the partial defects of ADH secretion among patients with pituitary tumors?

DR. FRASER: I would say it is a rare part of the clinical picture, in the order of 5 or 10 %.

DR. ROTH: I wanted to ask you about the peculiar test responses in acromegaly. It seemed to me that all patients who have high growth hormone levels from any cause seem to have these peculiar abnormal responses to the provocative and suppression tests. Since the etiology of these elevations in plasma GH is so different, it makes it harder for me to accept the uniqueness of the peculiar responses in acromegaly. I was wondering whether just high growth hormone levels do something which make the tests not work well.

DR. DAUGHADAY: In almost all these situations you are dealing with a hypothalamic pituitary system which does not appear to be subject to the usual controls. When the systems are 'go', the paradoxical, peculiar responses do not occur.

DR. HORWITH: We have been impressed with the so-called paradoxical response of growth hormone to L-DOPA. Also, we have noted hyperstimulation of growth hormone after glucagon in acromegalics.

DR. PEARSON: I would like to ask Dr. Daughaday and Dr. Fraser whether they have a shotgun test now for measuring all of the pituitary hormones at once such as using arginine, TRH, and LRH at the same time.

DR. FRASER: We haven't done it long enough to know whether it succeeds with all of these; but we now find that you can give the 2 releasing factors in the insulin tolerance test and get exactly the same responses as if you do them independently. So an insulin test combined with TRH and LHRH seems to be effective.

DR. UDVARHELYI: I would like to ask Professor Fraser how many of his cases with acromegaly showed a return of HGH to normal levels?

DR. FRASER: I think about 20 % come into the normal range. I cannot tell you the proportion, but more of these are hypopituitary than those with persistent abnormally elevated growth hormone levels.

DR. KLIMAN: I would like to turn to some emphasis on the Cushing's patients, to the use of dexamethasone testing to determine the adequacy of treatment after they have received pituitary irradiation or other procedures. I would be interested in Dr. Fraser's opinion as to whether dexamethasone suppression would be a worthwhile test to include in the follow-up of patients who have been treated for Cushing's disease, by pituitary radiotherapy.

DR. FRASER: I rather hastily gave my assessment of how best to assess Cushing's disease for obvious reasons. As I said, we feel the most useful test is the urinary-free cortisol level over 24 hours because you get an averaging of the performance throughout the day.

We have rather carefully assessed the usefulness of such basal measurement whether it be plasma cortisol at different times or urinary-free cortisol; but where urinary-free cortisol is abnormal, the suppression tests may not be normal.

Among the patients who have had a satisfactory remission, it is true, you can often confirm it with dexamethasone suppression, but I feel the metyrapone tests are better.

DR. KRIEGER: We have been following patients with Cushing's disease, not by measurement of free cortisol levels, but with determination of cortisol secretory rate. We have been following their response with regard to dexamethasone suppressibility, not by utilizing the midnight dose, but with the standard 2 mg and 8 mg courses of dexamethasone, using urinary 17-OHCS levels as the end-point. In our patients who have normal secretory rates following therapy, virtually none manifest normal dexamethasone suppressibility. In following other hypothalamic-pituitary-adrenal functions in both the patients with Cushing's disease and the patients with Nelson's syndrome, we have not used metyrapone as a test; rather, we have vasopressin more frequently as a stimulus. The marked hyperresponse of plasma corticosteroid levels following vasopressin administration in patients with active disease returns to normal in the patients with Cushing's disease in remission. However, again, in the majority of these cases, the plasma cortisol responses to an insulin test or a pyrogen test still remain abnormal (i.e. suppressed). We have observed this in patients who have been in remission for a period as long as 12 years following pituitary radiotherapy.

We have not used proton beam therapy, but conventional ^{60}Co irradiation (4000–4500 R) in these patients. We have yet to see any patient either with Nelson's syndrome or with Cushing's disease in remission who has shown a normal growth hormone response to several different parameters of testing for growth hormone (i.e. sleep associated increase, and response to insulin induced hypoglycemia or to vasopressin).

II. Neuro-ophthalmologic evaluation

Ocular manifestations produced by adenomas of the pituitary gland: analysis of 1000 cases

ROBERT W. HOLLENHORST and BRIAN R. YOUNGE

Department of Ophthalmology, Mayo Clinic and Mayo Foundation, Rochester, Minn., U.S.A.

The devastating effects produced on the visual apparatus by pituitary adenomas, while only part of the problem, are nonetheless of major importance in the proper management of these tumors. Decreasing vision is often the earliest symptom that alerts the patient to impending calamity. Since the dismal end-results of delay in diagnosis are in such marked contrast to the excellence of early treatment, the importance of prompt diagnosis and appropriate therapy cannot be overemphasized.

The following analysis of 1000 cases of proved and presumed pituitary adenomas is directed toward a quantitative appraisal of the problems as they relate to the visual apparatus. These problems include the presenting complaint in relation to the visual symptoms, the duration of the visual symptoms, the incidence of visual symptoms and of objective defects in the visual fields, the ophthalmoscopic abnormalities, and the occasional paralyses of the ocular muscles. Further, where available, the histologic features of the adenomas, the direction of growth, and the varieties and effects of treatment in this series are surveyed. As most of the 1000 patients were first seen more than 10 years ago and some as long as 35 years ago, a useful evaluation of the incidence and time of recurrence of the tumor is possible.

Materials and methods

Every patient underwent a perimetric and a tangent screen field examination before being treated at the Mayo Clinic. Those who returned for follow-up examination were re-examined in the same manner at each visit, usually annually. All were seen by a consultant in neuro-ophthalmology at each visit as a part of their systemic re-evaluation.

The compilation of the data was done with the help of the Computer Facility at the Mayo Clinic.

Our series

The clinic numbers and names of the patients were obtained from the record books in the perimetric field laboratory where all visual fields done since 1935 are listed. For 1935 through 1962 the cases are unselected, in that all cases are included if a visual field examination was recorded at the initial visit during that period; 867 of the 1000 patients were first seen during that period. An additional 17 patients, seen previously, were listed for re-evaluation during that period; 1 was seen initially in 1915, 1 in 1920, 9 in 1925–1929, and 7 in 1930–1934. We also included 116 patients seen first during the period 1963 through 1972.

There were 594 males and 406 females. Eight were less than 15 years old, 16 between 15 and 19, 36 between 20 and 24, 65 between 25 and 29, and 45 were 70 years old or older. The average age of the 228 patients who had evidences of acromegaly was 43 years, and the average age of the remaining 772 was 45 years.

Results of the survey

Presenting complaints

The most frequent primary complaint was loss of vision; next in order of frequency were headache and evidence of acromegaly (Table I). Among the 6 patients who had otolaryngologic complaints was 1 patient who had a huge nasopharyngeal tumor which proved to be a chromophobe adenoma, and another patient who had a mucocele of the sphenoid sinus diagnosed elsewhere.

Table I *Presenting complaints in 1000 cases of pituitary adenoma*

Complaint	Cases	
Visual	421	
Headache	137	
Acromegaly	136	
Related to hypopituitarism	95	
Amenorrhea	48	
Diplopia	7	
Others	156	
Pain unrelated to tumor		44
Cushing's syndrome		29
CNS signs or symptoms*		24
Diagnosis and treatment elsewhere		19
Tumor found on routine physical		10
Diabetes insipidus		10
ENT		6
CSF rhinorrhea		5
Enlarged sella (noted elsewhere)		5
Multiple adenomatosis		4
Total	1000	

* Syncope 5, seizures 5, dizziness 9, confusion 4, subarachnoid hemorrhage 1.

Among the 228 acromegalic patients, 136 presented with acromegaly as their chief complaint, whereas of the remaining 92, 32 complained of headache and 8 of amenorrhea.

Referral

Of the 1000 patients, 234 were referred by ophthalmologists, 11 by optometrists and 543 by other physicians; 212 came directly to our clinic without referral.

Duration of presenting complaint

In most cases a reasonably accurate estimation of the duration of the presenting complaint was possible (Table II). The most prolonged delays were for patients who suffered from one of the various manifestations of hypopituitarism.

Table II *Duration of presenting complaints in 1000 cases of pituitary adenoma*

Duration	Cases	
	No.	%
< 1 month	43	4.3
1–3 months	67	6.7
3–6 months	80	8.0
6–12 months	165	16.5
1–3 yr	321	32.1
3–5 yr	110	11.0
5–10 yr	122	12.2
> 10 yr	92	9.2

Duration of visual disturbances

Unexpectedly, the duration of visual disturbances was the same as the duration of the other complaints. In the series 613 patients had visual symptoms (Table III). In 346 cases the visual symptoms preceded the other manifestations; in 50 the visual and other symptoms began simultaneously; and in 217 the visual complaints occurred subsequent to other manifestations.

Table III *Duration of visual disturbances in 613 of the 1000 cases of pituitary adenoma*

Duration	Cases
< 1 month	46
1–3 months	74
3–6 months	80
6–12 months	136
1–3 yr	178
3–5 yr	38
5–10 yr	42
> 10 yr	19
Total	613

Subjective loss of vision

Many patients were unaware of their loss of vision or of the defects in their visual fields. Of the 1000 patients, 387 had no subjective loss, 116 stated that their right eye was affected, 194 complained of visual loss in the left eye, 282 complained of a visual loss in both eyes, and 21 had indefinite complaints or diplopia.

The objective findings, as shown by the results of perimetry and tangent screen examination, were difficult to tabulate, because although the typical loss involved the crossed fibers (therefore resulting in temporal or bitemporal defects in the visual fields), each case was different. To illustrate these general varieties, we employed 15 categories (Table IV). Some of these are illustrated (Figs. 1–9).

The miscellaneous group of 27 patients had defects in the visual fields that could not be assigned to any of the groups, although in general they too involved the crossing fibers.

Table IV   *Defects in visual fields in 1000 cases of pituitary adenoma*

Defect	Acro-megaly	No acro-megaly	Total
None	144	155	299
Bitemporal hemianopia (Fig. 1)	28	272	300
Superior bitemporal defect (Fig. 2)	31	70	101
Blind (1 eye), temporal defect (other eye)	3	78	81
Central or temporal scotoma (1 eye), superior temporal scotoma (other eye) (Fig. 3)	3	53	56
Homonymous hemianopia (Fig. 4)	3	39	42
Central or temporal scotoma (both eyes) (Fig. 5)	4	23	27
Superior temporal defect (1 eye) (Fig. 6)	4	29	33
Temporal scotoma (1 eye) (Fig. 7)	1	11	12
Central scotoma (1 eye) (Fig. 8)	0	8	8
Inferior temporal defect (1 eye)	0	4	4
Arcuate scotoma (1 eye)	0	4	4
Inferior temporal defect (both eyes) (Fig. 9)	3	0	3
Arcuate scotoma (1 eye), temporal defect (other eye)	0	3	3
Miscellaneous	4	23	27
Total	228	772	1000

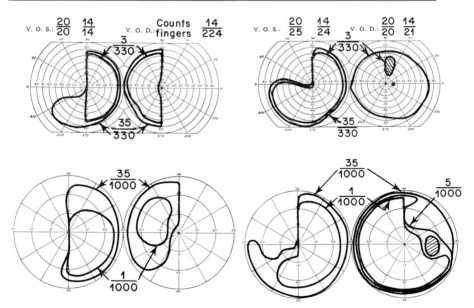

Fig. 1   Bitemporal hemianopia with loss of central vision of right eye. Major presentation of
(left)   tumor anteriorly and extending toward right optic nerve.

Fig. 2   Superior bitemporal defects. Major presentation of tumor anteriorly between the two
(right)   nerves and extending toward left optic nerve.

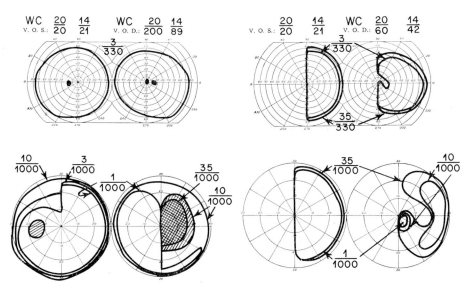

Fig. 3   Temporal scotoma of right eye and superior temporal defect of left eye (junction lesion).
(*left*)   Major presentation of tumor along right optic nerve, sparing chiasm and catching Wilbrand's knee in right optic nerve.

Fig. 4   Complete left homonymous hemianopia and temporal defect of right eye. Major presentation
(*right*)   of tumor under right optic tract, with extension along right side of chiasm and right optic nerve.

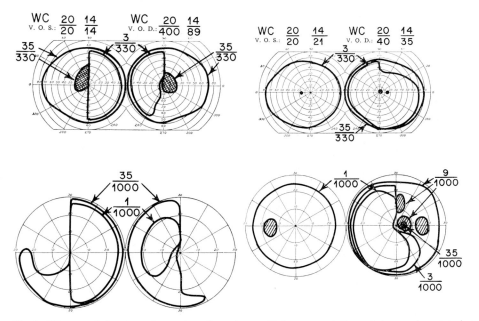

Fig. 5   Bitemporal hemianopia, scotomatous type. Major presentation of tumor in posterior
(*left*)   midline of chiasm, with extension along right optic nerve.

Fig. 6   Temporal scotomatous and superior temporal defects of right eye. Major presentation of
(*right*)   tumor along medial aspect of right optic nerve.

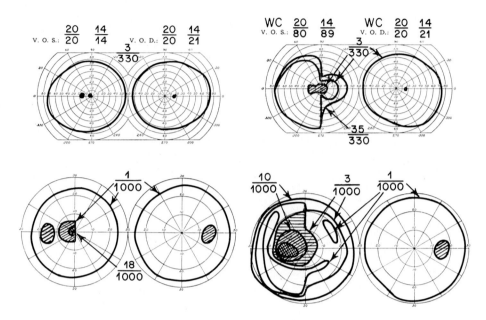

Fig. 7   Temporal scotoma of left eye. Major presentation of tumor along left optic nerve anterior
(*left*)   to Wilbrand's knee.

Fig. 8   Central scotoma with nasal anoptic defect of left eye. Major presentation of tumor along
(*right*)   lateral aspect of left optic nerve.

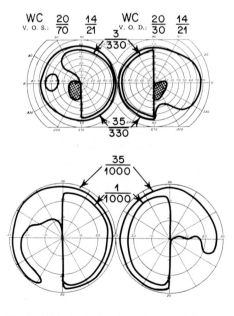

Fig. 9   Bitemporal hemianopia with inferior temporal scotomas. Major presentation of tumor
between the optic tracts, with suprasellar extension.

Of the 1000 patients, 701 (70.1 %) had defects in the visual fields: 149 of the right eye, 234 of the left eye and 318 of both eyes. Among the 228 patients with acromegaly, 84 (36.8%) had defects in the fields, and among the 772 non-acromegalic patients, 617 (80 %) had involvement of the visual pathways. Six of the acromegalic patients presented with normal visual fields initially but developed defects later: 3 after 2 years, 2 after 3–4 years and 1 during the 6th year. Among the 772 non-acromegalic patients, 53 (7 %) who had no defects initially developed them later: 14 after 2 years, 15 after 3–4 years, 17 after 5–8 years and 7 after 9 or more years.

Therefore, of the 701 patients who had involvement of the visual pathways as manifested by objectively demonstrable defects in the visual fields, 109 (15.5 %) were unaware of the visual involvement; of these, 33 overlooked the defect in the right eye, 40 that in the left eye, and 36 did not know they had bilateral defects.

Pallor of the optic disks

The more pronounced pallor, when present, was generally in the eye with the greater visual deficit. Pallor was observed in only 676 (34 %) of the 1995 eyes (Table V), which is considerably less than the 1336 (67 %) eyes that had demonstrable defects in the visual fields.

Table V   *Pallor of optic disks in 1000 cases of pituitary adenoma*

Degree of pallor	Eye	
	Right	Left
None	676	643
Grade 1	186	187
2	88	112
3	39	41
4	9	14
Eyes absent (other causes)	2	3

Only 3 patients in the entire series had papilledema; all 3 had large tumors, one invading the lateral ventricles, one invading the third ventricle, and one being a malignant adenoma.

Extraocular muscle palsy

At their initial examination, 12 patients had multiple palsies of cranial nerves III and IV or of III and VI; 2 patients had bilateral paralysis of nerve III and 32 patients had involvement of either nerve III or nerve VI (Table VI). Most of these patients had large tumors. In addition, 13 patients developed palsy of nerves III, IV or VI after operation, and 8 developed palsy at the time of the recurrence of tumor.

Pathologic aspects

Biopsy specimens were available only on 564 patients subjected to surgical extirpation of the tumor (Table VII).

Location of tumor

In most cases, the tumor could be classified as to its direction of growth on the basis of the surgical description, the type of involvement of the visual pathways, or the changes in the sellar region demonstrable by roentgenography (Table VIII).

Table VI   *Extraocular muscle palsy in 1000 cases of pituitary adenoma*

Palsy	Eye	At initial examination	Postop.	Recurrence
None	..	954	..	..
Total	..	62 (34)*	13	8
Nerve III	R	21 (12)	4	1
	L	23 (16)	3	0
IV	R	5 (0)	1	2
	L	0	1	2
VI	R	7 (4)	3	2
	L	6 (2)	1	1

* Numbers in parentheses refer to single palsy.

Table VII   *Histologic features in 1000 cases of pituitary adenoma*

Type	Acro-megaly	No acro-megaly	Total
Unknown	187	249	436
Known	41	523	564
Chromophobe	8	439	447
Eosinophil	13	6	19
Basophil	0	3	3
Mixed	15	28	43
Malignant chromophobe	0	3	3
Not specified	5	44	49
Total	228	772	1000

Table VIII   *Locations of lesions in 1000 cases of pituitary adenoma*

Location	Cases
Unknown	57
Intrasellar	320
Midline extension	422
To right optic nerve	54
To left optic nerve	63
Laterally right	33
Laterally left	33
Posteriorly right	9
Posteriorly left	7
Elsewhere	2

Results of treatment (Tables IX and X)

Of the 1000 patients, 140 were not treated at the Mayo Clinic (Table IX): some because the tumor gave no evidence of progression, some because the tumor had been treated previously elsewhere, and some because the patients refused treatment or went elsewhere.

Most of the 58 patients who had received radiation treatment and later surgery had been unsuccessfully treated elsewhere by X-ray prior to referral to the Mayo Clinic.

Table IX *Mode of treatment in 1000 cases of pituitary adenoma*

Mode	Cases
No treatment	140
Radiation alone	282
Surgery alone	280
Radiation, later surgery	58
Surgery, later radiation	240
Total	1000

Table X *Effect of treatment on pituitary adenoma*

Effect	Treatment									
	Radiation		Surgery		Radiation and surgery		Surgery and radiation		Total	
	No.	%	No.	%	No.	%	No.	%	No.	%
Visual field defects (648 cases)										
Improved	52	42.3	158	62.0	23	44.2	165	75.7	398	61.4
Unchanged	56	45.5	38	14.9	19	36.6	40	18.3	153	23.6
Worse	7	5.7	25	9.8	4	7.7	11	5.0	47	7.3
Died	2	1.6	32	12.5	6	11.5	1	0.5	41	6.3
Unknown	6	4.9	2	0.8	0	0	1	0.5	9	1.4
Total	123	100.0	255	100.0	52	100.0	218	100.0	648	100.0
Visual field defects and acromegaly (61 of 228 cases)										
Improved	11	44.0	15	71.4	2	50.0	10	90.0	38	62.3
Unchanged	14	56.0	2	9.5	2	50.0	1	10.0	19	31.2
Worse	0	0	1	4.8	0	0	0	0	1	1.6
Died	0	0	3	14.3	0	0	0	0	3	4.9
Total	25	100.0	21	100.0	4	100.0	11	100.0	61	100.0
Extraocular muscle palsy (41 of 46 cases treated)										
Improved	3		0		0		3		6	
Unchanged	3		0		8		0		11	
Worse	0		3		0		14		17	
Died	0		0		0		1		1	
Unknown	4		2		0		0		6	
Total	10		5		8		18		41	

Recurrence of treated pituitary adenomas (Table XI)

There was a significant risk of recurrence of a treated pituitary adenoma, regardless of the type of treatment. However, most of the patients were seen and treated more than 10 years ago and there have been remarkable improvements in surgical and anesthetic techniques, in instrumentation, in the application of vastly superior modes of radiation, and in the preoperative and postoperative treatment of hypopituitarism. Of the 1000 patients, 440 were treated before the corticosteroids became available in 1949. Thus, the statistics on mortality do not apply to patients treated during the past few years.

Table XI   *Recurrences in 1000 cases of pituitary adenoma*

	Total series (1000 cases)		Visual defects	
			Total (801 cases)	Acromegaly (84 cases)
None (> 10 yr)	568		349	54
Recurrence	186		176	8
Once		136	129	4
Twice		19	19	1
Three or more		4	4	0
Patient:				
Not followed or died postop.	79		48	8
Followed 2 yr (no record)	43		30	2
Followed 5 yr (no record)	48		41	3
Died of tumor		27*	24*	3*
Died of unrelated cause	64		48	4
Unknown	12		9	5

* Considered a recurrence.

Miscellaneous data

Large tumors

Of the 525 patients with pituitary adenomas treated by surgical means, 80 had 'very large', 'huge', or 'massive' tumors. Some of these lesions extended into the lateral ventricles[1], third ventricle[2], frontal lobe[2], cavernous sinus[3], hypothalamus and midbrain[2]. Of these 80 patients, 36 experienced improvement in vision, 18 had vision unchanged, 8 became worse, 1 died after radiation treatment, and 17 died after operation. In addition to these 18 deaths, 29 of the 80 patients ultimately died of the tumor.

Cushing's syndrome

Twenty-nine patients had both pituitary adenoma and Cushing's syndrome. Sixteen had lesions in which the histologic features were unknown. Of the 13 lesions with known histology, 8 were chromophobe adenomas, 1 was a basophilic adenoma, 1 was a mixed chromophobe-eosinophil adenoma, and 3 had features that were not specified.

Other tumors

Three patients had malignant adenomas; all 3 died with metastasis to liver, neck, or brain. One patient had no visual field defect, 1 had homonymous hemianopia, and 1 had arcuate defects in the visual fields. One patient had a large extension of tumor into the nasopharynx and had no visual defects.

Four patients, all females, had multiple adenomatosis, including parathyroid adenoma, thyroid adenoma or islet-cell tumor. Other neoplasms later developed in 7 patients: 1 meningioma in the posterior fossa, 1 parasagittal meningioma, 2 astrocytomas, 1 malignant melanoma of the ocular choroid, and 2 intracranial aneurysms.

Grooving of optic nerves and chiasm

At surgery in 25 patients, including 3 with acromegaly, the optic nerves or chiasm had evidence of grooving by the adjacent anterior cerebral artery. Eleven of the patients had bitemporal hemianopia, 3 had loss of vision in one eye and temporal anopsia in the other, and 11 had miscellaneous defects of the visual fields. All 25 had visual field defects at their initial examination. Fourteen improved after surgery, 4 were unchanged, 4 lost more vision, and 3 died after operation.

Glaucoma

Only 4 of the 1000 patients developed glaucoma, and none of the 4 had arcuate glaucomatous defects in the visual fields. Some authors have reported an increased incidence of glaucoma among acromegalics. Howard and English[1] found glaucoma in 7 of 70 acromegalics. In the age range of about 500 patients in our series, one might predict that at least 10 should have glaucoma, so our low incidence should dispel any but a chance relationship between pituitary tumor and glaucoma. None of the 228 patients with acromegaly in our series had glaucoma.

Pituitary apoplexy

Fifteen patients had significant hemorrhage within the tumor. Their presenting complaints varied: only 2 complained primarily of severe headache, 4 of visual deficit, 1 of severe weakness, 1 of amenorrhea, 4 of acromegaly, and 3 of non-related symptoms. Four had no visual defect, but 2 of the 4 had delayed loss of visual field within 2 years. Four had bitemporal hemianopia, 1 became completely and suddenly blind in both eyes, and the remainder had other defects. Surgical treatment produced improvement in vision in 5 and no change in 1, and surgery followed by radiation led to improvement in 5 and no change in 2. Two of these patients were lost to follow-up.

Discussion

The prompt diagnosis of pituitary tumor in a patient who has already lost a significant amount of vision, the referral for appropriate treatment, and the subsequent recovery of the vision to normal or near normal are some of the most gratifying experiences in ophthalmology. The relative rarity of chiasmal lesions, coupled with the complexity and diversity of possible visual symptoms from other causes, unfortunately may delay the diagnosis and result in the patient unnecessarily losing more vision. In our series, 421 of the 613 patients with visual symptoms had these as their presenting complaint; and in 346, nearly half of the 701 with objective loss of vision, the loss of vision preceded all other symptoms and signs. In 413 of the 613 the diagnosis was delayed from 6 months to 10 years from the time the loss of vision was first noted; and in 277 the delay was longer than 1 year (27.7 % of the 1000 cases). An additional 88 patients were unaware of the defects in their visual fields at the time of registration.

The major cause of delay in diagnosis was the failure to perform an adequate examination of the visual fields. In all but a few instances the diagnosis of a lesion involving the optic nerves or chiasm could have been made.

Rarely can the diagnosis of pituitary tumor be made simply on the basis of bitemporal field defects, because identical defects in the visual fields often occur in patients who have involvement of the optic nerves and chiasm by internal carotid aneurysm, chiasmal arachnoiditis, chordoma, craniopharyngioma, syphilis, metastatic carcinoma from breast or lung, or glioma of the chiasm.

Generally, pallor of the optic disks, which was present in 34 % of the 1995 eyes, is of little importance in establishing the diagnosis of a chiasmal lesion, as compared to the examination of the visual fields. Also, the lesser degrees of pallor give minimal prognostic assistance, because most patients with pallor of grade 1 or 2 seem to recover vision with appropriate therapy. However, the higher degrees of optic nerve pallor carry a poor prognosis for recovery[3].

The types of defects in the visual fields vary widely. Generally, the site of involvement of the visual pathways can be accurately localized by the pattern of the field defect. For example, a tumor in the presence of nearly symmetrical superior temporal defects in both eyes (Fig. 2) extends in the midline between the two optic nerves in a post-placed chiasm. A bitemporal hemianopia with a central field defect in the right eye (Fig. 1) localizes the tumor at the right side of the chiasm and involving the right optic nerve. A left homonymous hemianopia with a defect in central vision of the right eye (Fig. 4) localizes the tumor to the right optic tract, the right side of the optic chiasm, and the right optic nerve.

Among the 228 patients with acromegaly, 84 (36.8 %) initially had defects in the visual fields, comparable to those found in other smaller series of tumors[2]. Visual field defects were considerably more frequent among the 772 non-acromegalics, as they were present in 617 (80 %) of the group.

The importance of close observation of the visual fields is shown by the development of defects in the visual fields in patients who initially had no defects, i.e., in 6 (2.6 %) of the acromegalics and in 53 (7 %) of the non-acromegalics.

The analysis of the results of various modes of treatment as applied to the visual status is considerably out of date. Nonetheless, the improvement rates are impressive, ranging from 42 % in those treated by radiation alone to 75 % in those treated by surgery followed by radiation.

Hopefully, recurrences will be less frequent. Our figure of 18.6 % recurrence emphasizes the importance of the annual re-evaluation of the visual fields of patients who have pituitary adenomas. More than 15 % of all the patients who had defects in the visual fields at the initial examination were unaware of their defects. Therefore, it is not safe to rely on the patient's own observation to tell him if his tumor is recurring.

Summary

In the analysis of 1000 patients with pituitary adenomas, most of which were diagnosed between 1940 and 1962, 701 had defects usually of bitemporal type in the visual fields. Of these, more than 15 % were unaware of the defects. In some cases the diagnosis was not made for as long as 10 years after the initial complaint, and in most cases a delay in diagnosis was to the detriment of the patient. Paralysis of nerves III, IV, and VI was characteristic of large tumors that had extended out of the sella turcica into the cavernous sinus and adjacent structures. The overall immediate and long-term prognosis for patients with such large tumors is unfavorable. Of the 564 surgical specimens obtained, 447 were chromophobic, 19 eosinophilic, 3 basophilic, 43 mixed, and 3 malignant chromophobic adenomas. Among the 41 acromegalics, 8 had chromophobic, 13 eosinophilic, and 15 mixed adenomas. Treatment of 648 patients resulted in rates of improvement of vision that ranged from 42.2 % for radiation to 75.6 % for surgery followed by radiation. A total of 186 patients had recurrences; the duration between operation and recurrence ranged from 1 year to more than 21 years, the majority recurring within 8 years.

References

(1) HOWARD, G. M. and ENGLISH, F. P. (1965): Occurrence of glaucoma in acromegalics. *Arch. Ophthal.*, 73, 765.

(2) HUBER, A. (1971): *Eye Symptoms in Brain Tumors*, 2nd ed., pp. 189–211. C.V. Mosby Co., St. Louis, Mo.

(3) WALSH, F. B. and HOYT, W. F. (1969): *Clinical Neuro-Ophthalmology. 3rd ed., Vol. 3*, pp. 2130–2154. Williams and Wilkins Co., Baltimore, Md.

Discussion

DR. HOYT: This series of 1000 cases is a new 'landmark'. Dr. Hollenhorst has properly cautioned us about the problems of evaluating results of therapy from a series that includes patients treated 20 to 30 years ago. We need to know what is happening in this decade.

I have a few comments regarding some trends that I have observed in my work which is much like Dr. Hollenhorst's. I see these 'pituitary' patients during the diagnostic, surgical, radiation, and follow-up phases of their management.

1. *The diagnostic phase*:   Failure or delay of ophthalmologic diagnosis is a result not only of poor visual field examination, but also a failure to obtain skull films as soon as the ophthalmologist recognizes that his patient is progressively loosing vision in one or both eyes.

It should be recalled that no patient with a field defect has a small tumor. A possible exception to this rule is the adenoma that expands to compress an optic nerve against an anterior clinoid process. No matter how refined the perimetric technique employed, we are always searching for relatively large adenomas. Discovery of smaller tumors is not an ophthalmologic problem. Instead, it is a problem of educating the physicians who refer patients to endocrinologists.

2. *The surgical phase and immediate post-operative period*:   How fast can vision return after operation? Repeatedly, we have tried to document this point by doing visual field examinations earlier and earlier during the post-surgical period, even in the recovery room. As a result, we know that visual function can return immediately as the nerve and chiasm are decompressed.

3. *The radiation therapy phase*:   How often should visual fields be performed? Some enthusiasts have advocated daily fields during the first weeks of the radiation therapy.

If this policy is followed, you soon exhaust your perimetrist. I have never seen deterioration of visual fields during radiation therapy in spite of Harvey Cushing's admonitions to the contrary. The intervals between visual field examinations can be greatly extended, perhaps to monthly intervals for six months, and then yearly.

4. *The post-therapy phase*:   Three problems cause recurrent visual failure: (1) recurrence of tumor, (2) effects of the empty sella, and (3) radionecrosis. The latter two are rare.

Are visual field studies a good way to search for evidence of tumor recurrence? They are not. What we need is anatomic, not perimetric, information. We want to know when the tumor is regrowing and refilling the sella. This is a job for neurosurgery and neuroradiology. We need markers that will indicate refilling of the sella by tumor – perhaps a radiopaque marker which would be displaced by tumor regrowth, or the technique of comfortable small-exchange pneumoencephalogram as done by Rand.

DR. KJELLBERG: With respect to Dr. Hoyt's comment about a marker, for a number of years we have used gold foil for this purpose. The foil is folded in multiple segments and applied to the diaphragma, the cavernous sinuses, and the sella floor. We have assumed that we can recognize recurrence at an early time by simple AP and lateral skull films that could be done easily on an outpatient basis.

DR. HOYT: Does that mean you don't need to do visual fields?

DR. KJELLBERG: No, we always do visual fields. Until we are certain that the foil is reliable, we would not recommend abandoning established methods such as visual fields.

DR. FAGER: I am much more concerned about the patients with visual field defects who are candidates for radiation alone, and there are a large number of such patients. I think you would agree that your recommendation for follow-up within a month is not satisfactory.

When we elect to use radiotherapy alone in patients with pituitary tumors, we believe that their fields and acuity must be checked twice a week for the first week or two, and then once a week, and then once a month for the next few months.

DR. HOYT: When we treat patients primarily by radiotherapy, we do more frequent field examinations during the initial treatment period.

DR. HOLLENHORST: At our institution, whenever the tumor is being irradiated, we usually plot the visual fields at the beginning, at the middle, and at the end of treatment. I also have never seen a patient with pituitary tumor whose vision deteriorated during X-ray treatment.

DR. ZERVAS: Using visual fields, is it possible to discriminate patients having tumor recurrences from patients who might be having radiation damage?

DR. HOLLENHORST: Let me repeat that I have never observed significant diminution of vision during treatment of a pituitary tumor by irradiation. When a patient begins to lose vision 4 or 5 months after termination of radiation therapy, I would suspect that regrowth of tumor is more probable than radiation necrosis or vasculitis.

DR. HOYT: I agree fully with the statement by Dr. Hollenhorst. However, Dr. Zervas asked if we can use perimetry to differentiate among recurrence of tumor, radionecrosis, and the 'crimped nerve' of the empty sella. I am unable to make this distinction with perimetry. In my opinion, this is a neuroradiologic problem. I should note that with radionecrosis the discs become pale, the retinal arteries narrow, and the entire field is slightly decreased before a rather rapid loss of the visual fields takes place. Often the visual field loss suggests vascular involvement, but re-compression effects or empty sella effects are very similar.

DR. DI CHIRO: By pneumoencephalography the etiology of the visual changes in the empty sella has been demonstrated to be the result of the descent or perhaps 'pulling down' of the optic chiasma and/or optic nerves into the post-surgery or post-radiation empty sella.

DR. FAGER: I have seen visual fields deteriorate while patients were getting radiation therapy. I don't think there is any question about this. I think these patients have to be watched very closely. I insist that they be seen during the first week of their therapy two or three times and during the second week, at least once, and then once a week until the end of the month.

DR. RANDALL: We do not treat many patients having field defects with radiation therapy only, but we do follow such patients more carefully than patients who are decompressed at surgery and then given radiation therapy.

DR. KRAMER: I wonder if I might comment on this question of the visual fields and therapy as a practising radiation oncologist.

It is exceedingly unlikely for a tumor to enlarge significantly at the beginning of therapy and we need not worry about that.

As far as the visual field checks during therapy are concerned, I think it depends a little bit on the type of history and the evolution of the tumor that one is dealing with. A patient that has been relatively stable is not likely to change without complaining about it. Equally clearly a patient in whom there has been a rapid progression and where, as Dr. Fager might think, radiation therapy alone is the treatment of choice, it has to be checked very carefully.

Now, as to the interval between radiation therapy and improvement, I would agree that it is quite common to see improvement at least towards the end of radiation therapy. Sometimes we see it astonishingly rapidly, and the fact that changes have occurred so quickly induced many of our former colleagues to give very low doses and then repeat them frequently. This regimen produced the morbidity which we rarely see with a single extended course of radiation therapy.

Then again we see patients whose fields have remained stationary or who have begun to improve late in radiation therapy. All of these variants have to be taken into consideration before deciding whether further therapy is to be done.

DR. FAGER: What do you think happens when a patient worsens during radiation therapy? When I have operated on these, many of them look just like a pituitary infarction; like a hemorrhagic gland that has swollen and infarcted.

DR. KRAMER: I think you get hemorrhage whether you treat them or not. I don't think anybody has ever suggested that radiation therapy is a means of prevention of the hemorrhage.

DR. FAGER: No, but here is a patient who is getting slowly worse over a period of months, and then you subject him to radiation, and within a matter of a week or so, he becomes rapidly worse.

DR. KRAMER: I think it is impossible to say. I really cannot see any mechanism, because unless you give enormously high doses, it is exceedingly difficult to destroy vascular epithelium quickly.

DR. FRASER: I want to make a comment on this question of radiation worsening the field defect during radiation. When we put pituitary implants into patients, they will get intense radiation postoperatively over a period of about ten days. It is our practice, when they have field defects or evidence of a moderate upward extension, to watch very carefully for any field loss. If this occurs we put them on corticosteroids, and the field loss goes as the swelling shrinks.

So we would expect to get swelling in some tumors where you radiate them intensely and I don't see why you shouldn't when you radiate them more mildly with external irradiation. You should also be able to minimize this with corticosteroids.

VOICE: I would like to ask 2 questions. Does the degree of the defect in the visual fields influence the choice of therapy?

Secondly, I would like to ask whether the prognosis for improvement is related to the duration of the lesion.

DR. HOLLENHORST: There was, of course, some selection in choice of mode of treatment in our series in that radiation usually was not given to the patients with the more severe defects in the visual fields. In spite of this, the results from radiation alone were less favorable than from surgery plus radiation.

DR. HOYT: Duration of the lesion is a vital factor: if atrophy is already established, function in these fibers cannot return.

The obvious way to assess preoperatively the recovery that can be anticipated is to assess the amount of degeneration already present in the retinal nerve fiber layer. This can be seen funduscopically and photographed. We can now assess what is normal and to some degree, how much has been lost. This index provides a more direct parameter for assessment of nerve fiber attrition. If the nerve fiber layer is intact, it makes no difference whether the field defect has been present for six months; vision still can return, as exemplified frequently in the removal of sphenoid meningiomas. Reversible conduction block can persist for many months.

DR. BATZDORF: We have also looked at the question of duration of symptoms versus potential for visual recovery and found that long duration of a tumor is not necessarily incompatible with significant visual recovery.

In addition to duration, we have also examined the effect of tumor size on improvement. Substantial visual improvement can occur even with very large tumors extending above the sella and distorting the third ventricle.

DR. VAN BUREN: I had a question for Dr. Hollenhorst. When you found that your results from radiation were inferior to those of surgery plus radiation, were you not confounding the treatment with early low-voltage radiation to the more recent super-voltage radiation? I think the two are different.

DR. HOLLENHORST: I tried to emphasize in my paper that my data on the results of all types of treatment were long out of date and therefore invalid. We closed the series essentially in 1962, and 440 of my cases dated from longer than 20 years ago.

DR. ROSS: How long after treatment should one wait for the ascertainment of maximal improvement in a visual field that is impaired in the first instance?

DR. HOLLENHORST: Among surgical patients, I have seen some who have a practically complete recovery of vision almost immediately after they recover from the operative procedure. We plot the visual fields about five to seven days after the operation. We like to check it again in about three months, and then again about six months after the surgery; and then a year after that in order to have a baseline for recovery. Maximum recovery occurs usually by the third month, but there may be minimal further improvement during the entire first year. The improvement in vision brought about by irradiation is much slower; but probably, as with surgical treatment, the maximum recovery has taken place by the end of the third month. Some continue to recover vision for six or more months.

Usually recovery does not begin until four to six weeks after radiation is applied, but we have seen some recovery at times by the end of the second week.

III. Neuroradiologic evaluation

Radiographic and radioisotopic techniques in diagnosis of pituitary tumors

MICHAEL D. F. DECK

Memorial Hospital and New York Hospital, Cornell Medical Center, New York, N.Y., U.S.A.

The radiologic diagnosis of tumors of the pituitary gland and the differentiation from other sellar and parasellar lesions is based on standard techniques of plain skull films, tomography of the sella, pneumoencephalography and cerebral angiography. Recently, attention has focused on brain scanning as a method of detecting pituitary tumors and other sellar and parasellar lesions, and there has also been speculation as to the possible use of intrathecal scanning agents in attempts to delineate the cisternal encroachment of such lesions. Great interest has recently been aroused by a new method of diagnosing intracranial pathology using a system of transverse axial computerized tomography. An additional diagnostic method receiving increased attention is that of cavernous sinus venography to better delineate the size of the pituitary gland with particular reference to bilateral expansion.

Plain skull films

Evaluation of the sella turcica and adjacent structures is based primarily on its appearances in several projections of the skull. To detect the more subtle changes of sellar and parasellar lesions, a meticulous radiographic technique is required. A small focal spot X-ray tube (0.3 mm^2 or 0.6 mm^2) and low kvp (50–65) are used with a fine line grid. High detail intensifying screens and high contrast film ensures optimal bone detail and contrast. Rigid immobilization and accurate positioning of the patient are essential. In cases of questionable decalcification of the bony cortex lining the floor and intrasellar surface of the dorsum sellae (the 'lamina dura') magnification technique using a 0.3 mm^2 focal spot X-ray tube and primary radiographic magnification is often of great benefit. Stereoscopic views in lateral, frontal and axial projections may be of value although the usefulness of such views is somewhat limited by the subjective nature of the interpretation.

The routine radiographic study of the sella includes the lateral projection, the half axial or modified half axial projection ($+25°$ to $+30°$) to visualize the dorsum sellae and the anterior clinoid processes, the frontal projection (PA or AP 0°) to show mainly the sellar floor, the anterior clinoids and the lesser sphenoid wings, the inclined posteroanterior projections (PA $-25°$) for the sellar floor and superior orbital fissures and the axial projection (AP $-90°$) for the sphenoid sinus, floor of the middle cranial fossa, nasopharynx and basal foramina. (Skull projection angles are referred to Reid's base line.[11])

In addition to the projections just described, additional views to show the optic foramina and superior orbital fissure may be useful in asymmetric enlargement of pituitary tumors and in the presence of parasellar lesions, particularly aneurysms of the intracavernous carotid artery. The standard projection for the optic foramen ($-12°$, $+35°$) results in a true axial view of the optic canal which is projected into the inferolateral quadrant of the bony orbit. The 'optic strut view' is taken by turning the head less ($-12°$, $+20°$), thus giving a distorted view of the optic foramen but demonstrating the strut and the superior orbital fissure.

Tomography

Tomography of the sella turcica need not be performed routinely in patients with suspected pituitary tumors, but it should be used without hesitation to solve problems that are raised on the plain films. The use of complex motion tomographic units such as the Polytome (Philips Massiot) or the Stratimatic (C.G.R.) gives optimal definition with cuts slightly less than 1 mm thick and with very complete blurring of structures above and below the plane of section. The use of simpler apparatus allowing linear tomographic motion is, however, quite consistent with high quality studies. If it permits variation in the direction of the tomographic sweep, movement parallel to any linear structure of interest may be avoided and dense structures out of the tomographic plane may be smudged away from the area of interest. The indications for tomography include localization of parasellar and suprasellar calcification[2] and demonstration of defects in the sellar floor. In the case of asymmetric sellar enlargement, where the floor is not seen on the frontal projections, the side of the expansion may be shown (Fig. 1). In gross destruction of the sella, the inferior extension

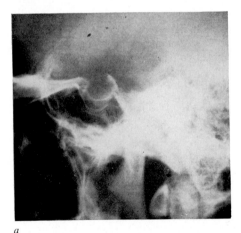
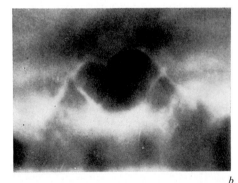

a   *b*

Fig. 1   (*a*) Lateral skull showing asymmetrical sellar enlargement with double floor.
          (*b*) Frontal hypocycloidal tomogram demonstrating the enlargement on the right side.

along the clivus may be obscured by the mastoid and petrous bone structures in which case tomography is indicated (Fig. 2). Any suspicion of sphenoid sinus opacity should be resolved by tomography; otherwise sphenoid sinus carcinomas and mucoceles may be overlooked.

If transsphenoidal surgery is contemplated, tomography in frontal and lateral projections gives a better demonstration of the anatomy of the sphenoid sinus septum and related structures, permitting more accurate preoperative planning.

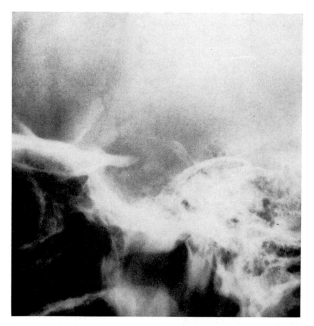

Fig. 2   Grossly enlarged sella turcica on lateral skull projection. Tomography is indicated to define the extent of the destruction inferiorly. Note the curvilinear calcification in the roof of the tumor. Operation revealed large chromophobe adenoma.

It should be remembered that if the patient is to undergo pneumoencephalography, there is no reason to perform tomography as a separate study as total delineation of the pituitary tumor will almost certainly require lateral and frontal tomography during the pneumoencephalogram.

Pneumoencephalography

While the size of the intrasellar component of a pituitary tumor can usually be accurately assessed from the sella enlargement on plain skull radiographs, a pneumoencephalogram is the study of choice to show the size and shape of the suprasellar portion of the tumor as well as the relationship of adjacent structures such as the optic nerves and chiasm and the foramen of Monro.

The use of tomography during the pneumoencephalogram is considered essential because the outline of the tumor is frequently obscured by overlying gas. Unfortunately, because of the cost of equipment, many centers are still performing the studies without tomography. The anterior recesses of the third ventricle may be visualized satisfactorily in the lateral projection by the use of autotomography, but this technique cannot be usefully employed in the frontal projection. The choice of a tomographic apparatus for pneumoencephalography is between the many units designed for this purpose, but capable only of linear tomography, and complex movement devices such as the Universal Polytome which give the best resolution and thinnest 'cut' available. While the latter unit provides the best detail, it is with considerable loss of convenience because of difficulty in obtaining tomographic cuts in other than horizontal or vertical planes. For greatest convenience, devices such as the Princeps and Neurocentrix (C.G.R.), Neurotome (G.E.) or Neurodiagnost (Philips) are available. These units use a linear tomographic motion the direction of which is variable through 180°, thus permitting orientation appropriate to the structure of interest. For example, it is of great value to orient the tomographic motion transversely across the head when studying a suprasellar mass because the lateral margins of the mass are of particular interest and because a vertical sweep smudges dense midline nasal structures over the midline suprasellar cistern. A probable additional advantage of linear tomographic motion during pneumoencephalography is that the contrast between air and soft tissue is somewhat greater than with hypocycloidal motion because the focal plane is somewhat thicker. While various workers have advised the use of the hypocycloidal motion[3-5] because of its superior resolution, McLachlan et al.[6] in 37 cases of pituitary tumor used a 10° circular motion, presumably because of greater contrast and thicker cut.

The technique of fractional pneumoencephalography for pituitary tumors is well described in standard works[7, 8] and differs little from that used for other intra-axial and extra-axial tumors. Adequate visualization of the whole ventricular system is necessary with particular attention to the anterior recesses of the third ventricle and the anterior horns of the lateral ventricles. Lateral and frontal tomography of the sellar region is performed when adequate filling of the ventricles and basal cisterns is achieved. Great care should also be taken to demonstrate the temporal horns, if necessary, with additional tomography as this may be the only means of showing a lateral extension of a chromophobe adenoma into the temporal lobe or Sylvian fissure (Fig. 3).

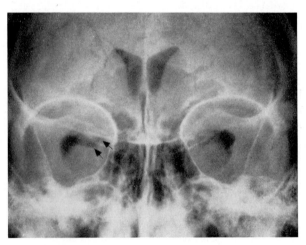

Fig. 3 Frontal temporal horn view showing lateral extension of tumor into the superior recess of the right temporal horn (arrows).

In the presence of a huge suprasellar extension with obliteration of the anterior part of the third ventricle, the foramen of Monro may be obstructed requiring air ventriculography for complete demonstration of the lateral ventricles. When the suprasellar cistern is well filled with air, demonstration of the optic chiasm and the optic and infundibular recesses of the third ventricle may be impossible without accurate lateral midline tomography. In fact small suprasellar masses may be partly obscured if the cistern is large. A thin-section tomogram is thus necessary to show slight bulging of the diaphragma sellae or a 2 to 3 mm extension through the infundibular hiatus.

If the anterior recesses of the third ventricle are obscured by cisternal air, it may be helpful to restudy the patient 3 to 5 hours later. By this time most of the cisternal air will have been reabsorbed.

Cerebral angiography

The main reason for performing carotid arteriography on patients suspected of harboring a chromophobe adenoma is to exclude an aneurysm which is usually not distinguishable from a pituitary tumor on plain radiographs or pneumoencephalography. Lombardi[9] recorded 2 operative deaths on patients incorrectly diagnosed by pneumoencephalography as having chromophobe adenomas. However, intrasellar aneurysms are relatively rare. They may arise from the cavernous part of the internal carotid artery in which case the sella is almost always enlarged more on the side of origin. Intrasellar aneurysms may also arise from the supraclinoid part of the internal carotid artery, the anterior communicating artery, the posterior communicating artery, posterior cerebral artery or rarely even the basilar artery.

Bilateral carotid arteriography, either by direct percutaneous puncture or using a femoral catheter, is necessary to rule out an aneurysm. Unilateral cerebral angiography with or without contralateral carotid compression may fail to opacify the lesion and occasionally aneurysms of the intracavernous part of the carotid artery may be bilateral.[10] Although the main reason for performing angiography is as stated, much useful information as to the size and nature of intra- and suprasellar masses may be obtained from high quality studies.

The cavernous part of the internal carotid artery, being in the cavernous sinus immediately lateral to the pituitary fossa, is usually displaced by an intrasellar mass (Fig. 4). On the lateral projection the 'siphon' may be displaced forward or backward or opened (Fig. 5), but on the frontal projection it is nearly always displaced laterally. Bull and Schunk[11] found the distance of the medial surface of the siphon to be 5 to 11 mm in 50 normal arteriograms and greater than 11 mm in 11 out of 12 cases of pituitary adenoma. These measurements have more recently been confirmed by Bergland et al.[12] who found a distance of 4

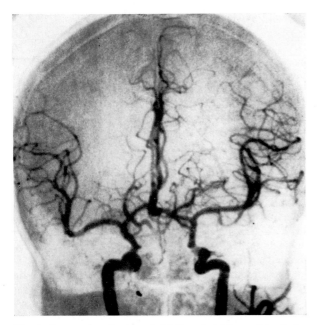

Fig. 4   Composite of subtracted left and right carotid arteriogram in frontal projection shows the lateral displacement of the carotid artery in the cavernous sinus and upward stretching of the precommunicating parts of the anterior cerebral arteries. The left middle cerebral artery is elevated.

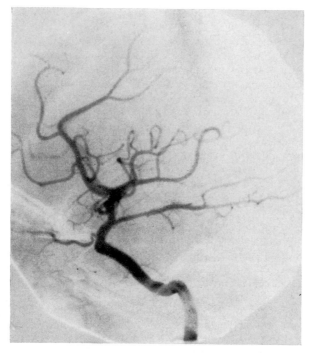

Fig. 5 Lateral carotid arteriogram demonstrates marked stretching of the cavernous portion of the internal carotid artery as well as stretching of the posterior cerebral artery and elevation of the supraclinoid part of the internal carotid artery.

to 23 mm between the cavernous parts of the carotid arteries in 225 autopsy specimens. The earliest changes may consist of flattening of the medial surface of the cavernous carotid artery, and this may be demonstrated best on an axial projection.[4]

It must be remembered that occasionally an intrasellar adenoma may extend through the cavernous sinus into the middle cranial fossa with little or no deformity of the 'siphon', but with elevation of the Sylvian part of the middle cerebral artery and an elevation of the anterior segment of the basal vein of Rosenthal.

Occasionally the cavernous part of the internal carotid artery may become surrounded by a pituitary tumor in which case the vessel will show irregular narrowing as well as displacement. Such a sign indicates a relatively poor prognosis[13] from a surgical point of view. It is more commonly seen in association with parasellar meningiomas, and its presence should lead to questioning of the diagnosis.

The angiographic signs of a suprasellar mass, whether of intrasellar origin or primarily suprasellar, have been described in detail in the literature and in standard texts.[7, 14, 15] The vascular displacements depend on whether the mass is anterior suprasellar, suprasellar or posterior suprasellar. They include elevation, lateral displacement and stretching of the terminal segment of the internal carotid artery (Fig. 5), elevation of the precommunicating parts of the anterior cerebral arteries (Fig. 4), lateral displacement of the posterior cerebral and anterior choroidal arteries and, if the mass is large, elevation of the anteroseptal and internal cerebral veins.

In many cases the angiographic findings correlate poorly with the findings at pneumoencephalography[16] in that the suprasellar mass is much larger than the arteriogram suggests. Gado and Bull[17] reviewed 27 cases of pituitary adenoma and found that in 11 cases the precommunicating part of the anterior cerebral artery (A1 segment) 'capped' the superior aspect of the suprasellar mass, thus accurately depicting its size, while in 6 cases the upward displacement was masked by opening of the carotid siphon. In 10 cases where the A1 segment was equivocal or grossly underestimated the size of the suprasellar mass, the lateral projection showed that there was anterior displacement of the medial end of the vessel

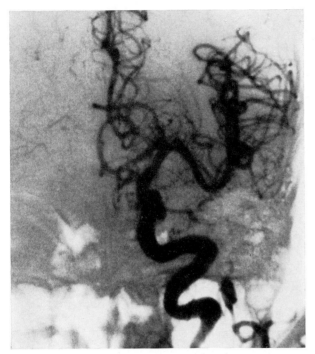

Fig. 6a Left carotid arteriogram frontal projection shows low precommunicating part of the anterior cerebral artery.

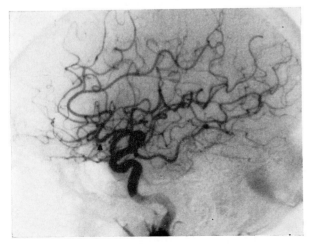

Fig. 6b Lateral projection shows the precommunicating part of the anterior cerebral artery to be displaced anteriorly (arrow).

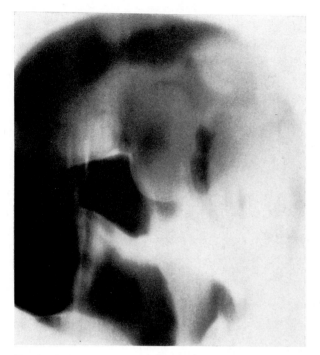

Fig. 6c   Lateral tomogram during pneumoencephalography shows the exact size of the suprasellar mass.

(point 2) at the anterior communicating artery (Fig. 6). Thus the tumor may slip posteriorly and extend high into the third ventricle even as far as the foramen of Monro, producing only slight anterior displacement of the anterior cerebral artery.

Many texts and older references indicate that most pituitary tumors are avascular while evidence of abnormal vasculature or 'blush' indicates malignant degeneration. There are, however, occasional examples of simple chromophobe adenomas, usually large, where abnormal vasculature is shown by standard angiographic techniques.[18-21]

The increasing use of subtraction and of radiographic magnification during cerebral angiography has resulted in reassessment of the importance of tumor vessels and blushes in pituitary tumors. The detailed anatomical descriptions of the blood supply to the sella turcica, pituitary gland, optic nerves and chiasm and the adjacent brain and dura[22,23] have stimulated the understanding of this region.

In a detailed description of the normal and abnormal anatomy of the sellar region using magnification and subtraction, Baker[24,25] found numerous abnormalities which had been ignored in the past. In all 76 cases of pituitary adenoma, the posterior pituitary blush was absent, while it was present in 68 of 75 normal magnified lateral angiograms. Small feeding arteries, usually from the meningohypophyseal trunk, were seen in 65 of the cases (Fig. 7), and tumor vascularities including abnormal irregular channels were present in 19 cases, a faint diffuse blush in 61 (Fig. 8) and capsular veins in 23. The circuminfundibular arterial plexus, seen normally in 71 of 75 cases, was a reliable indicator of superior extension of the tumor, being closely related to the optic chiasm.

One of the difficulties in the analysis of magnification lateral cerebral angiograms is the confusion caused by overlying blood vessels and brain blush in the basal ganglia, Sylvian

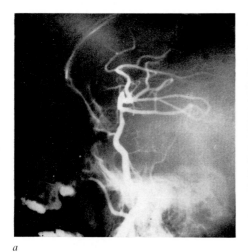
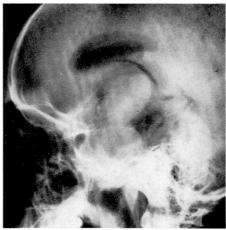

a   *b*

Fig. 7   (*a*) Lateral carotid arteriogram in a 16-year-old male demonstrates gross stretching of the internal carotid artery and enlargement of an artery from the internal carotid, probably the inferior hypophyseal branch. There is also gross elevation of the middle cerebral artery due to lateral extension into the temporal lobe.

     (*b*) Pneumoencephalogram shows massive suprasellar extension to the foramen of Monro as well as gross posterior extension into the prepontine cistern.

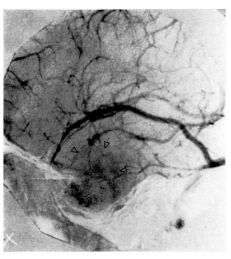
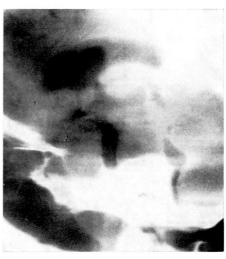

a   *b*

Fig. 8   (*a*) Lateral venous phase subtraction arteriogram shows faint tumor blush in the enlarged sella turcica and in the suprasellar cistern (arrows).

     (*b*) Pneumoencephalogram lateral tomogram brow-up shows actual size of the tumor.

fissure and temporal lobe. It is therefore possible that angiotomography may enhance the accuracy of cerebral angiography still further.

Angiography plays an important part in differentiating other suprasellar tumors from pituitary adenomas. Meningiomas in addition to hyperostosis usually exhibit a characteristic 'blush', and magnification should demonstrate hypertrophy of meningeal arteries. Metastatic tumors to the sphenoid, chordomas and sphenoid sinus carcinomas may be differentiated by the extent of the tumor stain and abnormal vasculature as well as by the plain radiographs and tomography, although difficulties may arise. Craniopharyngiomas, while usually avascular, may occasionally show tumor vessels and a diffuse blush. Optic chiasm glioma usually produces characteristic plain radiograph changes, but it may also result in marked angiographic abnormalities such as vascular blush, early venous filling and stretching of superior hypophyseal and premamillary arteries.

Technique of cerebral angiography

The choice between direct percutaneous cerebral angiography, selective catheter angiography from the femoral artery and retrograde brachial arteriography is based on the age of the patient and the particular skill of the angiographer. This author generally prefers selective catheterization from the femoral artery in patients under the age of 55 years. Attempts should be made to opacify the internal carotid artery selectively to obtain optimal contrast without overlying scalp vessels. Vertebral arteriography may be useful in evaluating retrosellar extension of a pituitary tumor and in excluding an aneurysm of the basilar artery.

Standard magnification serial angiography in inclined frontal and lateral projections may be performed in addition to routine non-magnification views. To obtain acceptable results with magnification technique, the focal spot of the X-ray tube must be no larger than 0.45 mm^2, the X-ray beam must be tightly collimated because the grid is removed and the mid-sagittal plane of the head should be placed equidistant between the focal spot and the film. Films should be taken at a minimum rate of 1 per second at least during the arterial and early venous phase.

Radionuclide techniques

It has been stated that brain scanning techniques play no important role in the diagnosis of pituitary tumors[4] because of their relative inaccuracy and insensitivity. In fact brain scans are performed infrequently on patients suspected of having suprasellar or intrasellar masses. In his analysis of 847 proven intracranial lesions, Burrows[26] studied 11 patients with pituitary adenomas, and there were 4 positive scans and 7 false negatives. Otto et al.[27] using their so-called multiphasic scintigraphy (views of the head taken 10 minutes, 60 minutes and up to 6 hours after the injection of 10 mc ^{99m}Tc pertechnetate) were able to detect 10 out of 14 pituitary tumors, while their review of the literature showed an overall success rate of slightly less than 50 % (80 positive, 85 false negative and 2 equivocal). These workers also found a surprising incidence of positive scans in craniopharyngiomas detecting all 6, with a review of the literature showing 38 positives and 19 false negatives. This high detection rate for craniopharyngiomas is confirmed by James et al.[28] who found scans to be positive in 12 out of 13 patients, concluding that the scans, when interpreted with the plain films, were almost diagnostic.

The problem with pituitary adenomas is their anatomic location in the sella turcica. The tumor is surrounded by blood in the carotid arteries and cavernous sinuses where the level of radioactivity is high with the sphenoid sinus immediately beneath it where selective excretion of ^{99m}Tc pertechnetate occurs. In addition, the temporalis muscles overlie the sella on the lateral view. Thus, even though the tumor may concentrate the isotope relative to the brain, there is no difference between it and the surrounding structures at the base of the skull.

It is possible that a tomographic scanning technique may reveal pituitary adenomas more reliably by removing the overlying activity in the temporalis muscles and temporal lobes.

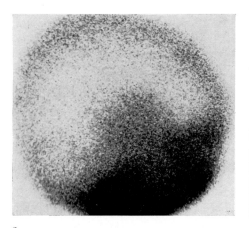
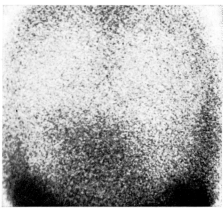

a   b

Fig. 9   (*a*) Lateral brain scan of 14-year-old female with gigantism showing large area of abnormal
activity in the suprasellar region.
(*b*) Frontal scan showing the slightly asymmetric mass with more activity to the right than
to the left.

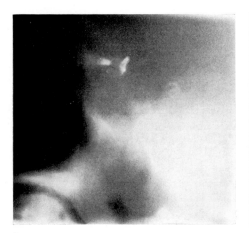
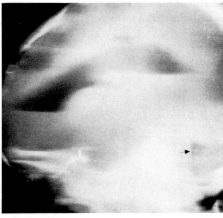

c   d

Fig. 9   (*c*) Lateral midline tomogram demonstrates destruction of the sella and sphenoid bone to
the level of the spheno-occipital synchondrosis. A soft tissue mass obliterates the nasopharynx
down to the level of the hard palate (arrow).
(*d*) Lateral tomogram during pneumoencephalography shows a suprasellar mass extending
to the foramen of Monro. There was also extension into the right temporal lobe and posteriorly into the posterior fossa with displacement of the fourth ventricle (arrow). Following
partial surgical resection and then external irradiation, the mass in the nasopharynx resolved
and a cerebrospinal fluid fistula led to recurrent episodes of meningitis.

Kuhl et al.[29, 30] demonstrated an optic chiasm glioma using their sectional scanning device
but attributed the difficulties in the region to the sphenoid sinus, cavernous sinus and carotid
arteries.

It may be predicted that pituitary tumors with suprasellar extensions greater than 2 cm
in diameter should be demonstrable (Fig. 9), while those confined to the sella or expanding
into the sphenoid sinus and nasopharynx would go undetected (Fig. 10).

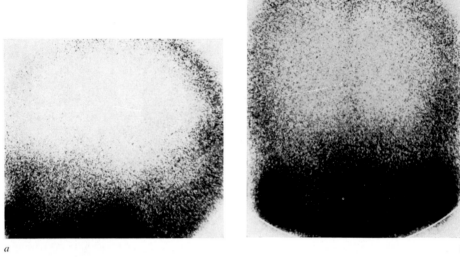

a   b

Fig. 10   (*a*) Lateral brain scan in a patient with gross enlargement of the sella turcica is normal.
(*b*) Frontal brain scan in the same patient is also normal.

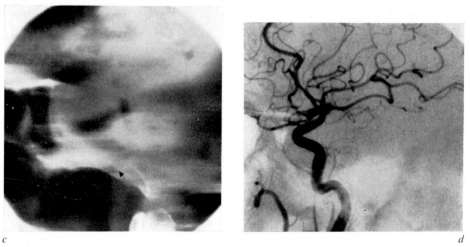

c   d

Fig. 10   (*c*) Lateral tomogram during pneumoencephalogram shows destruction of the clivus (arrow)
and extension into the sphenoid sinus but only slight suprasellar extension.
(*d*) Magnification carotid angiogram demonstrates enlarged branches supplying tumor.

RIHSA cisternography

Administration of labelled albumin or other large relatively non-diffusable substance into
the subarachnoid space is widely practised as a means of demonstrated disorders of the
cerebrospinal fluid circulation. The main use for such techniques is in the diagnosis of
communicating hydrocephalus due to obstruction of the distal cerebrospinal fluid pathways.[31-33] Another use for this technique is in the demonstration of cerebrospinal fluid
fistula[34] which may occur rarely in patients with pituitary adenomas after surgery or after
irradiation as in the case of the patient shown in Figure 8.

Potentially RIHSA cisternography may be useful in the diagnosis of pituitary tumors or other suprasellar masses. Di Chiro et al.[35] were able to demonstrate non-filling of the suprasellar cisterns in a patient with a craniopharyngioma, while in a patient with a hypothalamic glioma the cisterns appeared normal.

Isotope cisternography has also proved useful in demonstrating an 'empty sella' in a patient with gross sellar enlargement on plain radiographs.[36]

Computerized transverse axial tomography

A new system developed in England has been evaluated by Ambrose in various tumorous and non-tumorous conditions of the brain.[37] The scanning unit consists of an X-ray tube producing a tightly collimated X-ray beam with a pair of sodium iodide detectors on the opposite side of the head. The unit scans the head which is encased in a tightly fitting rubber cap which itself is contained in a rectangular box of water. The X-ray tube and detectors scan the head 180 times rotating 1° for each scan, and each scan is divided into 300 readings. The data, stored on a magnetic disc, are then processed in a computer, where 28,000 simultaneous equations are performed in approximately 5 minutes. The results are then reproduced as an axial tomographic section of the head, where each 'dot' represents a block of tissue $3 \times 3 \times 10$ mm, and the density of the 'dot' represents the coefficient of absorption for the tissue at that point. The technique gives a clear anatomical outline of the ventricles, dura and other intracranial structures as well as calcifications such as the pineal gland and the choroid plexuses of the lateral ventricles.

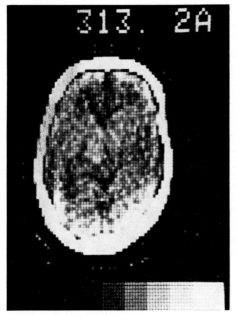 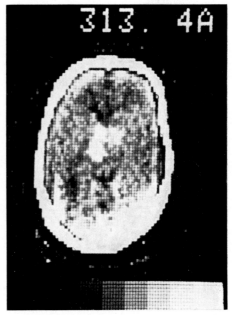

a   *b*

Fig. 11   (*a*) Computerized transverse axial tomogram of the skull in a patient with a chromophobe adenoma. There is a very slight increase in the absorption coefficient just to the left of midline in the suprasellar region.
(*b*) After intravenous injection of 40 ml sodium iothalamate there is obvious contrast enhancement of the chromophobe adenoma. (Courtesy of Dr James Ambrose, The Atkinson Morley Hospital, London.)

Tumors within the brain substance have a slightly lower absorption coefficient than normal brain and are therefore demonstrable. Deformities of the adjacent ventricles may also be seen. Intracerebral hematomas may be clearly seen because of their absorption coefficient which is greater than normal.

The device has demonstrated a suprasellar craniopharyngioma with great clarity because of the cholesterol content of the cyst fluid. It is becoming apparent that certain lesions which show up poorly initially may be demonstrated clearly after intravenous injection of iodinated contrast material such as is used for arteriography and intravenous pyelography. Figure 11 illustrates this contrast enhancement in a patient with a suprasellar extension of a pituitary tumor. The phenomenon is analogous to the 'blush' seen during carotid arteriography and is presumably due to leakage of contrast material through the capillary endothelium into the extracellular fluid.

Summary

The radiologic techniques used in the diagnosis of pituitary tumors include plain radiographs and tomography of the skull to demonstrate the size and shape of the sella turcica and any changes in adjacent bony structures. Pneumoencephalography remains the technique of choice to demonstrate the suprasellar component of a pituitary tumor, but carotid angiography is necessary to exclude the presence of an aneurysm and also to demonstrate the lateral extension of the intrasellar mass.

Radioisotopic techniques are not widely used because of their relative insensitivity. Routine brain scanning should demonstrate suprasellar extension of pituitary tumors if larger than 2 cm in diameter. Isotope cisternography may be of value in management of cerebrospinal fluid fistula and may demonstrate obliterations of the suprasellar cisterns by a large chromophobe adenoma. A new technique of computerized transverse axial tomography promises to be a major innovation as a non-invasive method for demonstrating intracranial pathology including pituitary tumors and craniopharyngiomas.

References

(1) NEWTON, T. H. and POTTS, D. G. (Eds.) (1971): *Radiology of the Skull and Brain, Vol. 1*, pp. 29-60. The C. V. Mosby Co., St. Louis, Mo.

(2) DU BOULAY, G. and TRICKEY, S. (1967): The choice of radiological investigations in the management of tumours around the sella. *Clin. Radiol. (Lond.), 18*, 349.

(3) METZGER, J. (1967): The sign of the chiasma from front view in hypocycloidal pneumotomography. *Rev. neurol., 117*, 666.

(4) DAVIS, D. O. (1970): Neuroradiological diagnosis of sellar and parasellar lesions. *Clin. Neurosurg., 17*, 160.

(5) HARWOOD-NASH, D. C. (1972): Optic gliomas and pediatric neuroradiology. *Radiol. Clin. N. Amer., 10*, 83.

(6) McLACHLAN, M. S. F., LAVENDER, J. P. and EDWARDS, C. R. W. (1971): Polytome-encephalography in the investigation of pituitary tumours. *Clin. Radiol. (Lond.), 22*, 361.

(7) TAVERAS, J. M. and WOOD, E. H. (1964): *Diagnostic Neuroradiology*. The Williams and Wilkins Co., Baltimore, Md.

(8) ROBERTSON, E. G. (1967): *Pneumoencephalography*, 2nd ed. Charles C. Thomas, Springfield, Ill.

(9) LOMBARDI, G. (1967): *Radiology in Neuro-Ophthalmology*. The Williams and Wilkins Co., Baltimore, Md.

(10) NOTERMAN, J., WARSZAWSKI, M., JEANMART, L. and BRIHAYE, J. (1972): Bilateral aneurysm of the internal carotid artery in the cavernous sinus: case report. *Neuroradiology, 4*, 63.

(11) BULL, J. W. D. and SCHUNK, H. (1962): The significance of displacement of the cavernous portion of the internal carotid artery. *Brit. J. Radiol.*, *35*, 801.

(12) BERGLAND, R. M., RAY, B. S. and TORACK, R. M. (1968): Anatomical variations in the pituitary gland and adjacent structures in 225 human autopsy cases. *J. Neurosurg.*, *28*, 93.

(13) EPSTEIN, B. S. and EPSTEIN, J. A. (1968): The angiographic demonstration and surgical implications of imbedding of the carotid syphons by a large pituitary adenoma. *Amer. J. Roentgenol.*, *104*, 162.

(14) CHASE, N. E. and TAVERAS, J. M. (1961): Cerebral angiography in the diagnosis of suprasellar tumors. *Amer. J. Roentgenol.*, *86*, 154.

(15) KRAYENBÜHL, H. A. and YASARGIL, M. G. (1968): *Cerebral Angiography.* J. B. Lippincott Company, Philadelphia, Pa.

(16) NADJMI, M., ENGELHARDT, F., MOLLADAWOUDI, A. and SONNTAG, I. (1970): The question of the discrepancy between angiographic and pneumoencephalographic findings in suprasellar space occupying processes. *Radiologe (Berl.)*, *10*, 466.

(17) GADO, M. and BULL, J. W. D. (1971): The carotid angiogram in suprasellar masses. *Neuroradiology*, *2*, 136.

(18) KRICHEFF, I. I. and SCHOTLAND, D. L. (1964): Tumor stain in a pituitary adenoma. *Radiology*, *82*, 11.

(19) BERKMEN, Y. M. (1967): Angiographically demonstrated abnormal vascular pattern in a pituitary adenoma. *Clin. Radiol. (Lond.)*, *18*, 197.

(20) WESTBERG, G. and ROSS, R. J. (1967): The vascular supply of chromophobe adenomas. *Acta radiol. (Diagn.)* 6, 475.

(21) HATAM, A. (1971): The vascular supply of eosinophilic and mixed pituitary adenomas in acromegalic patients. *Neuroradiology*, *3*, 4.

(22) PARKINSON, D. (1964): Collateral circulation of cavernous carotid artery: anatomy. *Canad. J. Surg.*, *7*, 251.

(23) BERGLAND, R. and RAY, B. S. (1969): The arterial supply of the human optic chiasm. *J. Neurosurg.*, *31*, 327.

(24) BAKER, H. L., Jr (1971): The clinical usefulness of magnification cerebral angiography. *Radiology*, *98*, 587

(25) BAKER, H. L., Jr (1972): The angiographic delineation of sellar and parasellar masses. *Radiology* *104*, 67.

(26) BURROWS, E. H. (1972): False-negative results in brain scanning. *Brit. med. J.*, *1*, 473.

(27) OTTO, H., FIEBACH, O., SAUER, J., BETTAG, W., LÖHR, E. and STRÖTGEN, M. W. (1972): Cerebral scintigraphy in relation to roentgenological methods for detection of tumours situated in the sellar region and the posterior fossa. *Neuroradiology*, *4*, 30.

(28) JAMES, A. E., Jr, DELAND, F. H., HODGES, F. J., III, WAGNER, H. N., Jr and NORTH, W. A. (1970): Radionuclide imaging in the detection and differential diagnosis of craniopharyngiomas. *Amer. J. Roentgenol.*, *109*, 692.

(29) KUHL, D. E., PITTS, F. W., SANDERS, T. P. and MISHKIN, M. M. (1966): Transverse section and rectilinear brain scanning with Tc^{99m} pertechnetate. *Radiology*, *86*, 822.

(30) KUHL, D. E. and SANDERS, T. P. (1971): Characterizing brain lesions with use of transverse section scanning. *Radiology*, *98*, 317.

(31) DI CHIRO, G. (1964): Movement of the cerebrospinal fluid in human beings. *Nature (Lond.)*, *204*, 290.

(32) BANNISTER, R., GILFORD, E. and KOCEN, R. (1967): Isotope encephalography in the diagnosis of dementia due to communicating hydrocephalus. *Lancet*, *2*, 1014.

(33) DI CHIRO, G. (1966): Observations on the circulation of the cerebrospinal fluid. *Acta radiol. (Diagn.)*, *5*, 988.

(34) DI CHIRO, G., OMMAYA, A. K., ASHBURN, W. L. and BRINER, W. H. (1968): Isotope cisternography in the diagnosis and follow-up of cerebrospinal fluid rhinorrhea. *J. Neurosurg.*, *28*, 522.

(35) DI CHIRO, G., ASHBURN, W. L., ZEIGER, L. S. and SCHALL, G. L. (1972): Radioisotope encephalo-cisternography and encephalo-ventriculography. *J. Neurosurg.*, *36*, 127.

(36) OVERBEEK, W. J., FRONT, D. and PENNING, I. (1971): Primary enlarged 'empty' sella. *Neurochirurgia (Stuttg.)*, *14*, 110.

(37) MEDICAL NEWS (1973): Britons develop non-invasive diagnostic system. *J. Amer. med. Ass.*, *223*, 7.

Relative merits of pneumographic and angiographic procedures in the management of pituitary tumors

JOHN R. BENTSON

Department of Radiological Sciences, UCLA School of Medicine, Los Angeles, Calif., U.S.A.

Though pneumoencephalographic and angiographic examinations have been the accepted means of radiographically demonstrating tumors of the pituitary and parasellar region for some time, improvements in equipment and refinements of radiographic techniques continue to occur and have sharpened the ability of the neuroradiologist to perform those tasks requested of him – namely, to determine whether or not a tumor is present in the sellar region, to determine its extent and to comment on its probable etiology. The available diagnostic procedures should be periodically compared to determine how helpful each is in providing answers to these questions.

Materials and methods

After some experience with sellar tumors, each investigator forms his own opinions regarding the relative merits of air and angiographic procedures. To determine whether or not these general impressions could be substantiated, the radiographs of those patients with proven tumors of the sellar region who had been studied by both angiographic and pneumoencephalographic techniques during the past 3 years at the UCLA Center for the Health Sciences were reviewed. These constituted 50 pituitary adenomas (13 with acromegaly), 15 craniopharyngiomas, 9 meningiomas and 10 other parasellar tumors. An extensive listing of all observations in each group would be cumbersome and will not be done, but some of the findings relevant to the topic of this paper will be given later.

All patients of this series had pneumoencephalograms. Ventriculograms are not satisfactory for the investigation of sellar problems because of the failure to fill the subarachnoid cisterns. The pneumoencephalograms performed on adults were nearly all done under sedation only and those patients with suspected pituitary insufficiency were given steroid premedication. There have been no complications. The oxygen injected was monitored fluoroscopically so that only that amount needed to visualize the desired structures would be used. Mechanical linear tomography* was used to take well coned serial anteroposterior and lateral laminograms of the sellar region in all cases. The temporal horns were filled simultaneously and filmed in the brow-up position so that they could be accurately compared.

---

* Mimer II.

Nearly all these patients had bilateral selective internal carotid arteriograms. The others, mainly acromegalics without marked sellar enlargement, were studied by cavernous sinus venography. Many also had selective vertebral arteriograms. The angiograms and venograms were subtracted, frequently in stereo pairs, this being of aid in localizing small vessels, distinguishing temporal lobe arteries from cavernous carotid branches and in appreciating stains. In former years, when bilateral neck catheters were used routinely, simultaneous anteroposterior carotid injections were done, allowing better comparison of the carotids and their branches without demonstrable increase in complications (Fig. 3).[1] In recent years, nearly all arteriograms are done by femoral catheter, so that simultaneous injections are no longer done. The arteriograms are generally done before the pneumoencephalograms, since this sequence is more acceptable to the patient and since the arteriogram will occasionally demonstrate a large distant tumor which has produced sellar erosion indirectly, in which case pneumoencephalography is unnecessary and may be potentially hazardous. Most of the cavernous sinus venograms have been performed by introducing catheters into the internal jugular vein and placing their tips in the inferior petrosal sinus.[2, 3] More recently, cavernous sinus studies have been done via the ophthalmic veins using a forehead vein catheter or by catheterizing the inferior petrosal sinuses using femoral vein catheters, since these approaches seem more comfortable to the patient and involve less radiation exposure to the operator.

Pituitary adenomas

Extension shown only by sellar changes

The pituitary tumor may extend in many directions, either singly or in combination. Extension anteriorly, posteriorly or inferiorly results in the well known changes in the sella turcica. If there is no suprasellar or lateral extension, contrast studies will generally be negative. Pneumoencephalography is valuable in these cases to identify the 'empty sella'. Arteriograms are generally normal in cases of 'empty sella' [4, 5] but occasionally the cavernous carotids are displaced laterally.[20]

Suprasellar extension

The tendency of a pituitary tumor to break through the diaphragma sellae and grow into the suprasellar region depends on many factors, such as the size and shape of the sella, the thickness of the sellar floor and the degree of competency of the diaphragma. The suprasellar tumor may then extend straight upward, upward and anterior, upward and posterior, or upward and to one side. The abilities of air and angiographic studies to detect these extensions will now be considered.

Minimal degrees of suprasellar extension may be detected on the pneumoencephalogram but generally not on the arteriogram. These minor suprasellar extensions will first be appreciated on the air study by noting a dome-shaped mass just above the diaphragma sellae. A slightly greater extension will cause impingement upon the shadow of the optic chiasm, which should normally be visible on nearly all lateral laminograms and some anteroposterior laminograms. Larger masses will cause nonfilling of the suprasellar portion of the chiasmatic cistern. The gas in the lateral extensions of the chiasmatic cistern about the carotid arteries may appear on plain films to be over the sella. This is one of the more common mistakes made on interpretation of the pneumoencephalograms of patients with sellar tumors and can usually be avoided when laminograms are taken. To be even more certain of the position of cisternal gas, it should be localized on both lateral and anteroposterior laminograms. Several conditions have been described which may mimic a suprasellar mass on the pneumoencephalogram.[6] The most important of these is retention of cerebrospinal fluid anterior to the arachnoid membrane of Liliequist,[7] which extends between the dorsum sellae inferiorly and the mamillary bodies superiorly. Repeating the gas injections when the patient's head is flexed backwards will nearly always overcome this problem, though occasionally, more often in children than adults, the chiasmatic cistern cannot be filled.

Greater degrees of suprasellar extension cause blunting of the anterior recesses of the third ventricle, followed by convex indentations into the ventricle (Figs. 1 and 2). Blunting of the recesses is more reliable than displacement of the anterior third ventricle, because of the normally great variation in the position of the latter. When displacement of the ventricle occurs, it gives information not only of the size of the suprasellar mass but also of its predominant direction of growth. Anteroposterior extension of a sellar mass will produce posterior displacement of the anterior third ventricle, while posterosuperior growth will

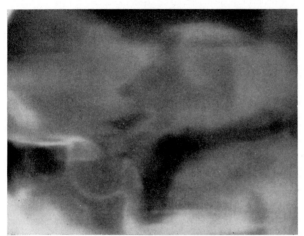

Fig. 1a   Chromophobe adenoma with suprasellar extension. Lateral midline tomogram of air study demonstrates superior and posterior borders of the suprasellar tumor, which indents the third ventricle.

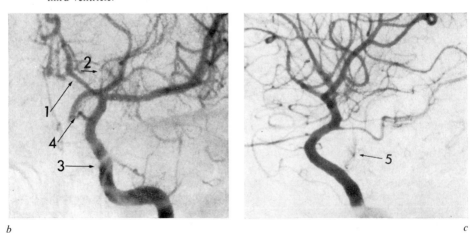

b   c

Fig. 1b   Subtracted AP projection of left internal carotid arteriogram shows elevation of anterior cerebral artery (arrow 1), lateral displacement of the anterior choroidal artery (arrow 2), but no definite displacement of cavernous carotid (arrow 3) or posterior communicating artery (arrow 4).

Fig. 1c   Lateral left carotid arteriogram. Patient faces reader's left on all arteriograms. The inferior hypophyseal artery is enlarged and gives rise to a stain (arrow 5).

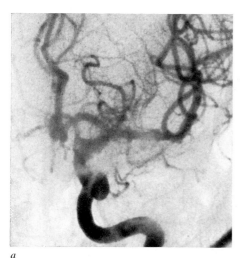 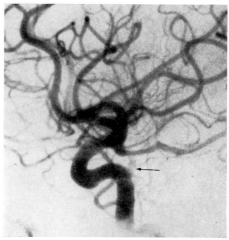

a   *b*

Fig. 2   Chromophobe adenoma with posterior suprasellar extension but normal carotid arteriogram. (*a*) Normal AP left carotid arteriogram. (*b*) On this normal lateral left carotid arteriogram, note the normal posterior pituitary blush (arrow). The pneumoencephalogram showed
suprasellar extension similar to that seen in Figure 1.

displace the ventricle straight upwards. Very large suprasellar tumors will elevate the anterior
horns of the lateral ventricles. This defect should not be confused with the normal indentation seen on the undersurface of the anterior horn just anterior to the foramen of Monro.
Anteroposterior projections are of help in this differentiation, since the indentation caused
by tumor will cause a flattening and medial elevation of the inferior surface of the anterior
horn. The anteroposterior projection will also demonstrate tilting of the inferior surface of
the effaced third ventricle, giving evidence of asymmetric extension of the tumor to one side.
Small collections of gas may outline the upper lateral boundaries of the suprasellar tumor.
The posterior border of the suprasellar mass is well outlined by gas in the interpeduncular
cistern but the anterior border is frequently not well seen (Fig. 1). One maneuver found to
be helpful in filling the anterior interhemispheric sulci just anterior to the tumor is to inject
gas with the head extended and then immediately obtain lateral and anteroposterior laminograms.

The principal angiographic signs of suprasellar extension are elevation of the first segment
of the anterior cerebral artery and straightening and elevation of the supraclinoid portion
of the internal carotid artery (opening of the syphon). Elevation of the anterior cerebral
artery is more accurately determined than changes in the position of the internal carotid
bifurcation, since the latter is subject to such wide normal variation.[8] More important
than simple medial elevation of the anterior cerebral artery is the associated stretching of
this vessel[9] (Figs. 1, 3 and 5).

In the series of cases reviewed, only about half the pituitary adenomas with suprasellar
extension demonstrated by pneumoencephalography showed elevation of the anterior cerebral arteries on arteriography. This discrepancy was related to the minor degrees of suprasellar extension in some cases. In others, the tumor extended superiorly and posteriorly,
thus causing no significant displacement of the anterior cerebral artery. Baker recently
described elevation of the arterial plexus about the infundibulum, seen on subtracted lateral
magnified arteriograms, to be a sign of suprasellar extension.[5] If there is gross suprasellar
extension, the arteriogram may show upward displacement of deep midline veins such as
the septal vein and venous angle and may demonstrate hydrocephalus secondary to blockage
of the foramina of Monro.

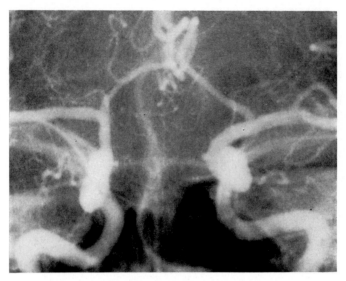

Fig. 3   Simultaneous AP internal carotid arteriogram showing asymmetric extension of a pituitary adenoma. The left cavernous sinus is normal, the right displaced laterally. There is elevation and straightening of the right carotid bifurcation and the right anterior cerebral artery is more elevated and stretched than the left.

Lateral extension

Unlike suprasellar extension, lateral extension of pituitary tumors is better demonstrated by angiographic means. The cavernous sinus venogram is more accurate than the carotid arteriogram in detecting small degrees of lateral extension, but large tumors may cause non-filling of the cavernous sinus, thus decreasing its usefulness. The cavernous sinuses are paired dural venous structures adjacent to either side of the sphenoid bone. The medial wall of each cavernous sinus forms the lateral limiting wall of the sella turcica. Together with their anterior and posterior intercommunicating sinuses, they surround the pituitary gland. The medial walls of the cavernous sinuses are normally straight and nearly parallel, so that laterally expanding tumors are easily recognized by the characteristic convex imprint they produce (Fig. 4). The basal projection is most useful, followed by a straight anteroposterior projection. Cases in which lateral extension was demonstrated by cavernous sinus venography but not by carotid arteriography have been found.[2, 3] This test is therefore done in cases of relatively small pituitary tumors for which transsphenoidal surgery, particularly cryo-surgery, is contemplated.[10] It is also valuable in those patients who have clinical evidence of cavernous sinus involvement, but in whom carotid angiography, pneumoencephalography and pituitary function studies have been negative. The cavernous sinus venogram in some of these patients will demonstrate partial or complete non-filling of the cavernous sinus which, together with painful ophthalmoplegia responding to steroid therapy, suggests the presence of non-specific granulomatous involvement of the cavernous sinus termed the Tolosa-Hunt syndrome.[11]

Lateral extension of the pituitary adenoma is detected on the carotid arteriogram by noting lateral displacement of the cavernous carotid. This is best seen on basal view but is satis-factorily demonstrated on the straight anteroposterior view.[9] An anteroposterior projection in which the petrous ridges are seen in the mid-orbits is better for evaluation of pituitary tumors than the standard carotid projection with the petrous ridges and orbital roofs super-

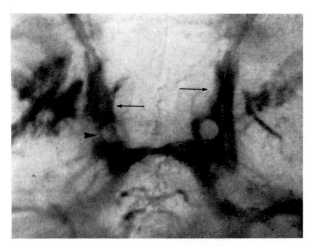

Fig. 4   Cavernous sinus venogram, basal projection. Anterior is at the top. The normally straight medial walls of the cavernous sinuses are curved laterally by the pituitary tumor (horizontal arrows). The carotid arteries are visible in the posterior cavernous sinuses and do not appear displaced (large arrowheads). The posterior intercommunicating sinus is filled but the anterior intercommunicating sinus is compressed and does not fill. The superior ophthalmic veins are seen passing from the anterior margins of the cavernous sinus obliquely to the top of the illustration.

imposed. The posterior portion of the cavernous carotid is normally more medial than the anterior portion. When laterally displaced by a pituitary tumor, the posterior segment will be in line with or lateral to the anterior segment and the cavernous carotid will be seen to be lateral to the precavernous portion (Figs. 3, 5 and 6). [9, 12]

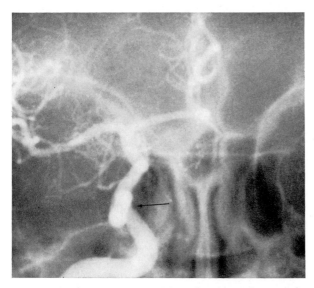

Fig. 5a   Pituitary adenoma with lateral and superior extension. The AP right carotid arteriogram shows marked lateral displacement of the cavernous carotid artery (arrow). The anterior cerebral artery is elevated and stretched.

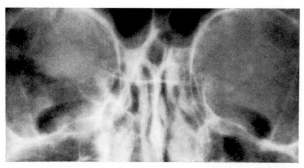

Fig. 5b Pituitary adenoma with lateral and superior extension. The pneumoencephalogram, however, shows no temporal horn displacement.

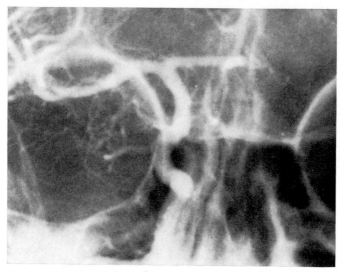

Fig. 6a This pituitary tumor has caused lateral displacement of the right cavernous carotid artery of
slightly less magnitude than that seen in Figure 5.

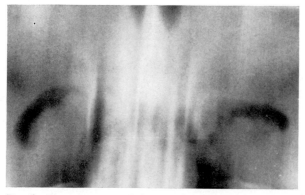

Fig. 6b The pneumoencephalogram shows tilting of the right temporal horn, indicating more extension of the tumor into the right middle fossa than the arteriogram indicates.

Though not as sensitive as the cavernous sinus venogram, the carotid arteriogram will identify lateral extension adequately for open surgical techniques or radiotherapy. It should be noted, however, that the amount of lateral extension of the pituitary tumor is not necessarily reflected in the amount of carotid displacement. In the case of large tumors, the lateral carotid projection will frequently show that the cavernous carotid artery has been straightened and depressed or, less commonly, elevated. Once this has occurred, considerable lateral growth of the tumor into the middle fossa may take place without further lateral displacement of the carotid (Figs. 5 and 6). The tumor may rarely encompass the artery and extend laterally without further displacement.[13] For these reasons, it is necessary to examine the temporal horns on pneumoencephalographic films carefully to detect gross lateral extension. The middle cerebral artery branches will be elevated by a large lateral tumor extension, but changes in the temporal horns will occur earlier. Of the 50 patients with pituitary tumors mentioned before, 47 had bilateral carotid arteriograms. Lateral displacement of one or both cavernous carotid arteries was found in 13, of whom pneumoencephalograms demonstrated temporal horn displacement in three cases.

Other aspects of arteriography in pituitary tumors

The possibility that a mass producing hypopituitarism or visual changes may be an aneurysm continues to be a significant reason for performing carotid arteriography. Aneurysms arising from the internal carotid artery at or near the origin of the ophthalmic artery may mimic tuberculum or planum tumors on the pneumoencephalogram. Aneurysms of the cavernous carotid artery occasionally project into the sella and may produce plain film findings typical of intrasellar tumors. One of the cases we studied in this series was an example of this second type. Though the possibility of aneurysm is often suspected because of the presence of such plain film findings as anterior clinoid erosion, enlargement of the superior orbital fissure or curvilinear calcification, these clues are not always present. Carotid arteriography should be done bilaterally, since the aneurysm may not fill with a unilateral injection, even with cross-compression.

There has been considerable interest in recent years in the blood supply of sellar tumors demonstrated by carotid arteriography. Several branches of the cavernous carotid artery supplying the sella and its contents have been well described in the radiologic literature.[14-17] The largest of these is the inferior hypophyseal artery which arises from the meningohypophyseal trunk, which in turn originates from the first (proximal) curve of the cavernous carotid artery. The inferior hypophyseal artery supplies the posterior pituitary gland, which is visible as a faint blush in the posterior sella in the majority of normal carotid arteriograms if good subtraction prints are made.[18] Enlargement of the inferior hypophyseal artery is seen in many pituitary adenomas (Fig. 7), and the tumor is seen to stain in some of these. Subtraction is usually necessary to demonstrate the stain, though it is occasionally pronounced on the unsubtracted arteriogram films (Fig. 8). The inferior cavernous artery and capsular arteries, which also arise from the cavernous artery distal to the meningohypophyseal trunk and which are almost never seen on normal arteriograms, may be visible in cases of pituitary tumors and contribute to the stain. It has been reported that the blush of the posterior pituitary is not seen if there is a pituitary tumor.[5] This would be helpful in differentiating pituitary tumors from cases of 'empty sella' if always true, since a normal posterior pituitary blush is found in the latter. However, in 2 cases of proven chromophobe adenoma in our series, subtraction prints of preoperative arteriograms had demonstrated an oval vertically oriented blush in the posterior sella, the typical appearance of the posterior pituitary (Fig. 2). In one of these, the inferior hypophyseal artery of the opposite carotid gave rise to a tumor stain. Enlarged branches of the meningohypophyseal trunk were apparent in 27 of the 50 pituitary adenomas in our series, with visible tumor stain in 13. Baker, using serial magnification and subtraction routinely, has recently reported visible arterial feeders of the capsule of the pituitary adenoma in 65 of 76 cases of pituitary adenoma

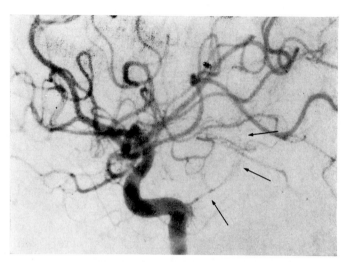

Fig. 7   Chromophobe adenoma. The lateral internal carotid arteriogram demonstrates an enlarged inferior hypophyseal artery which outlines the posterior border of the large, rounded suprasellar tumor (arrows). Later films showed a light stain.

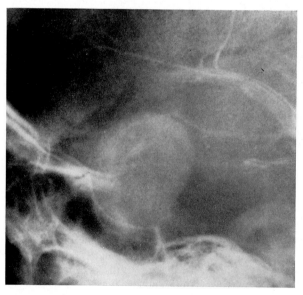

Fig. 8   Carotid arteriogram, venous phase, showing unusually heavy staining in a chromophobe adenoma.

and stain in 61. When enlarged vessels to the tumor capsule and stain are present, information regarding the posterior and superior extension of the tumor not otherwise apparent on the arteriogram may be gained (Fig. 7).

Other sellar and parasellar tumors

In the evaluation of the relative merits of contrast studies for pituitary tumors, some consideration must be given to how these tests fare in the detection and differentiation of other tumors of the sellar region which may mimic pituitary tumors both clinically and radiologically. Craniopharyngiomas and meningiomas are the most common tumors which may do this.

Craniopharyngiomas

Craniopharyngiomas may arise in the sella, resulting in enlargement of the sella identical to that caused by pituitary adenomas, but more commonly arise in the suprasellar region, typically causing depression of the dorsum sellae. The majority of craniopharyngiomas are calcified in children but not in adults. A significant minority of these tumors may be present without calcification and without sellar changes. There is a greater chance of missing craniopharyngiomas with arteriography than is the case with pituitary tumors, largely due to the posterior suprasellar location of most craniopharyngiomas. Lateral displacement of the anterior choroidal artery is not uncommonly the only angiographic sign of the presence of a craniopharyngioma. Tumor staining and enlargement of cavernous carotid branches have only rarely been reported in craniopharyngiomas, further increasing the difficulties in detecting these tumors arteriographically.[5, 19] Though the tumor illustrated by Figure 2 was a chromophobe adenoma, the radiographic findings are almost more typical of a craniopharyngioma.

Pneumoencephalography will nicely demonstrate the presence and extent of craniopharyngiomas. The tumor characteristically extends well upward into the anterior third ventricle, which tends to encompass the tumor to a greater extent than in the case of most suprasellar pituitary adenomas. Larger tumors will nearly obliterate the third ventricle and may block the foramina of Monro or efface the anterior horns. Occasionally the tumor will extend widely into the middle fossa. Craniopharyngiomas have a tendency to extend posteriorly and inferiorly behind the clivus into the posterior fossa. A craniopharyngioma we saw recently had extended to the second cervical vertebra level. Another was confined to the suprasellar space except for a small extension into one cerebellopontine angle. Because of this tendency, anteroposterior serial laminography of the posterior fossa should be done during the pneumoencephalogram when this tumor is suspected, for the posterior fossa extension may otherwise be missed at surgery.

Meningiomas

Most of the meningiomas resulting in symptoms similar to those of pituitary tumors arise from the tuberculum sellae and planum sphenoidale and grow posteriorly into the suprasellar space. Rarely meningiomas may be found within the sella. Plain films will usually show sclerosis and frequently irregular elevation of 'blistering' of the planum sphenoidale but may be negative. The internal carotid arteriograms of these presellar meningiomas generally show elevation and often posterior displacement of the anterior cerebral arteries, posterior displacement of the carotid syphons (closing) and the characteristic diffuse lingering stain (Fig. 9).

The typical pneumoencephalographic findings in these cases are obliteration of part or all of the chiasmatic cistern, posterior and occasionally downward displacement of the anterior third ventricle and sometimes elevation of the undersurfaces of the frontal horns. Capping of the anterior border of the tumor by gas seems to occur more often than is seen with pituitary tumors. If the meningioma arises from an anterior clinoid process of optic canal and is not large, it may not be detectable on arteriography or pneumoencephalography. We have

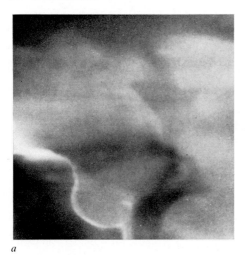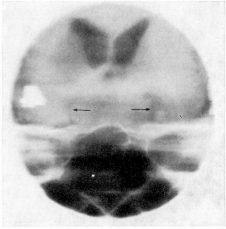

a   b

Fig. 9a,b   Typical planum sphenoidale meningioma extending posteriorly into the suprasellar space.
(*a*) The lateral tomogram from the air study shows posterior displacement of the anterior
third ventricle and bulging of the mass into the interpeduncular cistern. There is slight
thickening of the planum sphenoidale. (*b*) The anteroposterior tomogram demonstrates
the lateral margins of the tumor (arrows) and the 'blistering' of the planum sphenoidale.

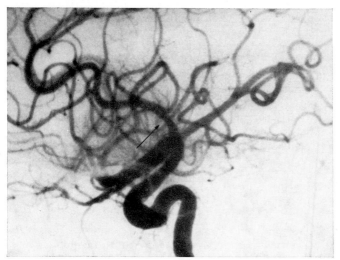

Fig. 9c   The lateral carotid arteriogram demonstrates closing of the carotid syphon, elevation and
posterior displacement of the first segment of the anterior cerebral artery (arrow) and early
diffuse stain.

had 2 such tumors which were only detected by sclerosis of adjacent bone. Meningiomas
arising from the walls of the sphenoid sinus or cavernous sinus may produce no pneumoencephalographic findings but usually induce enlargement of the intracavernous branches
of the carotid which, together with reactive enostosis, suggests the diagnosis.

Other tumors

Hypothalamic or optic gliomas may obliterate the chiasmatic cistern, produce defects in the

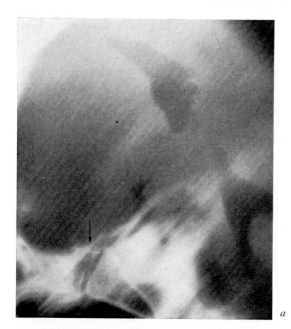

a

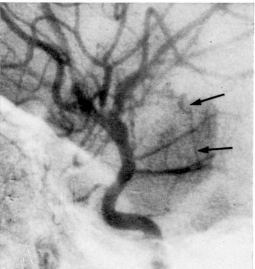

b

Fig. 10   Hypothalamic glioma. (*a*) The midline tomogram from the pneumoencephalogram demonstrates the huge suprasellar mass which nearly obliterates the third ventricle. Note the loss of the dorsum sellae (arrow) and extension of the mass dorsal to the upper clivus. (*b*) The carotid arteriogram gives clues to the origin of this tumor by showing tumor vessels, particularly a forward displaced premamillary artery (arrows), arising from the posterior communicating artery. An early stain is visible in the suprasellar region.

third ventricle and give other pneumoencephalographic signs typical of craniopharyngiomas or large suprasellar pituitary tumors. Arteriography may help differentiate these by demonstrating tumor vascularity originating from branches of the posterior communicating arteries which normally supply the hypothalamus and chiasm rather than from the cavernous carotid

(Fig. 10). Malignant tumors about the sphenoid and cavernous sinuses may cause enlargement of cavernous carotid branches but may be recognized by the pattern of bone destruction and by arterial encasement. Metastatic tumors of plasmacytomas within the sella may mimic pituitary tumors on all radiographic tests. The same may be true of pinealomas and histiocytosis X in the suprasellar region.

Summary

If a choice must be made, the pneumoencephalogram remains the most valuable radiographic test for the detection and delineation of pituitary tumors. The use of serial tomography allows confident demonstration of even minimal extension of tumors above the sella. Tumors extending into the posterior suprasellar space are well shown by the pneumoencephalogram but may be missed on arteriography. The arteriogram is better able to demonstrate lateral extension of a sellar tumor, may better show the anterior border of a suprasellar mass and will rule out aneurysms. The arteriogram also gives evidence of tumor vascularity which is very helpful in differential diagnosis. The most sensitive test for the determination of lateral extension of the small pituitary tumor is the cavernous sinus venogram. Because the merits of angiography and pneumoencephalography are complementary ones, both are recommended in the work-up of pituitary tumors. To reliably differentiate other tumors of the sellar and parasellar region, both angiography and pneumoencephalography are generally necessary.

References

(1)   BENTSON, J., WILSON, G. and HANAFEE, W. (1970): Simultaneous carotid angiography. *Nippon Acta radiol.*, *29*, 9.
(2)   WEIDNER, W., ROSEN, L. and HANAFEE, W. (1965): The neuroradiology of tumors of the pituitary gland. *Amer. J. Roentgenol.*, *95*, 884.
(3)   SHIU, P., HANAFEE, W., WILSON, G. and RAND, R. (1968): Cavernous sinus venography. *Amer. J. Roentgenol.*, *104*, 57.
(4)   KAUFMAN, B. (1968): The 'empty' sella turcica — a manifestation of the intrasellar subarachnoid space. *Radiology*, *90*, 931.
(5)   BAKER, H. (1972): The angiographic delineation of sellar and parasellar masses. *Radiology*, *104*, 67.
(6)   HANAFEE, W., BILODEAU, L., ALBERTI, J. and WILSON, G. (1967): Pseudo suprasellar tumors. *Amer. J. Roentgenol.*, *100*, 631.
(7)   LILIEQUIST, B. (1959): Subarachnoid cisterns. *Acta radiol. (Stockh.), suppl. 185.*
(8)   UDVARHELYI, G., LANGFITT, T. and COX, A. (1963): Neuroradiologic diagnostic procedures in suprasellar space-occupying lesions with special reference to angiographic measurements. *Acta radiol. (Stockh.)*, *1*, 485.
(9)   CHASE, N. and TAVERAS, J. (1961): Cerebral angiography in the diagnosis of suprasellar tumors. *Amer. J. Roentgenol.*, *86*, 154.
(10) RAND, R. and HANAFEE, W. (1967): Cavernous sinus venography and stereotaxic cryohypophysectomy. *J. Neurosurg.*, *26*, 521.
(11) WALSH, F. B. and HOYT, W. F. (1969): *Clinical Neuro-Ophthalmology*, pp. 398-399. Williams and Wilkins Co., Baltimore, Md.
(12) BULL, J. W. D. and SCHUNK, H. (1962): Significance of displacement of cavernous portion of internal carotid artery. *Brit. J. Radiol.*, *35*, 801.
(13) EPSTEIN, B. S. and EPSTEIN, J. A. (1968): The angiographic demonstration and surgical implications of imbedding of the carotid syphons by a large pituitary adenoma. *Amer. J. Roentgenol.*, *104*, 162.
(14) BERNASCONI, V. and CASSINARI, V. (1956): Un segno carotidografico tipico di meningioma del tentorio. *Chir. ital.*, *11*, 586.

(15) STATTIN, S. (1961): Meningeal vessels of the internal carotid artery and their angiographic significance. *Acta radiol. (Diag.)*, *55*, 329.

(16) WALLACE, S., GOLDBERG, H. I. and LEEDS, N. E. (1967): The cavernous branches of the internal carotid artery. *Amer. J. Roentgenol.*, *101*, 34.

(17) WESTBERG, G. and ROSS, R. J. (1967): The vascular supply of chromophobe adenomas. *Acta radiol. (Diag.)* *6*, 475.

(18) LEHRER, H. Z. (1970): Angiographic visualization of the posterior pituitary and clinical stress. *Radiology*, *94*, 7.

(19) GEORGE, A. E., LIN, J. P. and KRICHFFF, I. I. (1970): Craniopharyngioma with abnormal vasculature. *Radiology*, *95*, 93.

(20) KAUFMAN, B.: Recent personal communication.

Radiographic features of intrasellar masses and progressive, asymmetrical non-tumorous enlargements of the sella turcica, the 'empty' sella*

BENJAMIN KAUFMAN, OLOF H. PEARSON and WILLIAM B. CHAMBERLIN

Departments of Radiology, Medicine and Pathology, University Hospitals of Cleveland, Case Western Reserve University, Cleveland, Ohio, U.S.A.

The time has come to think in terms of evaluating the volume, shape and position of the pituitary gland, and with current radiographic techniques this is feasible. The concept of an enlarged sella turcica not being caused by a tumor, but resulting from interactions of the pressure and pulsations of the cerebrospinal fluid acting on the sella turcica walls through a deficient diaphragma sellae, was introduced by Kaufman in 1968.[1] The pituitary gland was shown to be remodeled and displaced, but functionally and histologically normal. The postsurgical 'empty' sella was described by Colby and Kearns in some patients who had their tumors surgically removed via a craniotomy approach and later developed eye symptoms with an enlarging sella.[2] The unifying physical factor in all cases of non-tumorous enlargement of the sella turcica, the 'empty' sella, is a deficiency in the diaphragma sellae, natural or acquired.[3-5]

With a high degree of accuracy, but certainly less than 100 %, one can distinguish between a pituitary neoplasm or intrasellar mass and non-tumorous enlargement of the sella turcica (NTEST). Any practical approach to the handling of the patient with an enlarged sella necessitates utilization of all clinical information and laboratory tests. Previous criteria for sella turcica changes of size and configuration are still valid when an enlarged pituitary neoplasm or cyst is present.[6-10] It should be stated clearly that normal size and configuration of the sella turcica do not exclude an intrasellar neoplasm or even suprasellar extension, and NTEST may be coincidental with an intrasellar pituitary neoplasm.

All changes associated with non-tumorous enlargement of the sella turcica occur below the plane of the diaphragma sellae. Plain film radiography supplemented with thin section laminography remain a good screening mechanism. However, the definitive diagnostic study is *pneumoencephalography with thin section laminography*,[11] demonstrating intrasellar air and, most importantly, the air-soft tissue interface with the pituitary gland or tumor. Arteriography has characteristic findings involving displacement of the intracavernous segment of the internal carotid artery (ISICA) and, in some, downward herniation of the anterior cerebral arteries into the sella turcica.

* Supported in part by grants from the United States Public Health Service, RR 80, CA 05197, the American Cancer Society T 46 I and the Frackleton Memorial Fund.

Meningeal relationships of the hypophysis

The macroscopic anatomy of the meningeal and pituitary gland relationships is now quite clear with 20–24 % of the diaphragma sellae being intact, although some are not considered effective barriers.[3, 12−17] Studies on newborns[17] show that the diaphragma sellae may be incomplete at birth with the gland fitting snugly, and no evidence of an infradiaphragmatic subarachnoid space. The development of a true infradiaphragmatic subarachnoid space (not merely visualization of air in the sella turcica) apparently correlates with age,[17] as does an increase in sella turcica size.[12, 18] Sunderland's comprehensive review of the subject gives credit to Key and Retzius (1876) for demonstrating an infradiaphragmatic subarachnoid space anatomically, and credit to Davidoff and Dyke (1937) for pneumoencephalographic demonstration of this space. Engels[19] demonstrated the space with positive contrast material and Ferner[20] demonstrated the microscopic characteristics of the infradiaphragmatic subarachnoid space. He stated that the infradiaphragmatic subarachnoid space may also be present along the lateral, anterior and posterior walls of the sella as well as along the inferior aspect of the pituitary gland. Visualization of contrast material on the radiograph within the confines of the sella turcica does not in itself indicate the presence of an infradiaphragmatic subarachnoid space.[3]

The pituitary gland

The average pituitary gland is bilobed, measures 13 mm in transverse diameter, 10 mm in sagittal diameter, 6 mm in vertical diameter, and weighs about 0.6 g (with dural coverings removed).[21] Actually, the shape of the gland is extremely variable, being influenced by the infradiaphragmatic subarachnoid space and the carotid arteries.[1, 3, 12−14, 16, 17, 19, 22, 23]

Many studies have been made attempting to correlate gland size with sella turcica size.[12, 14, 15, 24−27] Early workers discussed the very obvious variations between the bony sella turcica and the weight and volume of the pituitary gland.[21, 24, 25] When the gland is normal and the sella turcica is normal, the correlation is good; when the sella turcica is large and the gland is normal, the correlation is poor.[26] When the sella turcica is extremely small, part of the gland may be outside the sella.[26] This is the usual situation in infants.[17]

It has long been recognized that air will enter the sella turcica and be situated anteriorly, especially in slightly enlarged sella turcicas.[19, 22, 28−30] Practically, one should not call these cases 'empty' sellas, since the intactness and position of the diaphragma sellae have not been determined.[3] Indeed, the dura may be intact and displaced downward or definition of the tuberculum sellae (point of attachment of the diaphragma sellae) may not be possible.[3,14,15] A more accurate terminology would be intrasellar air and, in the case of an enlarged sella turcica, non-tumorous enlargement of the sella turcica with intrasellar air.[3]

In non-tumorous enlargement of the sella turcica, the usual position of the pituitary gland is posteriorly and inferiorly[1] and in pneumoencephalograms the hypophyseal stalk frequently is seen posteriorly.[31]

The anterior pituitary gland may be flattened to as little as 1 mm in height. The posterior pituitary gland may or may not be remodeled.[1] In vivo demonstration of intrasellar air in the slightly enlarged sella turcica may be associated with a non-remodeled gland.[3] A variation of the usual symmetrically remodeled and posteriorly-inferiorly displaced pituitary gland may be a bowl-shaped pituitary gland with the stalk entering in the center.[1] On the pneumoencephalogram the stalk may be seen in the center of the air-filled sella, suggesting this configuration. Asymmetrical remodeling of the pituitary gland in the normal or enlarged sella is not unusual[12−17] and we feel is causatively related to asymmetrical enlargement of the sella turcica.[1, 3]

The displacement of the pituitary gland leaves a portion of the infradiaphragmatic bone-dural complex exposed to the pressures and pulsatile forces of the CSF. From our preliminary studies it appears that this is the part of the sella turcica which remodels and enlarges to a greater extent than the remainder. Fenestration of the exposed and enlarging dura and discontinuity of the bone may occur with the development of spontaneous cerebrospinal fluid fistulas.[5, 31-36]

From our studies, no endocrine abnormalities have been attributed to the remodeled pituitary gland. We feel at present that endocrinopathy in most cases of NTEST is coincidental. Others have questioned the existing articles in the literature.[36-38] However, it is documented that a non-tumorous enlargement of the sella turcica may be present with a coincidental neoplasm, functioning or non-functioning.[39] Obesity is a factor in the development of NTEST, in that it leads to an elevation of the CSF pressures intermittently[40] or continuously as in pseudotumor cerebri.[41]

The sella turcica is not a sensitive indicator of the true size and configuration of the pituitary gland. No one has established whether the volume of the gland is decreasing in this remodeling process.

Arachnoid cysts, pituitary epithelial cysts and cysts of the pars intermedia

There has been no additional information available from our own or published work which would implicate congenital or acquired arachnoid cysts as the usual causative agent in the production of 'empty' sellas.[1, 5] There is no question that true arachnoid cysts of the developmental type, and also acquired arachnoid cysts following surgery and/or irradiation, will act as masses.[42] Epithelial cysts of the pituitary are characterized by a mass effect.[43, 44] Cysts of the pars intermedia are not rare[12] but we believe that they are coincidental rather than the cause of an 'empty' sella. Recently reported cases of cysts extending into the sella have also exhibited mass effects upon sellar structures above the plane of the diaphragma sellae.[45-47] As will be emphasized in the section on plain film findings, all the changes attributable to the infradiaphragmatic subarachnoid space will be confined to those structures below the attachments of the diaphragma sellae.

The arachnoid over the defective diaphragma sellae will bulge through the hole and this can readily be seen at the time of transsphenoidal hypophysectomy. This arrangement could be called an arachnoid diverticulum, but not a cyst since a cyst is a closed cavity.[11, 28, 45, 49] Whether a rupture of this arachnoid diverticulum is required to develop enlargement of the sella turcica is not known.

Radiographic plain film findings

The sella turcica (anterior clinoids, limbus sphenoidale, chiasmatic sulcus, tuberculum sellae, anterior wall, floor, dorsum sellae, and posterior clinoids)[50] is recognized on roentgenograms because it is bone responding as bone,[51] reflecting enlargements of the pituitary gland, metabolic processes of bone, adjacent encroaching perisellar processes, and altered cerebrospinal fluid states such as occur in increased intracranial pressure and decreased cerebrospinal fluid pressures and pulsations in diversionary neurosurgical procedures.[52]

In 1962, Di Chiro and Nelson published a comprehensive review of roentgenographic measurements of the sella turcica, covering linear, two-dimensional and volumetric approaches.[26] Busch (1951), in compiling his measurements of the bony sella turcica, excluded those cases of 'empty' sellas, some of which he recognized as slightly enlarged.[12] Camp (1923) pointed out the variations in size and configuration of the sella and the difficulty in establishing standards.[24]

Emphasis has been placed on correlating pituitary gland size (volume) with the volume of the sella turcica.[12, 15, 26] However, the point has been made very clearly that the larger the sella turcica, the less the correlation with gland size.[26] These authors and others[6, 10, 22] have recognized pragmatically that the larger sella turcica was frequently associated with visualization of an intrasellar subarachnoid space on pneumoencephalograms. The inability to assign numerical values to a given sella turcica and implicate an expanding mass has been appreciated by many.[7, 8, 22, 53]

In the past, progressive sella turcica enlargement, symmetrical or particularly asymmetrical (in the absence of increased intracranial pressure) has been attributed to an expanding mass in or around the sella turcica. The failure to have clinical involvement of the optic apparatus was thought to be due to an intact diaphragma sellae or simply to the tumor missing the pertinent nerves. In this paper, we wish to (1) stress that progressive, non-tumorous sella turcica enlargement, symmetrical or asymmetrical, is not rare, and (2) present an approach which may be helpful with the plain film differential diagnosis between non-tumorous enlargement ('empty' sella) and enlargement due to expanding masses. As will be evident, linear or volumetric measurements per se are not helpful in differentiating non-tumorous from tumorous enlargement, nor in estimating the size of the pituitary gland. All changes attributable to the mechanisms which produce non-tumorous enlargement of the sella turcica occur below the plane of the diaphragma sellae, and the bony margins of the sella are intact.

Various radiographic terms have been used to describe sella turcica enlargement attributable to expanding intrasellar or perisellar masses.[7–10, 53, 54] They are: undermining, ballooning, cupping, deepening, asymmetry, progressive enlargement and, pertaining to the dorsum sellae, displacement, ballooning, thinning, erosion and truncation. These terms are used in association with changes involving the anterior and posterior clinoids, limbus sphenoidale and chiasmatic sulcus.

The term 'remodeling' is used in this paper as meaning a change in the configuration of the sella turcica occurring at a rate slow enough to allow the lamina dura of the sella turcica to be visualized on radiographs.[1, 51, 54] Bone changes in non-tumorous enlargement of the sella turcica satisfy this definition, the changes occurring very slowly, so that the normal metabolic turnover of bone results in formation of new compact bone. 'Erosion' is used in the same manner, as described by Camp in 1924.[54] In essence, erosion and remodeling are the same phenomenon with an operative time factor. Camp[54] recognized that enlargement of the sella turcica may be produced by tumors situated elsewhere in the cranial cavity. Tönnis[55] described a large series of secondary sella turcica enlargements due to tumors and favored venous engorgement rather than increased CSF pulsations acting through a deficient diaphragma sellae as the basic mechanism. In enlargement of the sella turcica secondary to increased intracranial pressure caused by neoplasms at a distance, the dorsum sellae is never displaced backward although it may be markedly thinned.[6, 53] Obstructive hydrocephalus with dilatation of the third ventricle may cause destruction of the dorsum and enlarge the sella turcica.

Pneumoencephalography

The pneumoencephalographic examination is conducted in the usual manner, making sure that air is in contact with the dorsal surface of the sella turcica and that the sella is above the air.

The significant positive finding is a convex upward air-gland interface. As shown in Case 1 (see below), it is possible to have a non-tumorous enlargement of the sella and a convex upward air-tissue interface (Fig. 1); however, this is not very frequent.

It is well established that parasellar air may hide a large tumor. Intrasellar air may not be appreciated unless laminograms are taken. The edge of the dura may simulate the gland,[7] but fortunately it is concave upward. Air-fluid levels may occur within the sella, obscuring the true size of the pituitary gland. Thin section laminography in two planes is a necessity.

Occasionally air is in contact with the sella, but does not enter. With the proper warning to the patient and apologies for the discomfort, percussion of the head is done by rapping the back of the head with the heel of one's palm. It was while removing gross en bloc specimens of 'empty' sellas from formalin that it became apparent that fluid could be trapped within the 'empty' sella, even with the opening in a deficient diaphragma sellae pointing directly downward. The percussion of the head dislodges the intrasellar fluid and allows air to enter. Laminograms are taken in this position. It is also quite likely that a fenestrated diaphragma sellae may not allow air to enter initially and a diaphragma sellae with a small hole may also give difficulty.

When the sella turcica is small, it is possible to have the pituitary gland presenting with a convex upward surface. With a slightly enlarged sella turcica, one would expect the pituitary gland upper surface to be concave in non-tumorous enlargement.

Angiography

Enlarged 'empty' sellas may give angiographic findings usually attributed to intrasellar tumors or cysts. While the intracavernous portion of the internal carotid artery will reflect the position of the lateral walls of the pituitary fossa, when it is in contact, and cavernous sinus venography will also document the wall position, neither method adds any information as to the contents of the sella or hypophyseal fossa.

Again, the concept that all angiographic changes in non-tumorous sellar enlargements, as with plain film changes, occur below the plane of attachment of the diaphragma sellae, will be helpful. One valuable and helpful exception is that the anterior cerebral artery may approach or actually enter the sella turcica as a result of herniation of the anterior inferior portion of the third ventricle, the border of which is the hypothalamus and optic chiasm. Angiographic changes in non-tumorous enlarged sella turcicas are:

A-P projection: (1) outward bowing of the midsiphon segment of the intracavernous segment of the internal carotid artery; (2) a more lateral position of the posterior segment than of the anterior segment of the intracavernous segment of the internal carotid artery; (3) inward bowing of the intracavernous segment of the internal carotid artery, a change which may occur with any sella turcica;[13, 15, 23] and (4) downward dipping and actual herniation of the junction of the horizontal and vertical portions of the anterior cerebral artery.[5, 39, 60]

Lateral projection: (1) opening of the carotid siphon; (2) closing of the carotid siphon; and (3) downward course and actual herniation of the anterior cerebral artery to and into the sella turcica.

The lateral limits of the midsiphon segment of the internal carotid artery, as published by Bull and Schunk,[61] are easily exceeded in some cases of non-tumorous enlargement of the sella turcica. The qualitative relationship of the posterior segment of the intracavernous segment of the internal carotid artery, having a more medial position than the anterior part of the same segment, is frequently reversed in those cases of enlarged sellas in which the bulging lateral walls are in contact with the artery.[62] Space does not permit a more detailed description of the variations of arterial displacement in non-tumorous enlargement of the sella turcica. Figure 4 demonstrates midsiphon displacement.

Recent advances in angiography have resulted in visualization of the vascular blush of the pituitary gland.[63, 64] Baker[63] has shown the vascular pituitary blush in 2 of 3 patients who had slightly enlarged 'empty' sella turcicas.

Case reports with comments

The following cases will show the changes involving the bony walls of the sella turcica and non-tumorous enlargement of the sella turcica, emphasizing that all changes in non-tumorous enlargement are confined to those parts of the sella turcica which are below the attachment of the diaphragma sellae anteriorly, laterally and posteriorly, and that the dorsum, while thinned and slightly bowed, is intact and never displaced posteriorly.

Case 1 (D.D.)

The result of a defective diaphragma sellae and the CSF pressures and pulsations acting through the defect upon the inner surface of the hypophyseal fossa to produce an asymmet-

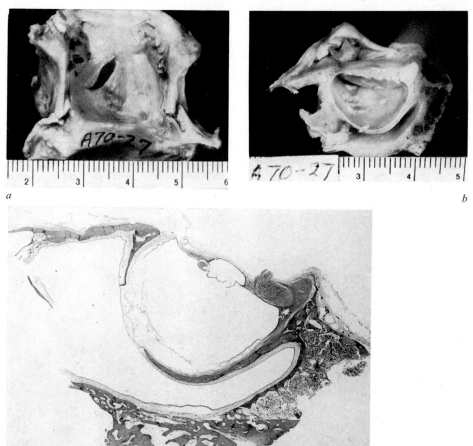

Fig. 1 Case 1 (D.D.): (*a*) Dorsal view of an en bloc section of sphenoid bone containing the sella turcica. A linear defect in the diaphragma sella is anterior and to the left of the hypophyseal stalk, which is completely surrounded by dense dura.

(*b*) Right side of a sagittal section of the sella turcica which is ballooned and contained CSF. The pituitary gland is displaced dorsally and posteriorly against the diaphragma sellae and dorsum sellae.

(*c*) Histological section of (*b*) showing a loss of bone anteriorly and inferiorly. Note the displaced pituitary gland.

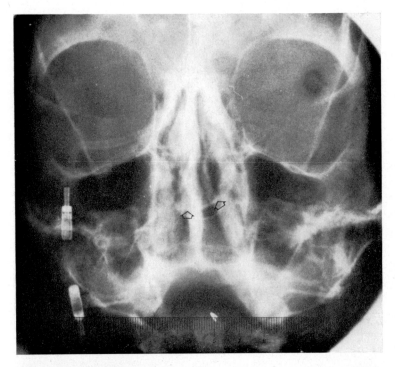

Fig. 1d

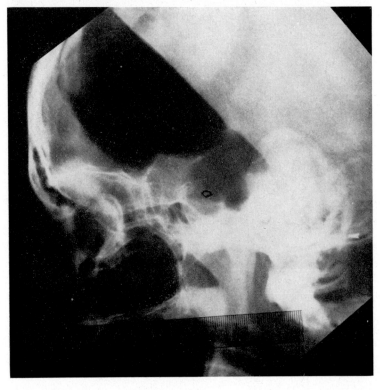

Fig. 1e

rical enlargement is seen in Figure 1a–e. This 44-year-old male had had varying degrees of hydrocephalus, secondary to aqueduct stenosis documented at age 14 years, and died of a septicemia. Whether the defect is congenital or acquired (no surgery done in region, but increased intracranial pressure may have caused a rent), it serves as a model to illustrate the principles that: (1) incompetency of the diaphragma sellae is necessary for the interaction of the CSF and the sella turcica walls, and (2) the size of the diaphragma sellae defect does not determine the size or shape of the remodeled sella turcica. The convex air-diaphragma sellae interface was discussed in the pneumoencephalographic section.

Case 2 (I.H.)

Figure 2a–d illustrates a classical 'empty' sella as viewed from above, and shows remodeling of the intact anterior wall of the sella turcica. 'Anterior remodeling' is probably a preferable term to 'undermining', which may or may not be associated by common usage with involvement of the planum sphenoidale. Again, note should be taken that the size of the hypophyseal foramen or absence of the diaphragma sellae does not reflect the extent or direction of the remodeling of the sella turcica. The remodeling of the anterior wall of the sella turcica may be asymmetrical in an anterior-posterior direction.[3] The patient was a 49-year-old

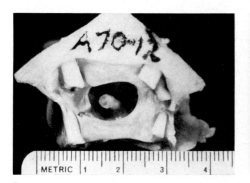 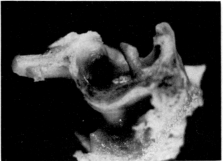

a   *b*

Fig. 2   Case 2 (I.H.) (*a*) Dorsal view of an en bloc section of sphenoid bone showing the classical appearance of an 'empty' sella with a deficient diaphragma sellae and non-visualization of the pituitary gland.

        (*b*) Right side of sagittal section of sphenoid bone showing the remodeled anterior and posterior lobes of the pituitary gland with the hypophyseal stalk in the middle. Note the ballooning of the anterior wall of the sella.

hypertensive female who died of a massive cerebral infarct. All endocrine studies were normal.

Minor asymmetrical change of the sella turcica is well described by Radberg[56] and it is becoming clear that asymmetry of the sella is not rare. We have entertained the thought that a common cause of a minimally asymmetrical sella is the 'empty' sella, particularly when the only change is a concave floor or a slight ballooning of the anterior wall. These are among the more common types of slight enlargement so well recognized and described by Taveras and Wood[10] and correctly attributed to an intrasellar subarachnoid space.

←——

Fig. 1   (*d*) Posterior-anterior view of skull showing asymmetrically enlarged floor of the sella turcica (hollow arrows).

        (*e*) Lateral head-hanging view of a pneumoencephalogram showing an air-soft tissue interface with a convex upward surface (arrow) representing the distended diaphragma sellae. The sella appears enlarged.

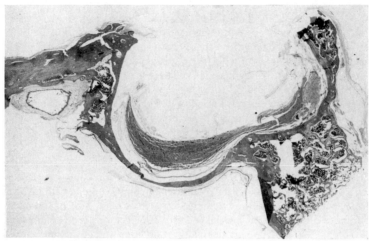

Fig. 2c   Histologic section of (*b*) showing a microscopically normal pituitary gland and intact bony walls.

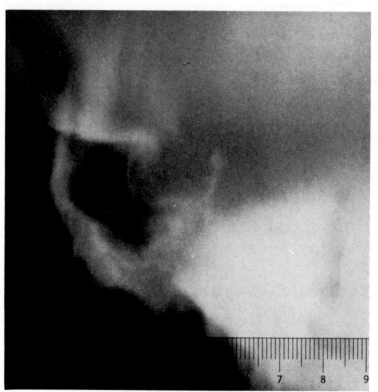

Fig. 2d   Lateral laminagram of sella showing the asymmetrical enlargement of the anterior part of the sella turcica, but with no involvement of the planum sphenoidale or limbus sphenoidale.

Fig. 3   Case 3 (J.S.): (*a*) Lateral view of the skull showing an unusual sella configuration with lack of definition of the sellar floor.

(*b*) Lateral laminogram demonstrating the deep type of sella characterized by a straight anterior wall directly joining the planum sphenoidale and an intact, non-displaced dorsum sellae. The floor of the sella is in contact with the floor of the sphenoid sinus (arrows ↑↑).

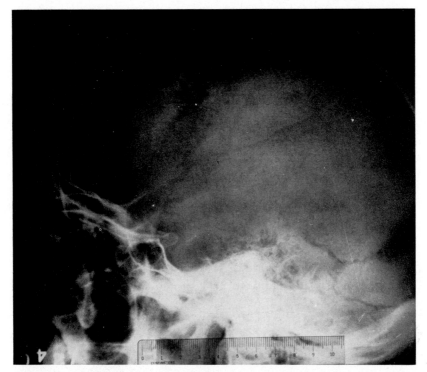

Fig. 3a

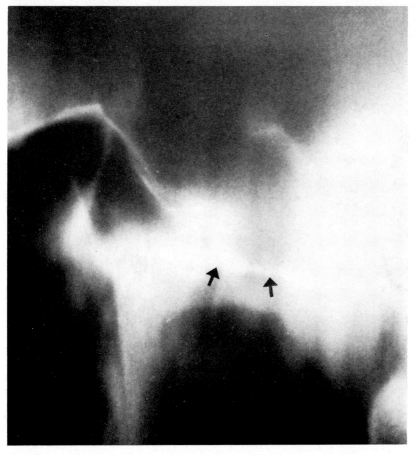

Fig. 3b

Case 3 (J.S.)

A deep and elongated type of remodeling of the sella turcica is seen in Figure 3*a* and *b*. The patient is a 56-year-old male who has for the past 25 years been followed for a seizure disorder and a suspected pituitary mass, despite normal endocrine studies. No therapy was instituted. The thinned dorsum is not displaced and is in line with the rest of the clivus. The anterior wall of the sella is continuous to the junction with the planum sphenoidale. Enlargement of the floor has extended downward causing obliteration of the sphenoid sinus. No appreciable change was noted in comparing films and linear laminograms over a 6-year period. This type of deep sella is not unusual and was previously described in a patient who was erroneously treated for acromegaly and had normal endocrine studies; at autopsy the bowl-shaped remodeled pituitary gland was histologically normal.[1]

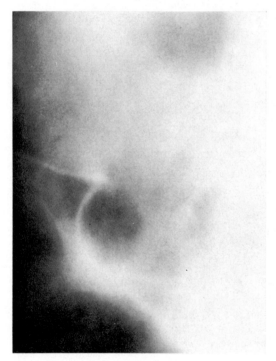

Fig. 4   Case 4 (E.G.): Lateral thin section (2 mm) laminagraphic view of the sella during a pneumo-encephalogram showing intrasellar air anteriorly in a markedly enlarged sella. All margins of bone are intact. The dorsum sellae is markedly thinned but intact and is in line with the clivus. The planum sphenoidale is normal. Note the apposition of the floor of the sella to the floor of the sphenoid sinus.

Case 4 (E.G.)

The significance of an enlarged sella occurring in a patient with endocrine symptoms is evident in this patient, who in retrospect was probably treated erroneously. Menstruation ceased at age 17 years and at age 23 her symptomatology and endocrine studies were consistent with panhypopituitarism. Sixteen years later, at age 39, the patient received super-voltage therapy, 3500 rads to the pituitary, with no change in her status. Ten years later a pneumoencephalogram was done and air was definitely visualized within the sella. Endocrine studies confirmed the previous findings of panhypopituitarism. The question at this time is whether the changes in the sella were due to a tumor which shrank following irradiation. This seems very unlikely, because changes in a sella in which successful therapy has reduced the size of the tumor show a slight decrease in the overall size and a thickening of the bony walls.[10, 57] The pneumoencephalogram has effectively excluded a cystic mass at this time. It is this type of sella which we would consider to be an 'empty' sella, satisfying all criteria of no involvement of any structure above the plane of the diaphragma sellae and a non-displaced dorsum sellae. We would insist on a pneumoencephalogram before instituting radiation therapy. A high index of suspicion is needed and adequate pneumoencephalography with thin section laminography is essential.

Case 5 (J.V.)

Progressive asymmetrical non-tumorous enlargement of the sella, failure to appreciate intra-sellar air on a pneumoencephalogram, misinterpretation of arteriographic findings, and over-emphasis on visual findings are illustrative of the diagnostic problems associated with 'empty' sellae, and are well demonstrated in the case of an obese (290 lb), 53-year-old, hypertensive black female. An acute visual loss in the left eye led to the observation that the sella turcica was asymmetrically enlarged. Five years later she was totally blind in her left eye, with questionable involvement of the right. Asymmetrical enlargement of the sella turcica with a volume of 3000 mm³ was documented (Fig. 5a–d). Arteriography showed lateral bowing of the midsiphon segment of the internal carotid artery. The pneumoencephalogram failed to show any suprasellar mass and, although intrasellar air was suspected (Fig. 5a), it was

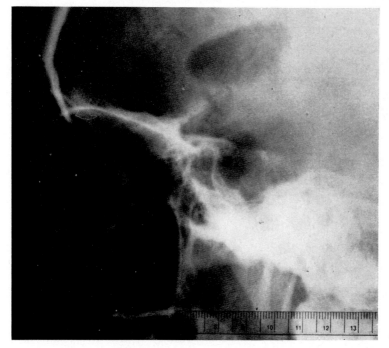

a

Fig. 5   Case 5 (J.Y.): (*a*) Lateral brow-up view of pneumoencephalogram showing intrasellar air and an enlarged sella turcica (3000 mm³).

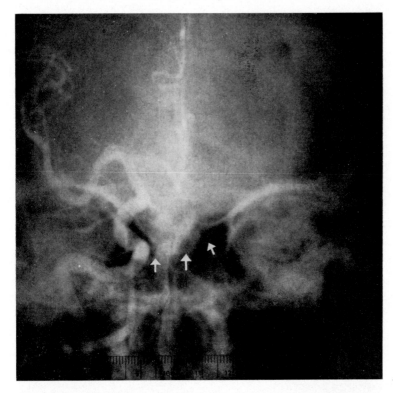

Fig. 5b

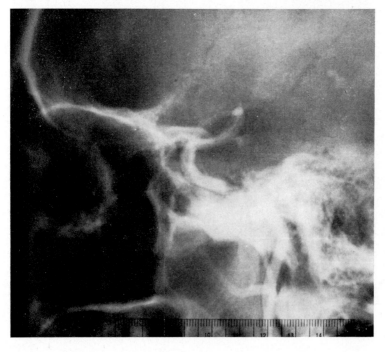

Fig. 5c

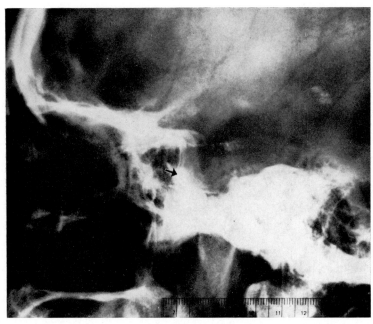

Fig. 5d

Fig. 5 (*b*) Anterior-posterior view of right carotid arteriogram showing lateral bowing of midsiphon part of the intracavernous segment of the internal carotid artery. Midsiphon-to-midline measurement is 15 mm. Note the sloping sellar floor (arrows ↑ ↑) proven with laminography.

(*c*) Lateral view of right carotid arteriogram showing opening of the carotid siphon secondary to a low position of the intracavernous segment of the internal carotid artery.

(*d*) Five years after the pneumoencephalogram shown in (*a*), the lateral skull shows an increase in sella turcica size. Laminograms documented the local bulge (arrow →) of the anterior wall. Note the progressive thinness of the dorsum without displacement.

felt that without laminograms (technically not feasible because of the patient's obesity) the visualized air could be parasellar. The above combination of events and findings led to external irradiation, 4000 rads, over a 5-week period. At all times and continuing to the present, pituitary function studies have been normal.

Three years later, at age 53, she presented with profuse spontaneous rhinorrhea. Her neurological examination was unchanged and endocrine functions were normal. The skull films showed a 1.5 mm increase in the A-P diameter of the sella to a total A-P dimension of 20.5 mm, and a 2.0 mm increase in the height of the sella to a total height of 18 mm. Laminography (2 mm sections) revealed a localized bulge of the anterior wall of the sella, immediately below the intact chiasmatic sulcus (Fig. 5*d*, arrow), but a definitive bone discontinuity was not demonstrated. A Pantopaque sinogram was unsuccessful, but maneuvering of Pantopaque from the lumbar subarachnoid space, introduced by a lumbar puncture, to inside the sella turcica did document a collection of Pantopaque anterior to the wall of the sella, strongly suggesting the site of the fistula (Weiss et al., in preparation).

At transsphenoidal surgery, the ballooned anterior wall of the sella had 8–10 1 mm perforations in it, corresponding to similar sized holes in the dura through which CSF was leaking. After going through a 0.5 mm rind of yellowish tissue, thought to be pituitary, the neurosurgeon observed 'a huge arachnoid and cerebrospinal fluid-filled 'empty' sella'. The diaphragma sellae was 'virtually absent' and a small amount of normal pituitary tissue could be seen on the left side of the inferior posterior portion of the sella, occupying about 10 %

of the sellar size or volume. No tumor tissue or irradiation effects were observed. Repair was accomplished, and 2 years later pituitary function continues to be normal without recurrence of the CSF leak.

Case 6 (A.D.)

The following case, which satisfied the criteria of a Forbes-Albright syndrome and had a large asymmetrical sella, is presented to illustrate the coincidental occurrence of 'empty' sellas in patients with galactorrhea (Fig. 6a–c).

The patient ceased menstruating at age 28 followed by a weight gain of 130 lb to 250 lb. At age 35, diabetes mellitus was discovered, as well as an adenocarcinoma of the endometrium which was treated with intrauterine radiation and subsequent hysterectomy and bilateral salpingo-oophorectomy. One year later galactorrhea occurred and skull films revealed an asymmetrically enlarged sella turcica. A pituitary tumor was suspected and, with the provisional diagnosis of a Forbes–Albright syndrome, supervoltage radiation therapy, 3500 rads tumor dose, was given to the sella. There was no visual field impairment or abnormal neurological signs.

Galactorrhea, headache, obesity and hirsutism persisted unchanged from the onset until the patient's demise. Endocrine studies revealed normal adrenal function and normal pituitary ACTH reserve, normal thyroid function, unmeasurable urinary gonadotrophins, and undetectable serum growth hormone even after provocative tests.

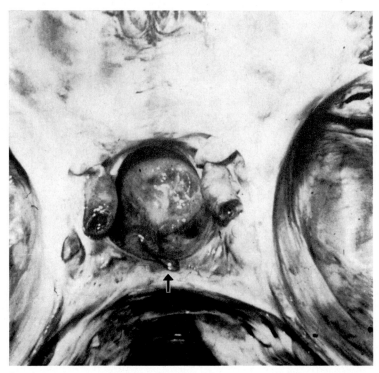

a

Fig. 6   Case 6 (A.D.): *(a)* Dorsal view of the sella turcica. The diaphragma sellae is deficient and the pituitary gland is asymmetrically displaced to the left and posteriorly. The hypophyseal stalk (arrow ↑) is posteriorly and to the left. Anteriorly on the right the dura on the floor of the sella is exposed.

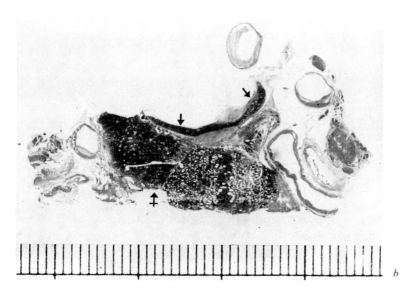

b

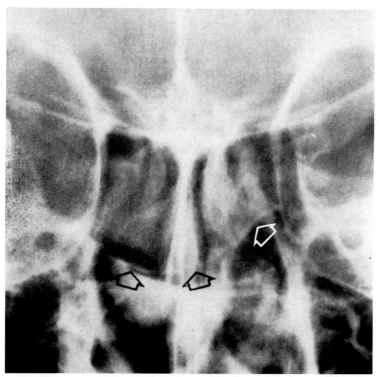

c

Fig. 6 Case 6 (A.D.) (*b*) Coronal section of the sella region showing the flattened anterior pituitary gland (arrows ↓↓) and the asymmetrical floor. The dense tissue (arrow ↕) is undifferentiated carcinoma of the sinus. (Scale: 1 div. = 1 mm.)

(*c*) The anterior-posterior view of the skull shows the floor of the sella (arrows) sloping downward on the right, corresponding with the configuration of the remodeled pituitary gland in (*b*).

At age 48 the patient developed a sudden dense flaccid left hemiparesis. Laminography documented the asymmetrical enlargement of the sella. On the left, the length of the sella was 20 mm and the depth 9 mm, and on the right the length was 30 mm and the depth 25 mm (uncorrected for 30 % magnification). No change had occurred in the sella in 9 years.

A right retrobrachial arteriogram revealed occlusive vascular disease. The carotid sulcus was closed, with elevation of the intracavernous segment of the internal carotid artery. There was lateral displacement of the posterior portion of the intracavernous segment of the internal carotid artery and an unusual downward deviation of the anterior cerebral artery.

At autopsy the optic chiasm was flattened against the porus of the anterior margin of the 'empty' sella turcica, sufficient to cause an indentation on its inferior surface. The low position of the chiasm probably explains the low position of the anterior cerebral artery. The diaphragma sellae was totally deficient and the pituitary gland was compressed to the left and posteriorly, but was histologically normal (Fig. 6a). An undifferentiated carcinoma was found extrasellar on the right side, probably arising from the lining cells of the sphenoid sinus and not affecting the sella. Marked atherosclerosis of the cerebral arteries was present and infarcts were documented in the right cerebral hemisphere.

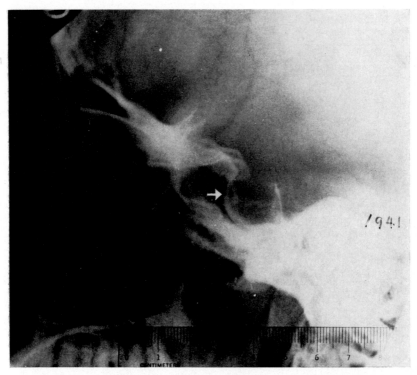

a

Fig. 7   Case 7 (M.J.): (*a*). Lateral view of the sella turcica which had shown a 2 mm increase in anterior-posterior dimension during a 1-year period. The slightly ballooned anterior wall is indicated by the arrow (→).

(*b*)   Lateral view of sella turcica 16 years later after enlargement had plateaued. Length 20 mm, depth 20 mm, and height 20 mm. Note the intact and unchanged chiasmatic sulcus. The dorsum is thinned but no displacement has occurred. (Scale: 1 div. = 1 mm)

(*c*)   Lateral view of sella 9 years later with no appreciable change (arrows →) of the anterior wall. Death occurred one year later.

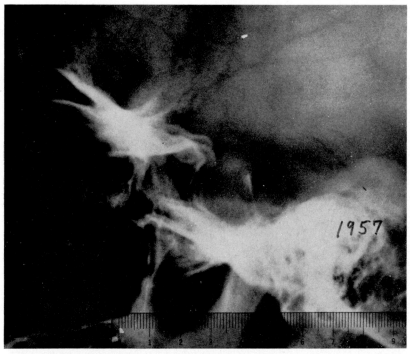

Fig. 7b

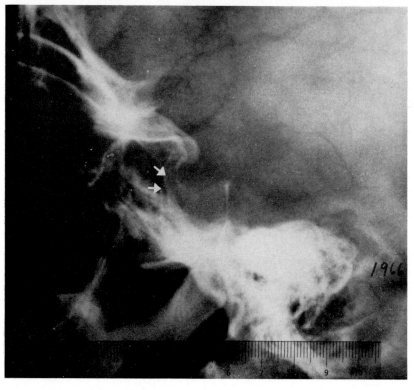

Fig. 7c

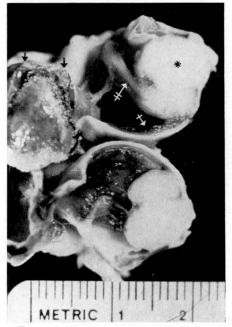

Fig. 7   (d) Sagittal section of the en bloc sella turcica specimen with half the specimen folded down 180 degrees. The diaphragma sellae is congenitally deficient, the planum sphenoidale and chiasmastic sulcus (between arrows ↓↓) are normal. Anteriorly the histologically normal anterior pituitary gland is remodeled and flattened (arrow ↥) and posteriorly the whitish mass is a chromophobe adenoma (asterisk *). There is disruption of the base of the dorsum sellae posteriorly and inferiorly. Anteriorly the changes involving the sella turcica are those of the 'empty' sella; posteriorly those of a classical pituitary neoplasm causing local destruction of the base of the dorsum sellae. The hypophyseal stalk is in the center (arrow ↦).

Case 7 (M.J.)

The concept of coincidence of 'empty' sella and pituitary adenoma is also illustrated in the next case, that of an obese, 250 lb female whose sella showed progressive enlargement, was erroneously treated, and at autopsy was found to harbor a chromophobe adenoma occupying a portion of the enlarged sella turcica (Fig. 7a–d).

She weighed 180 lb at age 18 and gradually increased her weight. At age 27 an X-ray of the sella turcica showed an increase in size from a normal 13 mm length and 14 mm depth to 15 mm length and 15 mm depth. Endocrine studies and neurological examinations were normal, but she received radiation therapy to the sella (dose unknown). Sixteen years later the sella turcica had increased to a length of 20 mm and a depth of 20 mm; the skull films were taken as part of a skeletal survey for adenocarcinoma of the breast. She died at age 47 of metastatic breast carcinoma.

At autopsy the gross appearance was that of an incomplete diaphragma sellae and an 'empty' sella, without evidence of arachnoiditis or radiation changes. On sagittal section the anterior portion of the enlarged sella exhibited a space occupied by CSF and a flattened anterior lobe with a pituitary gland shown histologically to be normal. Posteriorly a whitish mass was histologically proven to be a chromophobe adenoma.

We feel that the tumor is coincidental with an 'empty' sella, and indeed incidental pituitary tumors run as high as 25 %.[58] This figure includes nests of cells as well as gross adenomas. Films of the sella one year prior to death did not demonstrate a destruction of the base of the dorsum sellae. Either the bone change was not sufficient to appreciate on the radiograph, or the adenoma had not grown large enough to have caused a significant radiographic change. In any event, had original therapy caused a reduction in tumor size, one cannot implicate the reduced chromophobe adenoma as the cause of the progressive enlargement of the sella turcica. The appearance of the sella is compatible, as seen on X-rays, with progressive non-tumorous enlargement of the sella turcica.

The differentiation between non-tumorous enlargement of the sella turcica and intrasellar masses is illustrated in the next 2 cases. It should be clearly stated that at a certain stage in the growth of an intrasellar mass, the resultant plain film changes are identical with the 'empty' sella changes. Masses will cause bone changes above the plane of the diaphragma sellae and will displace the dorsum posteriorly. Asymmetry and progressive enlargement are changes common to both entities.

Case 8 (C.B.)

Figure 8 is a lateral film of a pneumoencephalogram showing dorsal displacement on one side of the dorsum sellae, posterior and upward displacement of the posterior clinoid, re-modeling of the floor, and a classical convex upward air-soft tissue interface so characteristic of an intrasellar mass extending beyond the sella. The anterior clinoid processes are not involved. The patient is a 22-year-old female with non-puerperal galactorrhea and is amen-orrheic. Therapy was transsphenoidal microsurgery with removal of a chromophobe tumor on the left side, leaving normal pituitary tissue on the uninvolved right side.

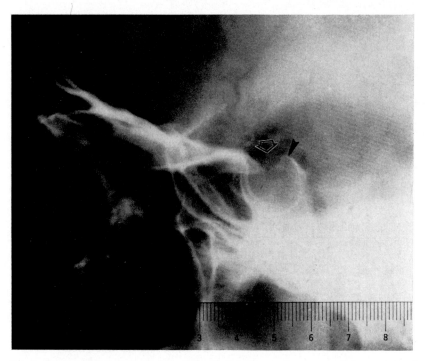

Fig. 8 Case 8 (C.B.): Lateral view of the skull during a pneumoencephalogram showing a convex air-soft tissue interface above the sella (hollow arrow), upward and posterior displacement of a posterior clinoid process (black arrowhead), dorsal displacement of one side of the dorsum sellae, and enlargement of one side of the floor and anterior wall of the sella resulting in a double contour. These findings are those of a classical intrasellar mass with suprasellar extension. The anterior clinoid processes are not involved.

Case 9 (C.W.)

Figure 9 illustrates the plain film findings of a pituitary mass with attenuation of an anterior clinoid process, asymmetrical enlargement on one side of the sella, and minimal posterior displacement of one part of the diaphragma sellae with its accompanying posterior clinoid process. From these findings one cannot predict whether there is extensive or minimal extension of the mass beyond the confines of the sella turcica. A pneumoencephalogram is necessary, and in these cases a convex upward air-soft tissue interface is evident, as was present to a minimal degree in this patient. Endocrine and neurological findings were normal and external radiation was the mode of therapy in this 21-year-old male, who has shown no change in 3 years.

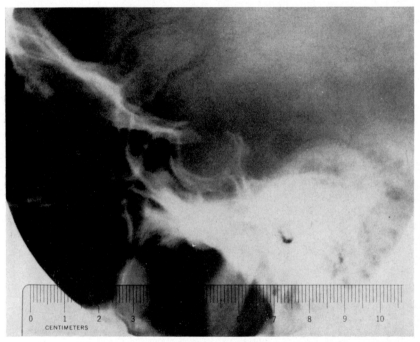

Fig. 9   Case 9 (C.W.): Lateral view of the sella showing the findings of an intra-sellar mass; elevation and attenuation of an anterior clinoid process; posterior displacement of the upper dorsum sellae and its accompanying posterior clinoid process; and a double contour of the floor and anterior wall.

In the plain film evaluation of non-tumorous enlargement of the sella turcica, the dorsum sellae may be thin, is not displaced, but may exhibit a very slight bowing in the larger globular sellas. There is no involvement of the posterior clinoid processes. One should therefore be aware of the normal variations of the dorsum and posterior clinoids, and the extensive works of Camp and Karlas[24, 25, 50] are extremely helpful. Our main point is that while asymmetry of the dorsum occurs normally, asymmetry occurs in the plane parallel with the slope of the clivus and not in an anterior-posterior direction.

In summary, therefore, symmetrical or asymmetrical remodeling occurs in non-tumorous enlargement of the sella turcica with predictable patterns. All the remodeling occurs below the plane of the diaphragma sellae, leaving the chiasmatic sulcus and the anterior and posterior clinoids intact. The bowing of the dorsum may be slight, but there is no posterior displacement as occurs classically with any large intrasellar tumor.[6–10, 51] The explanation which we offer is that the CSF forces are acting on the intrasellar side of the dorsum and are balanced by the CSF forces acting on the intradural side, resulting in a thinning with no displacement.

With current radiographic and endocrinologic techniques we feel that diagnosis of pituitary tumors can and should be made before the occurrence of these minimal, but definite, bony X-ray changes. The combination of asymmetrical sella turcica enlargement and endocrine findings do not in themselves justify therapy with the presumptive diagnosis of an intrasellar tumor. Pneumoencephalography remains the definitive diagnostic test and the air-soft tissue interface should be seen.

With the advent of transsphenoidal microscopic surgery for pituitary neoplasms, the identification of neoplasms before they become large is worthwhile and with our current radiographic techniques feasible, as illustrated in the next case.

Case 10 (M.R.)

Figure 10a–c shows the convex upward air-soft tissue interface of an enlarged or displaced pituitary gland in a normal sized, non-distorted sella turcica. The patient is a 25-year-old black male who has had galactorrhea for 11 years and gynecomastia for 7 years. Elevated prolactin levels were found (47–57 ng/ml), with no response to Thorazine or L-DOPA. The lateral view of the pneumoencephalogram appeared normal. Thin section laminography anterior-posterior and lateral views, in the head-hanging position with air maintained in contact with the sella, clearly demonstrate an abnormal air-soft tissue interface within the

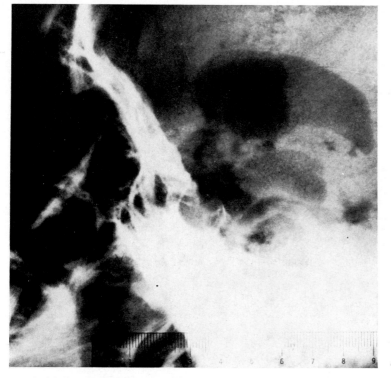

Fig. 10 (a) Case 10 (M.R.): *a* Lateral view of a pneumoencephalogram showing no evidence of a supra-sellar extension. Sella length is 13 mm and the dorsum is not thinned.

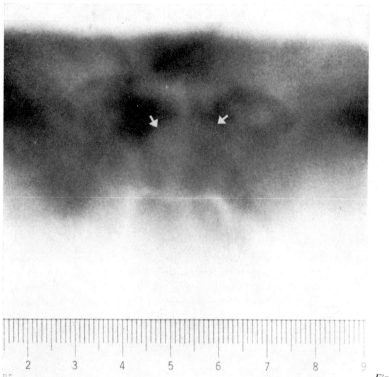

Fig. 10b

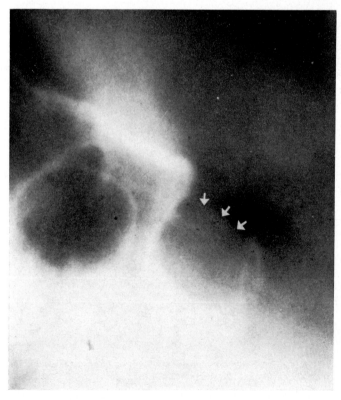

Fig. 10c

←

Fig. 10 (*b*) Thin section laminography (1 mm) in the A-P projection showing a symmetrical convex
upward air-soft tissue interface (arrows ↓). The stalk is in the midline and the hypothalamus
is contrasted with air in the suprasellar cisterns and third ventricle. The optic nerves and
carotid arteries are delineated with air. Note the intact sellar floor.

(*c*) Thin section laminography (1 mm) in the brow-up position shows a convex upward
air-soft tissue interface (arrows ↓) considered abnormal for a sella turcica of this size.

---

confines of the sella. The pituitary gland was felt to be either generally enlarged or displaced
upward by a mass. Surgery was by the transsphenoidal route (Dr. Jerald Brodkey) with
removal of an adenoma on the left side, leaving normal pituitary tissue on the right.

Case 11 (B.T.)

Illustrating the value of pneumoencephalography is the following case of an iatrogenic
Cushing's disease (Fig. 10*a–c*). The patient is a 43-year-old female presenting the classical
clinical findings of a florid Cushing's syndrome and an asymmetrically enlarged sella turcica
measuring 20 mm in length, an intact floor sloping markedly to the right, and a non-displaced
thin dorsum sellae with a central rarefaction which could be considered a normal variation.[50]
Because large sellas are unusual in Cushing's syndrome[59] and there was no bony involvement above the plane of the diaphragma sellae, a pneumoencephalogram was done. Based
on our experience of a coincidental chromophobe adenoma in an 'empty' sella (Fig. 7), the
possibility of a functioning basophilic adenoma in an 'empty' sella was also considered.
Figure 11 shows the intrasellar air, effectively excluding the asymmetrically enlarged sella,

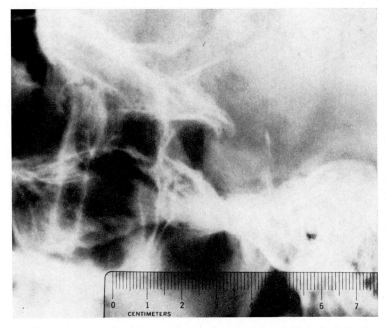

a

Fig. 11 Case 11 (B.T.): (*a*) Lateral view of an asymmetrically enlarged sella measuring 18 mm in
length. The dorsum sellae is thinned and there is no involvement of the anterior clinoids.
Probable dural calcification alongside the sella.

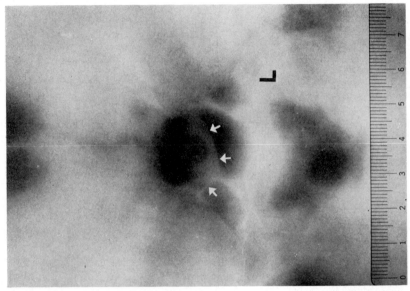

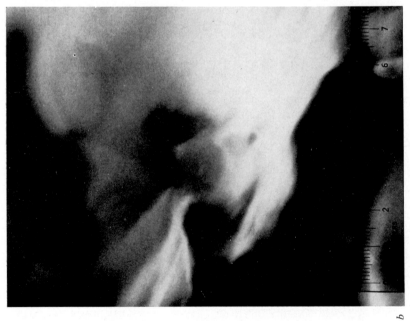

Fig. 11 (*b*) Brow-up lateral thick section laminographic view of sella during pneumoencephalography showing the low position of the anterior inferior third ventricle. Intrasellar air was suspected, but thick section laminograms did not resolve the question. (*c*) Anterior-posterior thin section laminograms (1 mm) taken at time of (*b*) show unequivocally the intrasellar air and also a central depression in the pituitary gland. The value of fine section laminography is evident. Note the intact asymmetrical sellar floor (arrows ↑).

as due to an intrasellar mass, but not excluding a small adenoma. The patient's florid Cushing's syndrome was subsequently determined to be caused by ingestion of excessive doses of cortisone, with which she was being treated for arthritis.

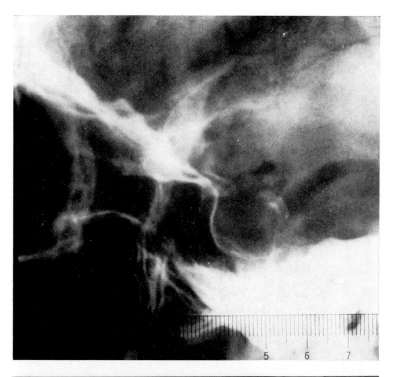

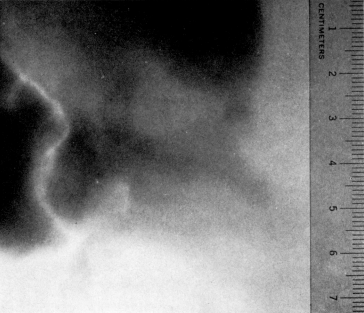

Fig. 12 Case 12 (O.H.): (*a*) Lateral view of skull in brow-up position during pneumoencephalo-graphy showing the sella at the upper limits of 'normal' measuring 16 mm in length and 14 mm in depth with a slightly asymmetrical floor (*c*). Intrasellar air was suspected. Note the lack of bony involvement above the plane of the diaphragma sellae.

(*b*) Lateral thin section laminograms (1 mm) during pneumoencephalography showing intrasellar air and the posterior position of the anterior inferior third ventricle. The need for thin section laminography is evident.

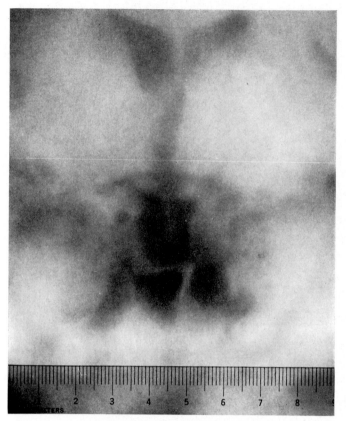

c

Fig. 12 (*c*) Anterior-posterior thin section laminograms (1 mm) showing intrasellar air, the stalk
and hypothalamus. On other sections a soft tissue density thought to be in the gland proper
was identified. Note the slight asymmetry of the sellar floor.

Case 12 (O.H.)

This patient had a moderately globular sella with an asymmetrical floor (Fig. 12*a–c*) still
considered within normal limits by existing standards in a patient with galactorrhea, demonstrating the value of pneumoencephalography and thin section laminography.

The patient is a 47-year-old female with galactorrhea. The globular sella measures 16 mm
in length and 14 mm in depth on routine skull films, with a slightly asymmetrical floor in
the A-P projections. The patient is obese (240 lb) and her CSF pressure was 425 mm of
water (H_2O) in a decubitus position. Pneumoencephalography with 1 mm thin section
laminography shows unequivocally that air is within the sella turcica and also illustrates
what can be accomplished with thin section laminography.

Summary

Differentiation between enlargement of the sella turcica caused by intrasellar masses and
non-tumorous enlargement, the 'empty' sella, can be accomplished with plain film radiography and pneumoencephalography. All bone changes attributable to non-tumorous enlargement of the sella turcica occur below the diaphragma sellae and the dorsum sellae is

not displaced posteriorly. Intrasellar neoplasms below the diaphragma sellae may present with the same radiographic findings as non-tumorous enlargement of the sella turcica, and pneumoencephalography remains the definitive diagnostic study. Diagnosis of intrasellar neoplasms within a non-distorted sella turcica is feasible with current radiographic techniques and desirable with the availability of newer microsurgical techniques. Non-tumorous enlargement of the sella turcica occurs not infrequently,[3] is and will be reported more frequently,[65] and can be expected to be coincidental with many disease entities, including endocrinopathies.

References

(1) KAUFMAN, B. (1968): The 'empty' sella turcica. A manifestation of the intrasellar subarachnoid space. *Radiology, 90,* 931.

(2) COLBY JR, M. Y. and KEARNS, T. P. (1962): Radiation therapy of pituitary adenomas with associated visual impairment. *Mayo Clin. Proc., 37,* 15.

(3) KAUFMAN, B. and CHAMBERLIN JR, W. B. (1972): The ubiquitous 'empty' sella turcica. *Acta radiol. (Stockh.), 13,* 413.

(4) KAUFMAN, B., CHAMBERLIN, W. B., Jr and PEARSON, O. H. (1971): Non-tumorous progressive asymmetrical enlargement of the sella turcica. Presented at: *57th Annual Meeting, Radiological Society of North America, Nov.-Dec., 1971.*

(5) MORTARA, R. and NORRELL, H. (1970): Consequences of a deficient sellar diaphragm. *J. Neurosurg., 32,* 565.

(6) DU BOULAY, G. H. (1965): *Principles of X-ray Diagnosis of the Skull,* p. 28. Butterworth and Co., London-Washington.

(7) LOMBARDI, G. (1967): *Radiology in Neuro-ophthalmology.* Williams and Wilkins Company, Baltimore, Md.

(8) NEWTON, T. H. and POTTS, D. G. (Eds.) (1971): *Radiology of the Skull and Brain. The Skull,* Vol. 1, Book 1, pp. 357-405. C. V. Mosby Co., St. Louis, Mo.

(9) ROSS, R. J. and GREITZ, T. V. B. (1966): Changes of the sella turcica in chromophobe adenomas and eosinophilic adenomas. *Radiology, 86,* 892.

(10) TAVERAS, J. M. and WOOD, E. H. (1964): *Diagnostic Neuroradiology.* Williams and Wilkins Company, Baltimore, Md.

(11) GABRIELE, D. F. (1968): The empty sella syndrome. *Amer. J. Roentgenol., 104,* 168.

(12) BUSCH, W. (1951): Die Morphologie der Sella turcica und ihre Beziehungen zur Hypophyse. *Arch. path. Anat., 320,* 437.

(13) BERGLAND, R. M., RAY, B. S. and TORACK, R. M. (1968): Anatomical variations in the pituitary gland and adjacent structures in 225 human autopsy cases. *J. Neurosurg., 28,* 93.

(14) MCLACHLAN, M. S. F., WILLIAMS, E. D. and DOYLE, F. H. (1968): Applied anatomy of the pituitary gland and fossa. *Brit. J. Radiol., 41,* 782.

(15) MCLACHLAN, M. S. F., WILLIAMS, E. D., FORTT, R. W. and DOYLE, F. H. (1968): Estimation of pituitary gland dimensions from radiographs of the sella turcica. *Brit. J. Radiol., 41,* 323.

(16) SCHAEFFER, J. P. (1924): Some points in the regional anatomy of the optic pathway, with especial reference to tumors of the hypophysis cerebri and resulting ocular changes. *Anat. Rec., 28,* 243.

(17) SUNDERLAND, S. (1945): The meningeal relations of the human hypophysis cerebri. *J. Anat. (Lond.), 79,* 33.

(18) ISRAEL, H. (1970): Continuing growth of the sella turcica with age. *Amer. J. Roentgenol., 108,* 516.

(19) ENGELS, E. P. (1958): Roentgenographic demonstration of a hypophyseal subarachnoid space. *Amer. J. Roentgenol., 80,* 1001.

(20) FERNER, H. (1960): Die Hypophysenzisterne des Menschen und ihre Beziehung zum Entstehungsmechanismus der sekundären Sellae-Weiterung. *Z. Anat. Entwickl.-Gesch., 121,* 407.

(21) RASMUSSEN, A. T. (1924): A quantitative study of the human hypophysis cerebri, or pituitary body. *Endocrinology, 8,* 509.

(22) DI CHIRO, G. (1961): *An Atlas of Detailed Normal Pneumoencephalographic Anatomy.*

Charles C. Thomas, Springfield, Ill

(23) KAUFMAN, B., LAPHAM, L. W., SHEALY, C. N. and PEARSON, O. H. (1966): Transsphenoidal Yttrium-90 pituitary ablation. *Acta radiol. (Stockh.)*, *5*, 17.

(24) CAMP, J. D. (1923): The normal and pathological anatomy of the sella turcica as revealed at necropsy. *Radiology*, *1*, 65.

(25) CAMP, J. D. (1924): The normal and pathological anatomy of the sella turcica as revealed by roentgenograms. *Amer. J. Roentgenol.*, *12*, 143.

(26) DI CHIRO, G. and NELSON, K. B. (1962): The volume of the sella turcica. *Amer. J. Roentgenol.*, *87*, 989.

(27) DI CHIRO, G. (1960): The width (third dimension) of the sella turcica. *Amer. J. Roentgenol.*, *84*, 26.

(28) CHYNN, K.-Y. (1966): Neuroradiologic exploration in intra- and parasellar conditions. *Radiol. Clin. N. Amer.*, *4*, 93.

(29) NADJMI, M. (1965): Bedeutung der sogenannten subdiaphragmalen Zisternen bei der gezielten Hypophyseneingriffen. *Radiologe (Berl.)*, *5*, 455.

(30) ROBERTSON, G. (1957): *Pneumoencephalography, 1st ed.* Charles C. Thomas, Springfield, Ill.

(31) ZATZ, L. M., JANON, E. A. and NEWTON, T. H. (1969): The enlarged sella and the intrasellar cistern. *Radiology*, *93*, 1085.

(32) DI CHIRO, G., OMMAYA, A. K., ASHBURN, W. L. and BRINER, W. H. (1968): Isotope cisterno-graphy in the diagnosis and follow-up of cerebrospinal fluid retinorrhea. *J. Neurosurg.*, *28*, 522.

(33) KAUFMAN, H. H. (1969): Non-traumatic cerebrospinal fluid rhinorrhea. *Arch. Neurol. (Chic.)*, *21*, 59.

(34) BRISMAN, R., HUGHES, J. E. D. and MOUNT, L. A. (1969): Cerebrospinal fluid rhinnorhea and the empty sella. *J. Neurosurg.*, *31*, 538.

(35) OMMAYA, A. K., DI CHIRO, G., BALDWIN, M. and PENNYBACKER, J. B. (1968): Non-traumatic cerebrospinal fluid rhinorrhea. *J. Neurol. Neurosurg. Psychiat.*, *31*, 214.

(36) HODGSON, S. F., RANDALL, R. V., HOLMAN, C. B. and MACCARTY, C. S. (1972): Empty sella syndrome. *Med. Clin. N. Amer.*, *56*, 897.

(37) BRISMAN, R., HUGHES, J. E. and HOLUB, D. A. (1972): Endocrine function in 19 patients with empty sella syndrome. *J. clin. Endocr.*, *34*, 570.

(38) CAPLAN, R. H. and DOBBEN, G. D. (1969/1970): Endocrine studies in patients with 'empty sella syndrome'. *Arch. intern. Med.*, *123*, 611 and *Psychiat. Dig.*, *31*, 59.

(39) OLSON, D. R., GUIOT, G. and DE ROME, P. (1972): The symptomatic empty sella. *J. Neuro-surg.*, *37*, 533.

(40) NULSEN, F. E.: Personal communication re ICP CSF in obese patients.

(41) FOLEY, J. (1955): Benign forms of intracranial hypertension, 'toxic' and 'otitic' hydrocephalus. *Brain*, *78*, 1.

(42) FRIEDMANN, G. and MARGUTH, F. (1961): Intrasellare Liquorzysten. *Zbl. Neurochir.*, *21*, 33.

(43) FAGER, C. A. and CARTER, H. (1966): Intrasellar epithelial cysts. *J. Neurosurg.*, *24*, 77.

(44) OBRADOR, S. (1972): The empty sella and some related syndromes. *J. Neurosurg.*, *36*, 162.

(45) CALKINS, R. A., PRIBHAM, H. F. W. and JOYNT, R. J. (1968): Intrasellar arachnoid diverticula. *Neurology (Minneap.)*, *18*, 1037.

(46) SANSREGRET, A., LEDOUX, R., PUPLANTIS, F., LAMOUREUX, C., CHAPDELAINE, A. and LE BLANC, P. (1969): Suprasellar subarachnoid cysts — radioclinical features. *Amer. J. Roentgenol.*, *105*, 291.

(47) WEBER, E. L., VOGEL, G. L. and ODOM, G. L. (1970): Cysts of the sella turcica. *J. Neurosurg.*, *33*, 48.

(48) Case Records of Massachusetts General Hospital — Case 45401 (1959): *New Engl. J. Med.*, *261/14*, 709.

(49) RING, B. A. and WADDINGTON, M. (1965): Primary arachnoid cysts of the sella turcica. *Amer. J. Roentgenol.*, *98*, 611.

(50) KARLAS, G. A. (1948): *Morphological Observations on the Superior Surface of the Body of the Sphenoid Bone in Human Adult.* Dissertation, University of Helsingfors.

(51) MAHOMOUD, M. S. (1958): The sella in health and disease: value of the radiographic study of the sella turcica in morbid anatomical and topographic diagnosis of intracranial tumours. *Brit. J. Radiol., Suppl. 8*, 1.

(52) KAUFMAN, B., SANDSTROM, P. H. and YOUNG, H. F. (1970): Alteration in size and configura-tion of the sella turcica as the result of prolonged cerebrospinal fluid shunting. *Radiology*, *97*,

537.
(53) Du Boulay, G. H. and El Gammal, T. (1966): Classification, clinical value, and mechanism of sella turcica changes in raised intracranial pressure. *Brit. J. Radiol.*, *39*, 422

(54) Camp, J. D. (1949): Roentgenologic observations concerning erosion of the sella turcica. *Radiology*, *53*, 666.

(55) Tönnis, W., Schiefer, W. and Rausch, I. J. (1954): Sellaveränderungen bei gesteigertem Schädelinnendruck. *Dtsch. Z. Nervenheilk.*, *171*, 351.

(56) Radberg, C. (1963): Some aspects of the asymmetrical enlargement of the sella turcica. *Acta radiol. (Stockh.) (Diag.)*, *1*, 152.

(57) Lewtas, N. A. (1966): Symposium on pituitary tumors. *Clin. Radiol. (Lond.)*, *17*, 149.

(58) Daughaday, W. H. (1968): The adenohypophysis. In: *Textbook of Endocrinology*, 4th ed., p. 67. Editor: R. H. Williams. Saunders, Philadelphia, Pa.

(59) Salassa, R. M., Kearns, T. P., Kernohan, J. W., Sprague, R. G. and MacCarty, D. S. (1959): Pituitary tumors in patients with Cushing's syndrome. *J. clin. Endocr.*, *19*, 1523.

(60) Kaufman, B. (1970): Angiographic findings in non-tumorous enlargement of the sella turcica — the enlarged 'empty' sella. *Invest. Radiol.*, *5*, 201 (abstract).

(61) Bull, J. W. D. and Schunk, H. (1962): The significance of displacement of the cavernous portion of the internal carotid artery. *Brit. J. Radiol.*, *35*, 801.

(62) Chase, N. E. and Taveras, J. M. (1963): Carotid angiography in diagnosis of extradural parasellar tumors. *Acta radiol. (Stockh.) (Diag.)*, *1*, 214.

(63) Baker, H. L., Jr (1972): The angiographic delineation of sellar and parasellar masses. *Radiology* *104*, 67.

(64) Lehrer, H. Z. (1970): Angiographic visualization of the posterior pituitary and clinical stress. *Radiology*, *94*, 7.

(65) Bernasconi, V., Giovanelli, M. A. and Papo, I. (1972): Primary empty sella. *J. Neurosurg.*, *36*, 157.

Discussion

DR. DI CHIRO: Dr. Baker will start the discussion.

DR. BAKER: Five years ago I was pessimistic about the arteriogram for the delineation of sellar and parasellar masses. I was also pessimistic because I thought all of the arteries of the brain had been described. It is true that many of them have been described, but the advent of serial direct magnification cerebral angiography has made visible some of the smaller arteries which in the past were not important to us in diagnosis but are now clinically important.

Some of my work, in the last few years, has been referred to by our essayists this afternoon and I would just like to give you a brief summary of this as it pertains to pituitary tumors.

Figure 1 is a drawing showing some of the arteries about the sella which have been described in the past, but which we have seldom been able to visualize before.

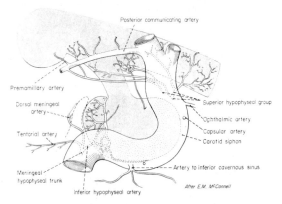

Fig. 1 Arterial vessels which vascularize the hypophysis, optic apparatus and parasellar structures. The upper carotid siphon and posterior communicating artery have been elevated to reveal the pituitary stalk. (Modified from McConnell, E. M.: The arterial blood supply to the human hypophysis cerebri. *Anat. Rec.*, 1953, *115*, 175-203.)

The meningo-hypophyseal trunk has been referred to several times. It is often seen when it is hypertrophied as with hypervascular tumors about the sella. It consists of inferior hypophyseal, dorsal meningeal, and tentorial branches.

The artery to the inferior cavernous sinus has been referred to in the radiologic literature when it is involved in the vascularization of perisellar meningiomas.

The inferior capsular artery and the anterior capsular artery of the pituitary have been described in the anatomic literature but since these pass directly across the sella turcica and arise on the medial wall of the siphon, they are not often seen or they have not been seen in the past in carotid arteriography.

The superior hypophyseal artery is usually hidden behind the upper limb of the carotid siphon and in Figure 1 (which is taken from McConnell's work with a few changes) the upper limb of the siphon has been raised so that the various branches of the superior hypophyseal artery are displayed. This vessel vascularizes the optic nerves, the chiasm and the optic tracts.

Now, the little plexus which encircles the infundibulum, called the circuminfundibular plexus, can be seen on most angiograms. It is a good indicator of the position of the optic chiasm.

At two times magnification, in the normal patient (Fig. 2) we see the meningeo-hypophyseal trunk and the posterior pituitary stain quite commonly. The little tangle of vessels superiorly is the circuminfundibular plexus which normally lies about a centimeter above the top of the dorsum sellae, or about two centimeters above in the magnified film. It is fed by the superior hypophyseal artery mostly hidden behind the upper limb of the siphon.

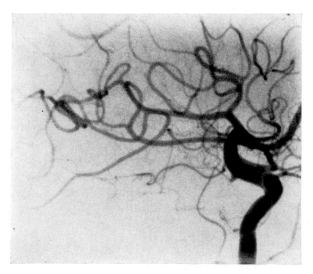

Fig. 2   Magnified lateral carotid angiogram — early phase (1.0 sec). Meningeo-hypophyseal trunk and posterior pituitary blush are clearly seen, inferiorly, and the circuminfundibular plexus, superiorly.

I would like to emphasize that it is often necessary to subtract the entire angiographic series in order to appreciate some of these structures. We make exposures at the rate of two per second. When we analyze magnified angiograms which have been subtracted we see that in 96 % of the cases, the meningeo-hypophyseal trunk is discernible, the circuminfundibular plexus in about 95 % of the cases, posterior pituitary blush in slightly less (86 %). Other small arteries, the main trunk of the superior hypophyseal, for instance, will be seen less often (11 %) (Table I). How does this apply to pituitary tumors? The blush of a tumor can be seen at certain phases of the arteriogram in over 80 % of the cases.

If you subtract the entire series, very often as you inject on one side, only half of the tumor is vascularized on the angiogram (Fig. 3). The other half of this tumor was vascularized, when the opposite side was injected, so that you might only see half of the tumor if you only do unilateral angiograms.

These stains are very subtle, as you can see. Fig. 4 shows a late arterial, early venous

Table I   *Visualization of vascular structures:*
110 'normal' magnified subtracted lateral carotid angiograms

Structure	%
Meningeo-hypophyseal trunk	96
Dorsal meningeal artery	92
Plexus	95
Posterior pituitary gland	86
Cavernous sinus	82
Posterior communicating artery	68
Premammillary artery	53
Tentorial artery	42
Mammillary bodies, chiasm, stalk	25
Artery to inferior cavernous sinus	16
Superior hypophyseal artery (main trunk)	11
Anterior pituitary	10
Pituitary capsular arteries	> 1

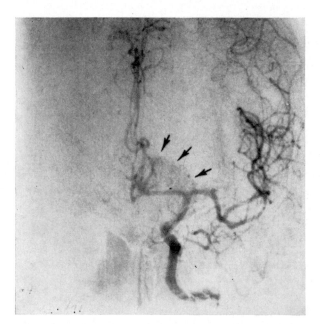

Fig. 3   Anteroposterior carotid angiogram (2.0 sec). Pituitary adenoma with parasellar extension. Only one half of the tumor (on injected side) has visible 'stain'. The opposite side of the mass was apparent when contralateral injection was made. (From Baker, H. L. Jr.: The significance of fine sellar, parasellar, and central cerebral arteries in diagnosis. In press.)

phase. The tumor does not extend above the diaphragm of the sella, but it is confined to the sella itself.

DR. FRASER: How do you minimize the side effects of pneumoencephalograms?

DR. KAUFMAN: High levels of cortisol may alleviate the pain of the pneumoencephalogram. In addition, gases other than air may be associated with less discomfort.

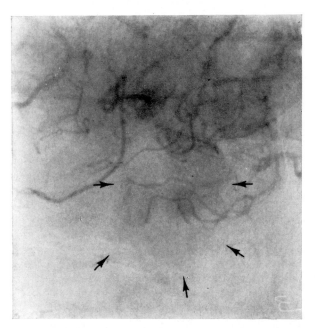

Fig. 4   Magnified lateral carotid angiogram (1.5 sec); a pituitary adenoma with slightly enlarged sella turcica. Capsular arteries and subtle diffuse 'stain' throughout the tumor are seen. The tumor is confined to the sella. (From Baker, H. L. Jr.: The angiographic delineation of sellar and parasellar masses. *Radiology*, 1972, *104*, 67-78.)

DR. BENTSON: We use glucocorticoids such as 100 mg of Solucortef coupled with something like Valium for sedation. Then we try to perform the first part of the test, during which the patient is sitting and uncomfortable, relatively rapidly. Finally, we usually give Demerol prior to the next stage where the patient is supine. Frequently, the patients go to sleep during this phase.

DR. A. LAWRENCE: Dr. Kaufman, I think that one has to appreciate that there is a spectrum of pituitary function in the so-called 'empty sella' syndrome, and that some patients do have bona fide hypopituitarism. Secondly, since tumors do occur in patients with the 'empty sella' syndrome, periodic follow-up examination is mandatory.

DR. KAUFMAN: I would like to emphasize 2 points: First, the 'empty sella' or non-tumorous enlargement of the sella is extremely common. I would estimate it is associated with enlargement of the sella in about 1 % of the population. Second, the occurrence of pituitary neoplasia in this syndrome is coincidental. Dr. Pearson can discuss the endocrine manifestations.

DR. PEARSON: I think it is very difficult to be sure whether there is an interrelationship between an endocrine abnormality and the presence of nontumorous enlargement of the sella turcica. We see so many patients with nontumorous enlargement that are perfectly normal endocrinologically when studied extensively. Thus, the presence of an endocrine disorder may be coincidental to the presence of nontumorous enlargement of the sella.

DR. LEBOVITZ: We have recently reviewed our experience with the so-called empty sella syndrome at Duke (*Medicine*, 1973, *52*, 73). Our findings are in agreement with Dr. Kaufman's; in 31 patients who have had extensive studies, our impression is that the endocrinologic abnormalities are just fortuitous. It is interesting to tabulate the reason why these patients had the initial skull X-ray done. Most had some type of neurologic symptom such as headache, seizures, papilledema, trigeminal neuralgia, trauma, syncope or vertigo. Relatively few presented with endocrine symptoms and those seem to have been coincidental.

On the other hand, there are several significant points that we felt came out of the appraisal of our data. One is that it is really hard to talk about the so-called empty sella syndrome after one has manipulated the sellar area, and so that we limited our analysis to patients who had never had radiotherapy, or surgery, or any other manipulation. And in the group that we looked at, it was interesting that there was a very high preponderance of women. Between 80 and 90 % were women.

There were also a very significant number of obese people, and I noted that some of Dr. Kaufman's patients weighed 230 pounds and 250 pounds. This brings out another point on the interpretation of the endocrinologic data. If you examine growth hormone responses in people with the empty sella syndrome who are obese, you find a rise in growth hormone to 6 or 7 ng/ml and one might be tempted to call this abnormal. However, this is the response that one would find in a group of otherwise normal obese people and therefore cannot be considered a sign of pituitary deficiency in the obese individuals with the empty sella syndrome.

DR. KAUFMAN: Obesity is an interesting phenomenon because many of our patients had a relatively sudden weight gain of 30 to 40 pounds and many were extremely obese. Some of the larger asymmetrical sellas are from patients with cerebrospinal fluid pressures of 425 mm H_2O, normal being up to 180 mm H_2O. Prolonged elevation of cerebrospinal fluid probably adds to the problem, although you can find people with normal CSF pressures who have big sellas.

I think the finding that the empty sella syndrome occurs more commonly in women than men is actually correct. Dr. Busch's series and Dr. Di Chiro's show the incidence is greater in females than males. This appears to be based on a congenital defect of the diaphragma sellae. One can see the same defect if sellas of infants are examined. Older age groups definitely will give you a higher incidence of big sellas.

Dr. Frank Nulsen, chief of Neurosurgery at University Hospitals of Cleveland, says obese patients have an elevated supine CSF pressure because of abdominal compression acting through Batson's plexus. Obese patients do have higher CSF pressures.

Saying that nontumorous enlargement of the sella is common means that they will be readily seen. I would estimate that in a 100 bed general hospital, two or three cases per week will be seen. If any one has any doubt, the easiest thing to do is to see consecutive autopsy cases, and the question will be solved for you very shortly.

In fact, the reason I became aware of the entity was when we were doing Yttrium-90 pituitary ablation and the question was the intactness of the diaphragma sellae. Four out of six autopsy cases had an incomplete diaphragm and the next one was a classical 'empty sella'.

We would also like to introduce the idea of stretching of the stalk or hypothalamus in patients with markedly enlarged sella turcicas. This stretching of the stalk or hypothalamus may in some way be causally related to galactorrhea in some patients with 'empty sella'. If the third ventricle, the floor anteriorly being the hypothalamus, does not move and the pituitary gland remodels downward, the length of the stalk has actually increased. No one knows the effect or what type of stretching mechanism occurs in any circumstance.

DR. DAUGHADAY: We have all been impressed by the demonstration of the inferior hypophyseal artery. Endocrinologists at the present time are increasingly interested in small and subtle lesions of the hypothalamus and its vascular supply.

What are the prospects for additional studies which would give us more detailed information of the region around median eminence and hypothalamus?

DR. DECK: We have been using a machine which is capable of doing circular angiotomography and to which we have recently added a film changer. This unit will give us four separate exposures, each exposure consisting of five tomographic cuts, half a centimeter apart. We are hoping to demonstrate the superior aspect of some of these suprasellar masses in frontal projections. This is going to make a very long and complicated study when routine bilateral carotid arteriograms plus lateral magnification series are performed in addition to the angiography. We will have to determine whether the additional effort is worth while.

VOICE: In those patients who are asymptomatic, but have what appears to be an enlarged sella with no evidence of encroachment upon the hypothalamus, the optic chiasm, nor evidence of endocrine insufficiency, what studies do the radiologists suggest we use?

DR. KAUFMAN: That is a very pertinent question. If we have a patient who has an asymmetrically enlarged sella and no particular evidence of any involvement above the plane of the diaphragm, we may be dealing with nontumorous enlargement of the sella. However, if there were any evidence of involvement above the diaphragm, even if the patient were asymptomatic, I would suggest that the patient has a growing tumor.

If clinically there are no endocrine symptoms, no eye findings, you could follow them with plain X-rays for three months, six months, one year. Demineralization of the sella wall would suggest tumor. Nontumorous changes occur very slowly, a millimeter over a couple of years or something of that order, unless it is associated with a rapid weight gain or elevated CSF pressure. If no X-ray or other changes occur, treatment should be withheld. Treatment should not be initiated prior to pneumoencephalography.

DR. BAKER: I would like to suggest that nothing radiological be done until symptoms occur in patients with a large sella with no endocrine dysfunction and no eye findings.

DR. BENTSON: Yes, that is what we do. A typical situation is that of the emergency room intern who took skull films for trauma and saw a questionably enlarged sella. He wonders if a pneumoencephalogram is necessary. I usually say it is not.

DR. DI CHIRO: I have to disagree with the other panelists. A large sella means pathology. We have to be sure, however, that we are confronted with a 'true large sella', i.e. one the size of which has been established in the three dimensions by a volumetric analysis. I don't believe that I have ever seen a case of true large sella not accompanied by or caused by underlying pathology. Abnormal clinical findings do not, of course, always accompany a large sella turcica. I agree with Dr. Baker and Dr. Bentson in not insisting on studies in asymptomatic patients. Incidentally, except perhaps for post-traumatic medico-legal reasons, I am not aware that skull X-rays are taken, in any center, just for routine check-up. The great majority of skull radiographs are taken in symptomatic patients.

I would insist that true large sella means pathology, which in certain instances may be at the subclinical level.

DR. KLIMAN: I think the timing of diagnostic radiographic tests has been totally reversed. The appropriate time to get a pneumoencephalogram and in most cases to treat the patient is before they have a pending visual loss, hypopituitarism and all the destructive changes you have demonstrated on pneumoencephalograms obtained late in the course of pituitary tumor growth.

I think the majority of persons with enlarged sella will have a pituitary tumor, and that the tumor should be treated by radiation before it destroys the pituitary and damages the optic chiasma.

IV. Surgical treatment of pituitary tumors

A. By transfrontal approach

B. By transsphenoidal approach

Indications for and results of surgical treatment of pituitary tumors by the transfrontal approach

COLLIN S. MacCARTY, E. JEROME HANSON Jr, RAYMOND V. RANDALL
and PAUL W. SCANLON

Mayo Clinic and Mayo Foundation, Rochester, Minn., U.S.A.

In 1886 Marie[1] suggested the etiologic relationship between acromegaly and aberrant function of the hypophysis. The evolution of modern neurosurgical techniques has permitted the development of alternate approaches to the hypophysis, some of which date back to the beginning of the twentieth century. According to Frazier,[2] Krause in 1905 suggested an approach through the anterior cranial fossa. In 1906 Horsley[3] exposed the area through the middle cranial fossa and in 1907 Schloffer[4] successfully approached the hypophysis by the extracranial, transsphenoidal route. Frazier wrote that Schloffer's operation was 'rather crude and disfiguring'. In 1910 Hirsch[5] reported 2 cases in which this particular tumor was treated successfully by the endonasal, transsphenoidal approach. Cushing initially favored the extracranial approach, but abandoned it, as did Adson, Naffziger and others, in favor of the intracranial transfrontal operation which until recently was the favored method of access to the hypophyseal area.[6]

The senior author, during his neurosurgical experience, has witnessed considerable advances in the surgical therapy of pituitary tumors. Many surgeons in the 1930s and 1940s were operating by an extradural, sphenoidal-wing technique which was accompanied by an appreciable incidence of postoperative epidural hematomas and resultant increased morbidity and mortality rates. With the advent of the use of small 'free bone flaps' and an intradural exposure, postoperative sequelae such as epidural blood clots almost entirely disappeared, and morbidity and mortality rates declined proportionately. Shortly thereafter, the historic isolation of cortisone by Kendall[7] and subsequent use of this agent as 'replacement' therapy for preoperative and postoperative loss of pituitary hormonal function allowed the neurosurgeon to operate upon the hypophysis with appreciable safety. It is our opinion that these 2 events – namely, improvement in surgical technique and the availability of steroid replacement – made pituitary surgery acceptably safe in the hands of the experienced neurologic surgeon.

The introduction of effective antibiotic agents and microsurgical techniques has brought the endonasal transsphenoidal approach very much into favor again, particularly because of the surgical skills and stimulation of interest in this technique as developed by my co-panelists, Guiot[8] and Hardy.[9]

Our surgical experience with all types of pituitary tumors in the 1960 decade was 263 cases with 9 hospital deaths, a hospital mortality rate of 3.4%. This compares with Troen and Rynearson's[10, 11] Mayo Clinic figure of a 6% hospital mortality rate accompanying all tumors operated upon which were situated in the region of the hypophysis, including mening-iomas, craniopharyngiomas, chiasmal gliomas, and pituitary tumors for which cortisone was given, and a hospital mortality rate of 17 % among those for which cortisone was not given.

Other series have been reported. Cushing reported an operative mortality rate of 2.4 % in his last 205 operations;[12] Krayenbühl[13] reported a rate of 5.9 % among those patients operated upon by the transfrontal approach from 1955 through 1960; Ray and Patterson[14] reported upon 80 patients operated on between 1950 and 1960 via the frontal route with no operative deaths. Svien and Colby,[15] from our clinic, reported an operative mortality rate of 6.8 % among 117 patients for whom the frontal route was employed, 31 % of whom had 'excessively enlarged sellae'. They stated that 'cases in which massive extrasellar extension has occurred carry a higher risk of death, perhaps of the order of 25 %. Postoperative bleed-ing or edema, or both, require reoperation in 3 to 4 % of cases. Wound infections prolonging hospitalization and care do occur, and in perhaps 2 to 3 % of cases necessitate revision of the wound with loss of bone flap requiring subsequent cranioplasty. Convulsive disorder re-sults from surgery in 3 to 4 % of the cases with operation by the frontal route'.

Indications for the transfrontal approach

In the past we rarely operated upon pituitary tumors which had not caused field defects. However, as surgical morbidity and mortality rates declined abruptly, we have operated upon 'functioning' adenomas not causing field defects, proceeding by either the transfrontal or the transsphenoidal approach. Prior to this, irradiation therapy usually was administered. Generally, however, surgical treatment has been utilized when field defects have been present and the patient's general status would allow major surgical intervention. Occasionally, hemorrhage into pituitary adenomas, with sudden and marked loss of vision, demanded emergency surgical treatment. In the rare instances when dysfunction of the optic nerve, chiasm and extraocular motor nerves have complicated aggressive pituitary tumors pro-ducing Cushing's syndrome, transcranial operation has been performed. Large chromophobe tumors which produce increased intracranial pressure by obstructing the third ventricle, foramina of Monro or occasionally the subarachnoid pathways in the vicinity of the tento-rium have been operated upon to relieve the increased pressure and to preserve life.

Material

The patients reported here represent: (1) the first 100 pituitary tumors operated upon 2 decades ago, after the advent of adrenal steroid therapy; and (2) the last 100 tumors operated upon prior to 5 years ago. Data in our selected 100 cases in each series have been analyzed as to preoperative status, postoperative morbidity and mortality rates as well as long-term results for those patients treated by operation alone and for those who received surgical treatment plus prophylactic postoperative irradiation. We are aware of the problems in-herent in such a retrospective analysis. Still, we hope that this review will contribute to clari-fication of the status of transfrontal surgery for adenomas of the pituitary gland.

Results: first 100 cases, January 1952-March 1954

Hospital deaths

Initially, we reviewed data on 100 successive patients operated upon by the transfrontal route for pituitary adenomas between January 1952 and March 1954, shortly after adrenal steroid substances came into use to supplement surgical therapy (Table I).

Table I *100 Cases of pituitary tumor: group 1, January 1952–March 1954*

Hospital deaths	5
Death from tumor	20
Death from unrelated causes	22
Alive	42
Lost to follow-up	11

Five patients died of complications occurring in the immediate postoperative period. These included 2 who had infarction in the midbrain secondary to postoperative hematomas. Two other patients died 1 day and 12 days postoperatively of massive right hemispheral infarcts. Another died of hypernatremia, hyperchloremia with acidosis and renal failure.

Postoperative survival

Twenty patients died of recurrent tumors, secondary endocrine deficiencies or postoperative causes and complications related to subsequent operations for their tumors.

Twenty-two patients died of causes unrelated to their pituitary tumors. One of these died of suppurative parotiditis and respiratory obstruction following operation for a postoperative hematoma secondary to an aneurysm of the circle of Willis 3 weeks after having been dismissed from the hospital after surgical treatment of a recurrent chromophobe adenoma. The other 21 patients died during the past 17 to 20 years.

Eleven patients have not responded to recent inquiries. At last contact 7 were suspected of having recurrent tumors, while 4 were considered to be without recurrent tumors.

At the time of this report 9 patients are still alive, although known to have had recurrent tumors which subsequently were operated upon by us or surgeons elsewhere. Thirty-three patients are still living without recurrences.

Thus, of the 100 patients operated upon, 5 died in the hospital and 20 subsequently died of recurrences, making a total of 25 patients who died of their pituitary tumors. Twenty-two patients have died of unrelated causes and without clinical evidence of recurrence. At the time of writing 42 patients are known to be living, and follow-up data are incomplete concerning the remaining 11 patients.

Irradiation therapy

Only 42 of the 100 patients received significant irradiation therapy either preoperatively or postoperatively or for recurrent tumors. For the purposes of this study we have arbitrarily considered a tumor dose of 2500 rads or more to be 'significant irradiation therapy'. Currently, however, we routinely give a tumor dose of 4000 to 5000 rads.

Fifteen of the 33 patients who are surviving without recurrent tumors have received significant postoperative irradiation. Five of 9 surviving patients who have recurrent tumors received significant doses of radiotherapy after the recurrence. Two other patients, lost to follow-up several years ago, received radiotherapy for recurrent tumors and were alive when last heard from. Thus, of the 42 surviving patients from this series of 100 patients, 20 received significant irradiation therapy as an adjunct to the operation.

Eleven of the 20 patients who died of their tumors or of associated endocrine deficiency received significant doses of irradiation at some time during their illness. Nine of the 22 patients who died without clinical evidence of recurrence received significant irradiation therapy.

Summary, first 100 cases, 1952–1954

The hospital mortality rate among the 100 patients operated upon 2 decades ago was 5 %. Twenty patients later died of their tumors. Endocrine failure played a prominent role in the death of several of these 20 patients, and may have been contributory to the death of others. Twenty-two patients later died of unrelated causes, and 42 are known to have survived. Eleven patients have been lost to follow-up inquiry. The significance of irradiation therapy in this group of patients is unclear because of so many variables. Fifteen, or 45 %, of the 33 patients who have survived without clinical evidence of recurrence received this form of therapy, and 11, or 55 %, of the 20 patients who died of recurrence also received significant irradiation therapy.

Results: second 100 cases, January 1964-May 1968

Hospital deaths

Data about the second group of 100 successive patients operated upon by the transfrontal route between January 1964 and May 1968 (Table II) show that 3 died in the immediate

Table II   *100 Cases of pituitary tumor: group 2, January 1964–May 1968*

Hospital deaths	3
Death from tumor	2
Death from unrelated causes	9
Alive	73
Lost to follow-up	13

postoperative period, one of a postoperative hematoma with infarction in the midbrain and another of a parasellar hematoma with hypothalamic compression and rupture into the third ventricle. The third patient died of refractory diabetes insipidus with marked hypernatremia and cerebral edema.

Postoperative survival

Two patients died of recurrent tumors, one within a year of operation and the other within 2 years after operation. It should be mentioned that both patients were operated upon twice and both patients received several courses of radiotherapy. In each instance the tumor extended beneath the chiasm, into the third ventricle in one case and into the interpeduncular fossa and down the clivus in the other.

Recurrent tumors have occurred in 7 patients and have been operated upon again by us or by surgeons elsewhere. These patients are known to be alive. These 7 did not receive radiotherapy after their initial operation, but have received therapeutic irradiation after their subsequent surgical treatment.

Nine patients are known to have died of unrelated causes during the 4- to 8-year follow-up period. None of these patients had clinical evidence of recurrence.

Thirteen patients have been lost to follow-up inquiry. Two patients may have recurrences of their tumors, but in the other 11 recurrence seems unlikely.

Sixty-six patients are known to be alive and without evidence of recurrence of their tumor.

Of the 100 patients, 5 died of their tumor. Three died postoperatively and 2 died of subsequent recurrences. Nine died of unrelated causes and 7 are still living after being successfully treated for recurrent tumors. Sixty-six patients are alive and without evidence of recurrence of their tumor. Thirteen patients are lost to follow-up inquiry at present, but 11 are thought to be alive without recurrent tumor.

Irradiation therapy (Table III)

Table III *Total patients receiving irradiation: group 2, January 1964–May 1968*

Total patients	74		
Irradiation before initial operation		2	
Irradiation after initial operation		65	
Recurrence (with death)			2
Irradiation after operation for recurrence		7	
Recurrence (to date)			0
No irradiation after initial operation	22		
Recurrence (survival after subsequent irradiation)			7

Of the 100 patients in this group, 74 eventually received significant (2500 rads or greater) radiotherapy either preoperatively or postoperatively. Twenty-two patients did not receive therapeutic doses of irradiation. Of the remaining 4 patients in the group, 3 died in the immediate postoperative period and 1 patient was to have received radiation therapy elsewhere but documentation of this is not present in our records.

Of the 74 patients who received significant irradiation therapy, 65 received it after their initial operation. Two patients were initially treated with radiotherapy and operated upon at a later date when defects of visual fields developed. Seven patients did not receive radiotherapy until after surgical treatment for a subsequent recurrence. All 7 remain free of recurrence to date.

Of the 65 patients receiving radiotherapy after operation, only 2 subsequently had recurrences and both died. One died 2 years after the initial surgical procedure despite the administration of 2 courses of irradiation (a total of 7500 rads) and a second surgical attempt to remove the tumor. The other patient died despite irradiation with 3500 rads and a second attempt to remove the tumor as well as a subsequent shunting procedure.

Of the 13 patients about whom follow-up data are incomplete, 8 received irradiation and 5 did not.

Summary of second 100 cases, 1964–1968

In this group the hospital mortality rate was 3 %. Two patients subsequently died of recurrent tumors. Thus, of the 100 patients, 5 are known to have died. Thirteen have been lost to recent follow-up inquiry, but 11 are thought to be alive without recurrence and 2 are alive, probably with recurrent tumors. Seven patients who were operated upon and who did not receive postoperative irradiation therapy had recurrent tumors. They have been operated upon again, and given postoperative irradiation, and are living without known recurrences of their tumor. Nine patients have died of unrelated causes without clinical evidence of recurrence of their pituitary tumors. Sixty-six patients are alive without clinical evidence of recurrent tumors.

Irradiation therapy may be effective in preventing recurrence of pituitary tumors, in view of the fact that recurrent tumors developed in only 2 of 67 patients who received this form of therapy. Twenty-two patients did not receive irradiation therapy postoperatively and 7 were operated upon again for recurrent tumors. However, it is obvious that not enough time has elapsed for adequate evaluation of the efficacy of either surgery or irradiation in this second group of patients.

Endocrine insufficiency played little if any role in the mortality rates within this second group of 100 patients as opposed to these rates in the 1952–1954 group.

Need for long-term follow-up

Table IV   *Interval between initial operation and death from recurrence or treatment for recurrence: group 1, January 1952–March 1954*

Years	Interval between initial operation and	
	Death from recurrence (No. of patients)	Treatment for recurrence (No. of patients: all living)
0–1	3	
1–2	2	
2–3	2 (2)*	
3–4	2 (1)	
4–5	4 (4)	1 (1)
5–6	1 (1)	
6–7		
7–8		1 (1)
8–9	1	
9–10	1	
10–11		1 (1)
11–12		
12–13	1 (1)	
13–14		2
14–15	1 (1)	1
15–16		
16–17	2 (1)	1 (1)
17–18		1 (1)
18–19		1 (1)
Total	20	9

* Numbers in parentheses indicate those who received irradiation therapy.

Table IV demonstrates the need for long-term follow-up of patients before one can draw conclusions about survival and efficacy of treatment. Two groups of patients from the 1952–1954 series are represented. The first group consists of the 20 patients who died from recurrence of their tumors. The second group of 9 patients are those who subsequently had treatment for recurrence of their tumors and are known to be living at this time. While death or treatment for recurrence may occur within the first 5 years after initial operation, these events may not take place for 10 or more years after the initial operation.

References

(1)   MARIE, P. (1886): Sur deux cas d'acromégalie: hypertrophie singulière non congénitale des extrémités supérieures, inférieures et céphalique. *Rev. Méd. (Paris)*, 6, 297.
(2)   FRAZIER, C. H. (1913): An approach to the hypophysis through the anterior cranial fossa. *Ann. Surg.*, 57, 145.
(3)   HORSLEY, V. (1906): Diseases of the pituitary gland. *Brit. med. J.*, 1, 323.
(4)   SCHLOFFER: Cited by Frazier [2].
(5)   HIRSCH, O. (1910): Endonasal method of removal of hypophyseal tumors: with report of two successful cases. *J. Amer. med. Ass.*, 55, 772.

(6) LOVE, J. G. (1956): Operative approach to the pituitary gland. *Clin. Neurosurg., 4*, 75.

(7) KENDALL, E. C. (1949): Some observations on the hormone of the adrenal cortex designated Compound E. *Mayo Clin. Proc., 24*, 298.

(8) GUIOT, G. and THIBAUT, B. (1959): L'extirpation des adénomes hypophysaires par voie trans-sphénoidale. *Neurochirurgia (Stuttg.), 1*, 133.

(9) HARDY, J. (1971): Transsphenoidal hypophysectomy. *J. Neurosurg., 34*, 582.

(10) TROEN, P. and RYNEARSON, E. H. (1955): The prophylactic use of cortisone for surgery of the pituitary (abstract). *J. clin. Endocr., 15*, 857.

(11) TROEN, P. and RYNEARSON, E. H. (1956): An evaluation of the prophylactic use of cortisone for pituitary operations. *J. clin. Endocr., 16*, 747.

(12) HENDERSON, W. R. (1939): The pituitary adenomata: a follow-up study of the surgical results in 338 cases (Dr. Harvey Cushing's series). *Brit. J. Surg., 26*, 811.

(13) KRAYENBÜHL, H. (1961): Hypophyseal adenomas and craniopharyngioma. In: *Abstracts, II International Congress of Neurological Surgery, Washington, D.C.*, pp. E10–E12. ICS 36, Excerpta Medica, Amsterdam.

(14) RAY, B. S. and PATTERSON JR, R. H. (1962): Surgical treatment of pituitary adenomas. *J. Neurosurg., 19*, 1.

(15) SVIEN, H. J. and COLBY JR, M. Y. (1967): *Treatment for Chromophobe Adenoma*, p. 17. Charles C. Thomas, Springfield, Ill.

Indications for and results of surgical treatment of pituitary tumors by the intracranial approach

CHARLES A. FAGER, JAMES L. POPPEN* and YOSHIRO TAKAOKA

Department of Neurosurgery, Lahey Clinic Foundation, Boston, Mass., U.S.A.

The indications for intracranial surgery of pituitary tumors were more simply stated before so many other techniques were available. If this conference is to achieve any success, it will hopefully be in the direction of resolving some of the confusion of a rapidly expanding methodology.

The tendency to become preoccupied with the technical aspects of approaching the pituitary (above or below, stereotactic or open) has overshadowed a more important question. Should it be approached at all? It is quite clear that every case of an enlarged sella turcica does not require treatment.

Once treatment has been decided upon, what is the best approach in each patient? It is our belief that radiation remains the safest method of treating the uncomplicated pituitary tumor. Its objective is clear in definitive therapy, but its usefulness has also been documented[1-5] in the prevention of recurrence as an adjunct after operation. Our 22-year experience at the Lahey Clinic Foundation with the 2 million electron volt unit has been most gratifying. A dose of at least 4000 roentgens is delivered to the tumor by a rotational method with estimated radiation falling off to 75 % at 1.5 cm from the central 4 cm sphere.

Other factors to influence indications for intracranial surgery at this institution include the refinements in transsphenoidal surgery. It is not possible to remove selectively a microadenoma from above. The skillful demonstration of adenoma excision from below by Guiot and Thibaut[6] and Hardy and Wigser[7] is an accomplishment that also limits, to a degree, the indications for craniotomy. This technique will have an even greater effect in the future as more surgeons gain experience with microsurgery.

Indications for surgical treatment

It was once believed that hemorrhagic infarction constituted the clearest possible mandate for surgical intervention, but several patients have now been seen who weathered the storm of so-called pituitary apoplexy quite well without requiring operation. This does not imply an advocacy of conservative treatment when vision is threatened since the indication for surgery is clear in such a situation. However, it does suggest another area where previous criteria for operation may be open to question.

---

* *Present address*: 110 Francis Street, Boston, Mass. 02115, U.S.A.

What then are the indications for intracranial surgery? Two categories exist: the clear and unmistakable indication presented by large adenomas, and the equivocal indication imposed by the threat of permanent visual loss in smaller sellar and suprasellar tumors.

Large pituitary adenomas

In a patient with evident erosion of the sella, marked visual loss and a sizable suprasellar projection of the lesion, little doubt exists that operation will be necessary. The same can be said of the parasellar adenoma associated with early third nerve paresis on one side. There would be little argument that temporal adenomas require temporal craniotomy as initial treatment; therefore, no question arises about the mandate for surgical intervention in these patients.

Cerebrospinal fluid rhinorrhea.   This rarely occurs spontaneously in pituitary tumors but does at times develop in the course of treatment. It usually appears many months or years after surgery or radiation or both and presents a clear indication for intracranial surgery to close off the fistula in the sphenoid sinus.

Visual changes

In regard to the smaller adenomas, if a patient has visual acuity in a range worse than 20/70 in each eye with severe bilateral visual field defects, it would obviously be hazardous to consider radiation as initial therapy. In the lesser grades of visual loss, the decision can be more difficult because radiation therapy has successfully restored vision to many patients.

One cannot set arbitrary levels of vision in developing the criteria for operation. All factors should be weighed from a clinical and radiologic standpoint. If temporal field defects and diminished acuity have developed slowly over many months or years and if no sizable extension is present above the sella, then, in the authors' experience, little or no harm results in trying a course of radiation, which means only another 3 to 4 weeks, and is performed under close observation. Failure of visual fields or acuity to show some improvement in the next month is clearly an indication for operation.

Rapid onset of signs.   If the visual loss and field defects have developed quickly within a month or two, this certainly suggests a rapidly growing adenoma and possibly a good-sized tumor outgrowing its blood supply. One must then be more cautious about delaying operation, but radiation may be just as effective as with the slower growing lesions with the help of steroids, providing no large suprasellar extension is present and vision is not in serious jeopardy. Of course pneumoencephalography and bilateral carotid arteriography must be completed on all patients prior to radiation therapy.

Size of tumor

The location of the tumor in relation to the optic chiasm is also probably of some importance. Often one can predict if the suprasellar part of the tumor has expanded anterior to the chiasm (so-called postfixed chiasm). This seemed clearly so in the patient with definite elevation of the anterior cerebral complex whose air study is shown in Figure 1. It proved to be the case at operation which resulted in successful restoration of vision. This patient had a short history of moderately severe visual loss in each eye and bitemporal hemianopia.

On the other hand, the patient whose encephalogram is shown in Figure 2 had a 1-year history of visual loss as a result of partial bitemporal hemianopia with no significant reduction of visual acuity. The absence of anterior cerebral elevation with bitemporal hemianopia here suggests anterior placement of the chiasm (so-called prefixed chiasm) or posterior extension of tumor beneath the chiasm. At any rate, operation in this patient resulted in a complete bitemporal hemianopia *and* the diplopia that comes as a result of such a visual defect. This type of adenoma would have been more suitable for radiation therapy as initial treatment. The patient also had some evidence of arteriosclerosis, an additional factor complicating whatever vascular changes may have been present in the chiasm. The contrasting results of these 2 cases illustrate how a patient with more impairment of vision and a larger adenoma may at times be a better candidate for operation than one with less visual loss and a smaller tumor.

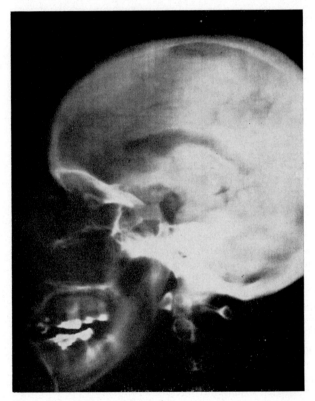

Fig. 1   Suprasellar extension of tumor.

The patient whose vascularized adenoma appears in Figure 3 had a very stormy course after operation and eventually made a good recovery with vision no better or no worse than before operation. This is also a situation where one could reasonably argue in favor of radiation therapy as the primary method of treatment if time and vision permit.

Results of surgical treatment

In several of our previous communications,[8-11] the results of treatment of pituitary adenomas have been presented. The present study brings experience up to date from the last paper 9 years ago and summarizes our overall results. A number of other series[2-4, 12-16] of pituitary adenomas with almost comparable follow-up periods have already been reported

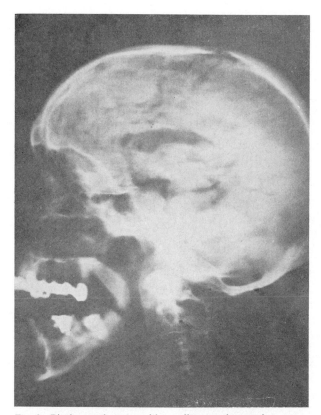

Fig. 2   Pituitary adenoma with small upward extension.

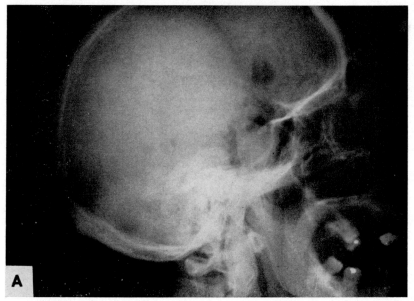

Fig. 3a   Small suprasellar extension shown by air study. Mild visual loss and field defects.

in the literature – some of the results have been comparable and others have been differing, especially in their emphasis upon one modality of treatment or another.

From a total of over 450 patients, we were able to select 382 for adequate study. Of these, 197 patients underwent operation. While the intention of this paper is to survey the results of surgical treatment, the philosophy of treatment at our institution has been so oriented

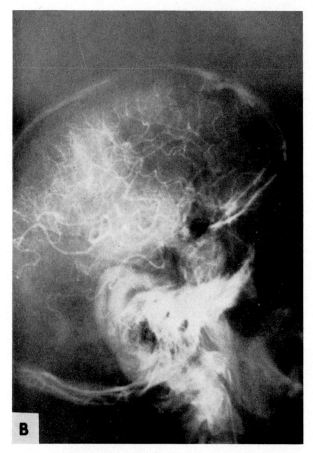

Fig. 3b   Lateral carotid angiogram discloses vascular adenoma.

toward radiation therapy, especially since 1950, that it has been difficult to isolate the *two* modalities of therapy and arrive at meaningful results. Furthermore, because of our interest in radiation, there have been many occasions, especially in recent years, when surgical ex- tirpation was conservative, with the knowledge that radiation would follow.

Tables I through IV list a few of the important data in the total series of 382 patients including 197 who had operations of one type or another. The overall surgical mortality rate is 13 %; in the last 22 years, it has been only 2 %. Among the surviving patients, 12 (6 %) had worsened visual acuity and 6 (3 %) had visual fields made worse by operation. A poor survival rate resulted in 14 patients, though most of these were also before 1950.

The only reasonable way to analyze our results of treatment, since so many patients had combined therapy, was to divide the entire series into 2 groups – those whose initial treat- ment was radiation (273 cases) and those whose initial treatment was operation (109 cases).

Table I   *Pituitary adenomas: periods of follow-up (total patients 382)*

Period of follow-up (yr)	No. of patients
< 1	25
1–5	60
6–10	65
11–20	148
21–30	68
> 30	16
Total	382

Table II   *Pituitary adenomas: general results of treatment (total patients 382)*

Results of treatment	No. of patients
Poor	14
Fair	30
No change	14
Very good	215
Full recovery	82
Deaths	27
Total	382

Table III   *Pituitary adenomas: survival and mortality (382 patients)*

	No. of patients
Surgical deaths	26 (22 before 1950)
Poor survival (hypothalamic syndrome, etc.)	14 (13 before 1950)
Subsequent deaths (unrelated)	90
Unknown cause	12
Now alive	240
Total	382

Table IV   *Pituitary adenomas: surgical* morbidity (197 patients)*

Visual fields		
Worse	6	(3 %)
Visual acuity		
Worse	12	(6 %)
Poor survival	14	(7 %)

* Surgical approach: frontal 184, frontotemporal 4, temporal 4, transsphenoidal 5.

Tables V and VI indicate the general results, including all patients in each group, that is even those who were treated because of endocrine dysfunction (mainly acromegaly), cranial nerve palsy, severe headache, or intracranial pressure when visual fields and acuity were not affected. Tables VII through X deal specifically with results as far as vision is concerned.

Table V   *Pituitary adenomas: initial treatment radiation (273 patients)*

```
273    Radiation ─────────────── Improved──►178  (65 %)
          │  Unimproved
          │     95
          ▼
88     Radiation+surgery ─────── Improved──►58   (21 %)
          │  Unimproved
          │     30
          ▼
12     Radiation+surgery+radiation── Improved──►9   (3 %)
          │  Unimproved
          │     3
          ▼
       Unimproved                 Improved
            Total    28   (11 %)       Total   245   (89 %)
```

Table VI   *Pituitary adenomas: initial treatment surgery (109 patients)*

```
109    Surgery──────────────── Improved──►26   (24 %)
          │  Unimproved
          │     83
          ▼
57     Surgery+radiation ────── Improved──►29   (26 %)
          │  Unimproved
          │     27
          ▼
20     Surgery+radiation+surgery ── Improved──►12   (11 %)
          │  Unimproved
          │     8
          ▼
       Unimproved                 Improved
            Total    42   (39 %)       Total   67   (61 %)
```

Table VII   *Initial treatment radiation: total patients 273, abnormal visual fields 208 (76 %)*

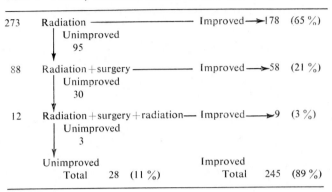

```
208    Radiation ─────────────────── Normal or ──►124   (59.6 %)
          │                            improved
       Worse  Death  Unimproved
       or       1       5
       unimproved
       78 │
          ▼
78     Surgery   or   surgery+radiation ──── Normal or ──►47   (22.6 %)
          │                                   improved
       Worse  Death  Unimproved
       or       5      19
       unimproved
       7  │
          ▼
7      Surgery   or   radiation ──────── Improved ──►5   (2.4 %)
          │
          ▼
       Death              Unimproved
         1                    1

       Visual fields unimproved or worse      Visual fields improved or normal
       Total  32   (15.4 %)                    Total  176   (84.6 %)
```

Table VIII *Initial treatment radiation: total patients 273, decreased visual acuity 216 (79 %)*

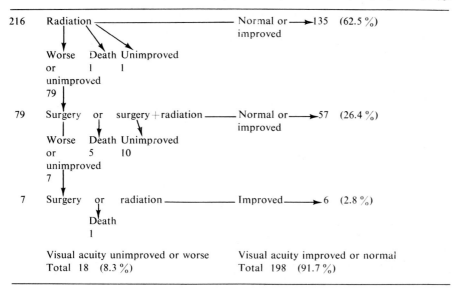

216   Radiation ——————————————— Normal or ——►135   (62.5 %)
                                                          improved

       Worse   Death Unimproved
       or   1   1
       unimproved
       79

79   Surgery   or   surgery + radiation ——— Normal or ——►57   (26.4 %)
                                                          improved
       Worse   Death Unimproved
       or   5   10
       unimproved
       7

7   Surgery   or   radiation ——————————— Improved ——► 6   (2.8 %)

                 Death
                  1

       Visual acuity unimproved or worse   Visual acuity improved or normal
       Total 18   (8.3 %)   Total 198   (91.7 %)

Table IX *Initial treatment surgery: total patients 109, abnormal visual fields 106 (97 %)*

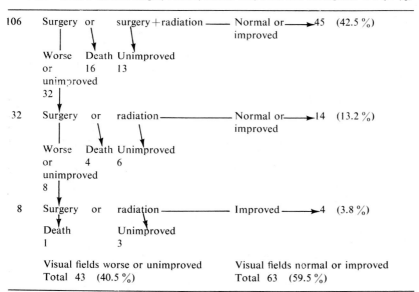

106   Surgery or   surgery + radiation ——— Normal or ——►45   (42.5 %)
                                                          improved
       Worse   Death Unimproved
       or   16   13
       unimproved
       32

32   Surgery   or   radiation ——————————— Normal or ——►14   (13.2 %)
                                                          improved
       Worse   Death Unimproved
       or   4   6
       unimproved
       8

8   Surgery   or   radiation ——————————— Improved ——► 4   (3.8 %)

       Death   Unimproved
       1   3

       Visual fields worse or unimproved   Visual fields normal or improved
       Total 43   (40.5 %)   Total 63   (59.5 %)

In each category, some of the patients who were not improved after initial treatment received no additional therapy. Thus, of 273 patients who underwent initial radiation, only 88 of the 95 who were not helped subsequently had operation and only 12 of the additional 30 who were not helped went on to either another operation or radiation (Table V). A summary of the general results indicates 89 % improvement among those patients whose initial treatment was radiation, and only 61 % of those whose initial treatment was operative. It

Table X   *Initial treatment surgery: total patients 109, decreased visual acuity 107 (98 %)*

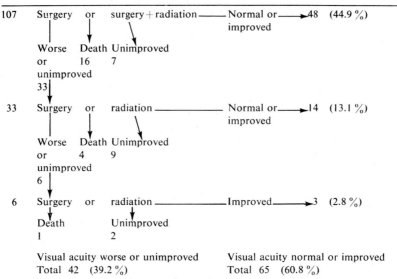

107   Surgery   or   surgery + radiation ——— Normal or ——→48   (44.9 %)
                                            improved

      Worse   Death Unimproved
      or   16   7
      unimproved
      33

33   Surgery   or   radiation ——————— Normal or ——→14   (13.1 %)
                                       improved

      Worse   Death Unimproved
      or   4   9
      unimproved
      6

6   Surgery   or   radiation ——————— Improved ——→3   (2.8 %)

      Death   Unimproved
      1   2

      Visual acuity worse or unimproved   Visual acuity normal or improved
      Total   42   (39.2 %)   Total   65   (60.8 %)

should be clear, however, that the patients subjected to operation first were usually those with larger tumors, more visual loss and generally poorer risks from the endocrine standpoint as well.

As Tables VII through X show, a similar correlation exists in the results of surgery, radiation and combined therapy as far as visual fields and acuity are concerned.

Summary

Large suprasellar, parasellar and temporal adenomas constitute a clear indication for operation. Smaller tumors with mild or moderate visual loss must be studied individually from a clinical and radiologic standpoint. The rapidity of their growth and location in relation to the optic chiasm are important factors in determining whether operation or radiation should be the initial method of treatment.

In our entire series 382 patients with pituitary adenomas have been found suitable for follow-up study; 197 of these underwent operation with a mortality rate of 13 %. In the last 22 years the mortality rate has been 2 %. Fourteen patients had a poor survival, most of these also before 1950. As a result of operation, visual fields were worse in 3 % and visual acuity was worse in 6 %.

In this series so many patients have had combined radiation and surgery that it is difficult to isolate the 2 methods of treatment. Among the patients whose initial treatment was radiation, general and visual improvement occurred in over 60 %, requiring no further treatment. An additional 25 to 30 % improved after operation, further radiation, or both. Of the patients whose initial treatment was operation or operation followed by radiation, about 45 % improved, but only an additional 15 % were helped by further operation or radiation.

References

(1) HAYES, T. P., DAVIS, R. A. and RAVENTOS, A. (1971): The treatment of pituitary chromophobe adenomas. *Radiology*, **98**, 149.

(2) RAY, B. S. and PATTERSON, R. H. (1971): Surgical experience with chromophobe adenomas of the pituitary gland. *J. Neurosurg.*, *34*, 726.

(3) SVIEN, H. J. and COLBY, M. Y. (1969): Pituitary chromophobe adenomas: comparative results of surgical and roentgen treatment. *Behav. Neurol.*, *1*, 35.

(4) CHANG, C. H. and POOL, J. L. (1967): The radiotherapy of pituitary chromophobe adenomas. *Radiology*, *89*, 1005.

(5) SHELINE, G. E., BOLDREY, E. B. and PHILLIPS, T. L. (1964): Chromophobe adenomas of the pituitary gland. *Amer. J. Roentgenol.*, *92*, 160.

(6) GUIOT, G. and THIBAUT, B. (1959): L'extirpation des adénomes hypophysaires par voie trans-sphénoidale. *Neurochirurgia (Stuttg.)*, *1*, 133.

(7) HARDY, J. and WIGSER, S. M. (1965): Trans-sphenoidal surgery of pituitary fossa tissues with televised radiofluoroscopic control. *J. Neurosurg.*, *23*, 612.

(8) POPPEN, J. L. (1963): Changing concepts in the treatment of pituitary adenomas. Charles A. Elsberg Lecture. *Bull. N.Y. Acad. Med.*, *39*, 21.

(9) HORRAX, G., HARE, H. F. and POPPEN, J. L. (1952): Chromophobe pituitary tumors. II. Treatment. *J. clin. Endocr.*, *12*, 631.

(10) HORRAX, G. (1951): The chromophobe pituitary adenomas: surgical and radiation treatment. *Surg. Clin. N. Amer.*, *31*, 877.

(11) HORRAX, G., SMEDAL, M. I., TRUMP, J. G., GRANKE, R. C. and WRIGHT, K. A. (1955): Present-day treatment of pituitary adenomas. Surgery versus X-ray therapy. *New Engl. J. Med.*, *252*, 524.

(12) HENDERSON, W. R. (1939): Pituitary adenomata: a follow-up study of surgical results in 338 cases (Dr Harvey Cushing's series). *Brit. J. Surg.*, *26*, 811.

(13) RAY, B. S. and PATTERSON, R. H. (1962): Symposium on pituitary tumors. – I. Surgical treatment of pituitary adenomas. *J. Neurosurg.*, *19*, 1.

(14) SVIEN, H. V., KENNEDY, W. C. and KEARNS, T. P. (1963): Results of surgical treatment of pituitary adenoma: the factor of the excessively enlarged sella. *J. Neurosurg.*, *20*, 669.

(15) BAKAY, L. (1950): Results of 300 pituitary adenoma operations (Prof. Herbert Olivecrona's series). *J. Neurosurg.*, *7*, 240.

(16) GERMAN, W. J. and FLANIGAN, S. (1964): Pituitary adenomas: a follow-up study of the Cushing series. *Clin. Neurosurg.*, *10*, 72.

Discussion

DR. VAN BUREN: Dr. Randall's comment about the duration of follow-up needed for evaluation of the effects of treatment is very pertinent. As I recall, it was some 10 years before approximately half of the recurrences declared themselves. This behooves us all to take a rather long look at any type of treatment, surgical or radiation, in our final evaluation.

I would ask Dr. Hardy and Dr. Guiot what their feeling would be about the surgical approach for the patient with a nonsecreting tumor with severe visual field and acuity difficulty, who has a significant elevation of his anterior cerebral artery, suggesting a post-fixed chiasm and a considerable suprasellar growth.

Is this type of patient suitable for a transcranial approach or do you feel that the trans-sphenoidal approach would be superior?

DR. GUIOT: The volume does not really influence the choice of the route. The important thing is the morphology of the tumor. Even if there is a large suprasellar extension, it could be approached from below because the consistency of the adenoma is usually soft, sometimes fluid, sometimes that of a hematoma and thus extremely easy to curette or to aspirate.

DR. FRASER: What do the speakers believe to be appropriate treatment for a tumor, extruding behind the chiasm, and inside the optic tract? In particular, what about the usefulness of pre-operative radiation?

DR. FAGER: In general, those tumors that extend behind the chiasm are the most difficult with which we deal. If they are sizeable, we would prefer to use a temporal approach.

I think that radiation should certainly be given first. Professor Guiot and Dr. Hardy may have a different answer.

DR. HARDY: For any route, either intracranial or transsphenoidal, the major goal is maximal access to the tumor. Coming from above, you have the optic nerves and the chiasm in front of the lesion. When the sella is very large and the dorsum sellae and the clivus partially eroded, these tumors have been easily accessible by the transsphenoidal approach.

DR. FRASER: Even if you have a sausage-like extension?

DR. HARDY: Yes.

DR. SHERINS: I would like to ask the panel if pre-operative radiation significantly affects the difficulty of the operation or if surgery in any way modifies the required dosage for effective radiation.

DR. FAGER: Yes, I think it does. I have operated on a number of pituitary tumors which have been radiated. I think we do get some infarction, and to me, that helps tremendously.

DR. HARDY: It has been my experience, particularly with acromegalic patients, that radiotherapy given about a year before surgery produced a softening of the tumor making it milky and easy to remove. However, pre-operative irradiation makes it more difficult to differentiate normal gland from the pathological tissue.

In contrast, radiotherapy given several years before, results in scarred fibrotic tissue in the sella with retraction of the diaphragm producing a so-called 'empty sella'. In these cases good dissection and selective excision of the lesion is impossible so that we have to be radical.

DR. HORWITH: Could we have some indication as to whether or not an attempt was made at total hypophysectomy in any of the patients treated?

DR. FAGER: Our aim has always been total hypophysectomy when we are dealing with functioning adenomas. We have always adhered to this philosophy. We have been so impressed with the value of radiation that, in general, we do not attempt to strip a so-called capsule or a diaphragm away from the optic chiasm. Hence, our total hypophysectomy has been reserved for those cases of small tumors that were hyperfunctioning.

DR. OMMAYA: I had a question about two presenting signs: first, papilledema, particularly in patients who have large sellas but no X-ray evidence of suprasellar extension; and second, cerebrospinal fluid rhinorrhea in patients who have had no treatment.

DR. FAGER: There are only six or seven cases in the literature of spontaneous rhinorrhea from pituitary adenomas. It just doesn't occur. I think the tumor acts as a stopper, so that you don't get rhinorrhea until you remove the tumor. I have not seen papilledema without suprasellar extension, except in the massive parasellar tumors – or adenoma extending toward the temporal fossa.

DR. HARDY: I would like to comment on spontaneous rhinorrhea that occurs in a patient in whom incidentally you find an enlarged sella. Most of these patients have invasive adenomas.

You have to operate to cure the fistula first, but you find that the tumor is destroying the floor, the dura, and has to be treated further with intensive radiotherapy.

DR. NOEL: Dr. Fager, in those patients who had radiotherapy first, or only radiotherapy, how many had minimal or no visual field impairment, or minimal or no endocrine abnormality. To what extent are the results you have shown biased by inclusion of patients who had neither visual nor endocrine deficits at the time of their treatment?

DR. FAGER: I think there were 45 or 50 patients who had no visual field defect or decreased acuity whom we radiated.

DR. PEARSON: What will be the indication for intracranial surgery for pituitary tumors in the future?

DR. FAGER: Large adenomas in the temporal fossa and large suprasellar extensions above the chiasm will remain prime indications for intracranial surgery. A patient who presents with severe visual loss, either of acuity in one eye or the other or severe visual field loss with loss of visual acuity, is a candidate for transfrontal operation.

DR. A. LAWRENCE: Does anyone have any experience in long-term follow-up of untreated patients with recognized pituitary adenomas?

DR. SHELINE: I reported 32 such patients in my paper. To examine the question of what happens to the untreated lesion, I went over our hospital records and succeeded in identifying 32 patients in whom the pituitary lesion had been diagnosed as a chromophobe adenoma but no therapy had been given. Of the 32, 8 were diagnosed at autopsy and obviously did not require therapy. They did have large sellas, but I know nothing about their endocrine status. There were another 8 in whom there was no follow-up.

Of the remaining 16 patients, half had visual field defects and half did not. As these patients were watched for periods of time varying up to 20 years, 14 of the 16 eventually showed signs of growth of the presumed chromophobe adenoma.

I should emphasize that these lesions were not the little marginally enlarged or the slightly remodeled sella that were discussed earlier.

Of the 16 patients, 14 finally came to therapy and the end result in 7 was an increased visual field deficit over that originally present, and 1 patient ended up with a permanent cerebrospinal fluid rhinorrhea. The latter patient was a boy, about 16 years of age when initially seen, who had a lesion extending into the sella but with normal visual fields. During the next 6 years, the lesion gradually eroded through the floor of the sphenoid, but his fields remained normal. By the time therapy was instituted the chromophobe adenoma presented in the nasopharynx.

At least in this limited group, there was hazard involved in watching without treatment.

Transsphenoidal approach in surgical treatment of pituitary adenomas: general principles and indications in non-functioning adenomas

G. GUIOT

Department of Neurosurgery Foch Hospital, Suresnes, France

The times when supporters of either the intracranial or transsphenoidal approach to pituitary adenomas confronted each other are over. Nowadays, the validity of the transsphenoidal route can hardly be denied, and those who were reluctant to accept this route did not really understand it. However, it is also clear that neither this route nor the intracranial route is appropriate for surgical removal of all pituitary adenomas. In fact, each approach has its particular indications. The choice depends on a consideration of indications, operative risk, the functional results, and the patient's future.

This will be our subject of discussion.

General principles of transsphenoidal surgery of pituitary adenomas

The surgical technique of the transsphenoidal approach for removal of pituitary adenomas has remained almost identical to the one Cushing[2] initially performed with the addition of improvements by Kanavel[18] and Hirsch[15] and as modified by Halstead,[10] who first used the sublabial incision. As he developed intracranial surgery, Cushing abandoned the transsphenoidal route. Thus it had been forgotten by most, but one of his pupils, Dott,[4] continued to use the transsphenoidal approach and taught us its benignity and efficiency (Tables I and II).

Several recent innovations have increased the versatility, safety and precision of this technique. These include intraoperative radioscopic control, first with the image intensifier[9] and then with television;[12] the angular endoscope which enables observation of the corners of the sella;[8] and, most importantly, the operative microscope applied for the first time to transsphenoidal hypophysectomy by Hardy.[11] These innovations, particularly the use of the microscope, have enabled us to approach the true objective of the surgery for pituitary adenomas. This goal consists not only in the elimination of tumor tissue, but also in the preservation of functioning normal hypophyseal tissue.

In order to fully understand the varying difficulties in achieving the ideal therapy, a fundamental distinction must be made between the two major types of pituitary adenoma: the chromophobe or 'non-functioning' adenomas and the group of 'hormone-secreting adenomas'. The technical problems are quite different in each case; our paper deals mainly with the non-functioning adenomas while the paper by Hardy will deal with the secreting adenomas.

The need for the distinction between non-functioning and secreting adenomas, and the influence of this distinction as a determinant of therapeutic goals, must be explained. This can be understood better by digressing for a moment to consider the role of irradiation treatment for pituitary adenomas. Indeed, radiotherapy is complementary to surgery and the two modalities are often combined in the treatment of the same patient.

Surgical statistics on postoperative recurrence[1, 5, 13, 19, 20] emphasize the importance of external irradiation. Without postoperative irradiation, 15–20 % of pituitary adenomas will recur; whereas with postoperative radiotherapy the rate of recurrences decreases, as Henderson[14] first showed in a paper concerning 338 patients of Cushing. Currently, improvements in radiation techniques have reduced the rate of recurrences to a very low level when postoperative irradiation is used. However, increasing experience with irradiation has demonstrated both the limits of its efficiency and the difference in its impact upon the growth potential and upon the secretory potential of pituitary adenomas.

Irradiation therapy may reduce the volume of a pituitary adenoma and some histologic varieties are even particularly sensitive.[6] In general, radiation therapy may be expected to impede or abolish the process of cellular multiplication. The fact that tumor recurrences are rare among patients with non-secreting adenomas receiving postoperative irradiation suggests that the residual fragments of adenomatous tissue usually become unable to proliferate following irradiation. In contrast, residual fragments of a secreting adenoma, although usually unable to proliferate, frequently retain their ability to secrete hormones. In acromegaly, for instance, if the postoperative level of growth hormone remains excessive, demonstrating the persistence of pathologic tissue, irradiation will rarely lower it to normal. In spite of improvements in the technical formula, irradiation at the usual doses frequently does not cure acromegaly, although it may inhibit further tumor growth.

The cure of a secreting adenoma can only be ensured by radical removal or destruction of all the adenomatous tissue. A small amount of residual adenoma is enough to produce an excessive hormonal secretion and persistent endocrine and metabolic symptomatology. The surgical problem is therefore to achieve this total removal without at the same time endangering healthy hypophyseal tissue. Depending upon the adenoma's stage of evolution (Fig. 1), this goal can be possible, problematic or illusory.

During the first or intrahypophyseal stage of development, the adenoma is only a small nodule within the gland. Theoretically this is the ideal time for a complete and selective removal of the tumor. For this purpose the transsphenoidal approach should be the treatment of choice, provided that the adenoma is located in the inferior part of the pituitary as seems to be the rule.

At the second stage, the adenoma has increased in volume, enlarging the sella. The normal pituitary tissue is compressed and reduced to a thin layer of tissue adherent to the dura. The adenoma is still tightly enclosed by the dural envelope of the hypophysis and may be separated from it. The complete extirpation of the adenoma is still possible and again the transsphenoidal approach is indicated. However, the difficulty at this stage is to distinguish the normal pituitary from the pathologic tissue. Since a pituitary adenoma has no proper capsule, tissue of doubtful nature poses a dilemma. If questionable tissue is left behind, there is risk that the disease will not be cured. On the other hand, removing it carries the risk of postoperative pituitary insufficiency. The risk must be calculated in relation to the age and sexual capacities of the patient, the importance of clinical disorders, and the predictable course of the disease.

At the stage when the pituitary adenoma has extended above the sella, even if it seems well encapsulated, the dural envelope and particularly the diaphragm are very often infiltrated by the adenoma. Accordingly, this envelope has to be removed as completely as possible. In this case, we think that the intracranial route gives a better chance of complete removal of all the tumor tissue. Even so it is not always technically feasible. Also it is difficult to find and save the remaining normal hypophyseal tissue, and the result is therefore problematic.

Table I *Foch Hospital - Neurosurgical Department. Transsphenoidal operations (from 1957 until 1972, Oct. 30)*

1.	Pituitary tumors	504
	Adenoma	485*
	Craniopharyngioma	12
	Varia and unclassified	7
2.	Functional hypophysectomy	22
3.	Transsphenoidal rhinorrhea Intrasellar cysts Symptomatic empty sella	24
4.	Clivus chordoma	13
	Various sphenoidal tumors	13
	Sphenoidal mucoceles	6

*Including 10 cases of recurrences Total 582

Table II *Foch Hospital - Neurosurgical Department. Pituitary adenomas*

	→	1957 → 1972 (Oct. 30)	
Intracranial route:	34	56	90
Transsphenoidal route:	0	475	475
		Total of cases:	565

At the last stage of its evolution, the pituitary adenoma has become an 'invasive adenoma'. Not only has it penetrated but it has also traversed its dural envelope at one or more points. Then endocrine cure is no longer possible, since radical removal of an invasive adenoma is practically impossible.[16]

Such complicated problems do not arise with non-secreting adenomas. In the absence of an endocrine problem, the tumor can be treated effectively by combined surgery and radiotherapy. The surgical goal is essentially to eliminate the tumor's compressive effects without risk to function or the patient's life. Postoperative radiotherapy will prevent proliferation of tumor residues which escaped excision or which were left deliberately for reasons of safety.

In summary, the surgical objectives are very different in these two groups of pituitary adenomas. In the case of a chromophobe adenoma, the objective is an excision ensuring vital and functional safety. In the case of a secreting adenoma, the objective is radical excision with a risk which has to be calculated. This simplified formulation sums up our present concept of the treatment of pituitary tumors.

Non-functioning adenomas

In view of its benignity, the transsphenoidal route has been selected when it seemed feasible. The removal of a non-functioning adenoma is always possible by the transsphenoidal route when the tumor has a regular round or ovoid shape, providing there is no intracranial transcapsular extension, i.e. in all cases of 'global' and 'encapsulated' adenomas (Figs. 2 and 3).

The volume of a non-secreting adenoma does not really influence the choice of the route from above or from below. Even an adenoma with substantial suprasellar extension can be approached from below if the suprasellar portion communicates widely with the intrasellar portion, in spite of a slight narrowing at the level of the carotids. This wide communication makes it possible for the instruments to reach the higher portion of the tumor without risks,

Stages of Development	Approach	Endocrinal cure
INTRA-HYPOPHYSEAL 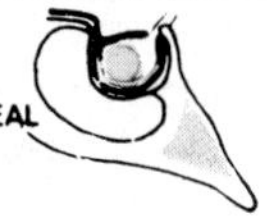	T. Sph.	Possible
INTRA SELLAR 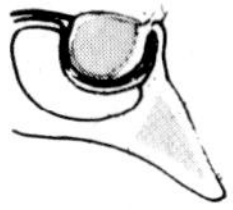	T. Sph.	
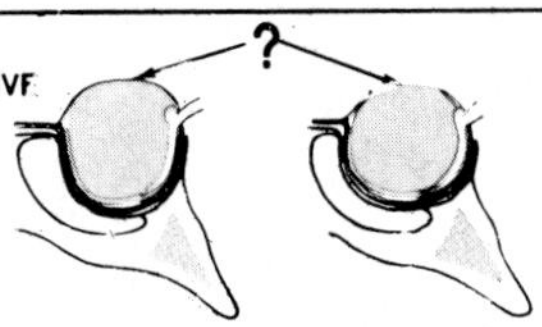 EXPANSIVE	Intra CR. preferably	Uncertain
INVASIVE	T. Sph.	Exceptional
	Intra CR	

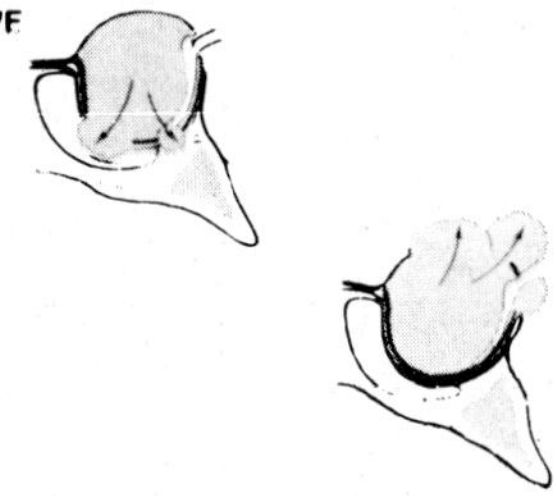

Fig. 1   Surgical approaches to and prognosis of secreting pituitary adenomas according to the stage of development of the tumor.

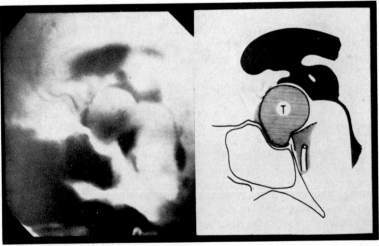

Fig. 2   Global and encapsulated chromophobe adenoma. Large suprasellar extension (here, without significant enlargement of the sella).

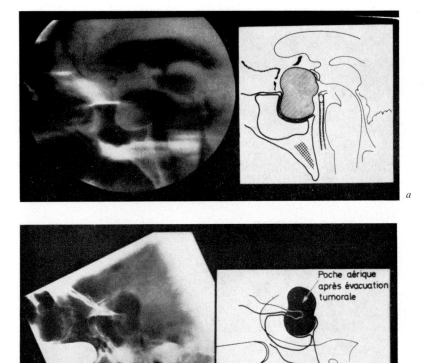

Fig. 3 (*a*) Chromophobe adenomas of 'global' type. Large communication between suprasellar and intrasellar parts of the tumor.
(*b*) Air has filled the tumor cavity, demonstrating the evacuation of the entire adenoma.

since the adenoma is encapsulated and allows the suprasellar portion to descend to the intrasellar floor after the sella has been evacuated.

This descent, which may be assisted or provoked by means of jugular compression, occurs because most tumors are soft in consistency, dense ones being unusual (ca. 6 %). As a rule adenomatous tissue is soft and easy to scrape or even suction. Often the fluid adenoma literally 'flows' into the sphenoidal sinus as soon as the dura is incised. In about 15 % of cases, the tumor consists of one or several liquid cysts. Tumor tissue may also be infarcted and turned into a red pulp (12 %) or into a circumscribed hematoma (7 %) which can be completely evacuated by simple transdural puncture (Fig. 4). This soft, fluid or cystic consistency of adenomas greatly facilitates evacuation by curettage or suction, and it explains the usual efficiency of the transsphenoidal route.[7]

Obviously all these global and enclosed adenomas (about 60 % of our cases) could be approached from above with probably the same success and with the very low mortality which is now possible with intracranial surgery (Fig. 5). One can only say that if the results are equivalent, then the simpler operative procedure is better.

Beside these *ad libitum* indications, there are unequivocal indications for both the intracranial route and the transsphenoidal route:

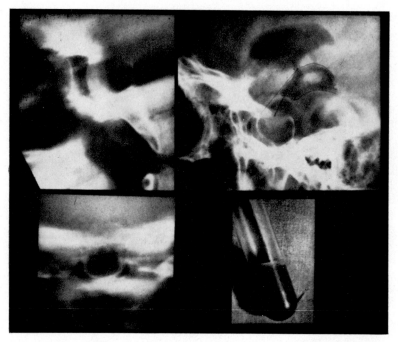

Fig. 4 Chromophobe adenoma completely transformed into a hematoma. No clinical suggestion of infarction.

Non-secreting pituitary adenomas
Intracranial or transsphenoidal approach?

'Ad libitum'	61.5 %
Absolute indications for intracranial approach	10.5 %
Absolute indications for transsphenoidal approach	28 %

Fig. 5   Intracranial or transsphenoidal approach for non-functioning adenomas?

1. The intracranial route is absolutely indicated when the adenoma has invaded and traversed the diaphragm and, generally speaking, when an extrasellar intracranial extension (subfrontal, retrochiasmatic or temporal) is separated from the intrasellar portion by a narrow neck (Figs. 6–12). We have withheld transsphenoidal surgery for this indication in 10.5 % of our cases (a figure which now appears too restrictive).

2. Absolute indications for the transsphenoidal route include: (*a*) cases where the intracranial route is associated with an unacceptable risk, and (*b*) intrasphenoidal tumor extension (Fig. 13).

(*a*) *Risk of intracranial route*. The benignity of the transsphenoidal route makes it the route of choice in the following 4 situations:

(i) Elderly patients (37 of our patients were over 65 years old, including 13 over 70) or patients in poor general condition (Fig. 14).

(ii) Patients rendered almost blind by an optic chiasmal compression of long duration, whose optic nerves would probably not tolerate the slightest additional trauma. The fibrous cupola covering the adenoma separates and protects the optic tracts from the instruments

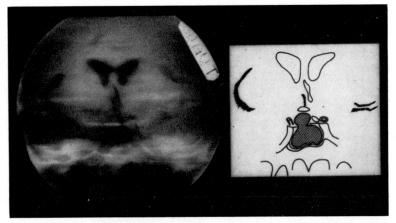

Fig. 6 Small transdiaphragmatic extension on the right, a contraindication for the transsphenoidal route.

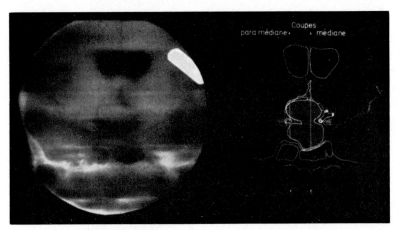

Fig. 7 Dumbbell-shaped pituitary adenoma with a narrow neck between supradiaphragmatic and intrasellar part of tumor: a positive indication for intracranial approach.

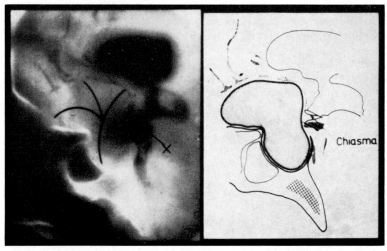

Fig. 8 Prechiasmatic and subfrontal extension: an absolute indication for the intracranial route.

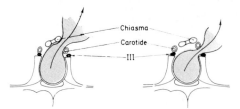

Fig. 9a Extension of the adenoma towards the frontal chamber through a passage situated either between optic nerve and carotid artery or between carotid and cavernous sinus, involving the third cranial nerve at the same time.

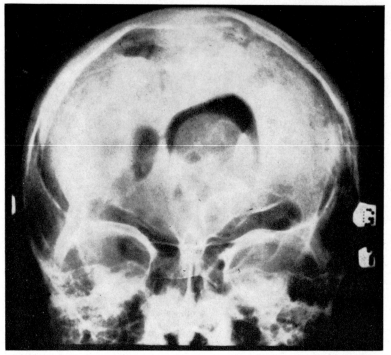

Fig. 9b   Compression of the frontal horn of the ventricle by the ballooning tumor.

introduced from below. This probably explains why, generally speaking, the visual results have been better after our transsphenoidal than after our intracranial operations. Following transsphenoidal surgery, recoveries have been more frequent, more rapid and more complete.[3]

(iii) Severe cases of intrasellar hypertension with sudden headaches, oculomotor palsies and rapid decrease of vision. In addition to this symptomatic trilogy, a syndrome of meningitis and/or an acute syndrome of adrenal insufficiency may occur. These syndromes may also be complicated by a spasm of the basilar arteries beyond surgical possibilities.

(iv) Paninvasive adenomas. The combination of large sphenoidal destruction and multidirectional intracranial extensions of adenoma exclude an intracranial operation. Seven patients with this type of adenoma have been referred to us. Five of them had recurrences of adenomas operated from above and not irradiated postoperatively. Spontaneous rhinorrhea was a complication in 3 of them and a second intracranial operation had been ruled out. All had surgery by the transsphenoidal route and all accessible tumor tissue (partially hemorrhagic

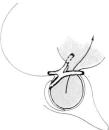

Fig. 10a Retrochiasmatic extension of a pituitary adenoma.

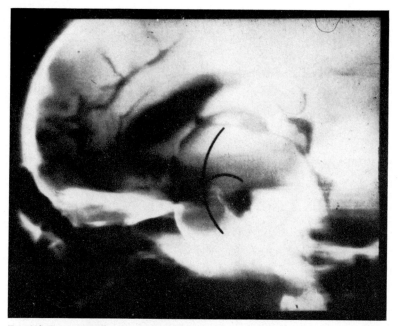

Fig. 10b Demonstrative encephalography.

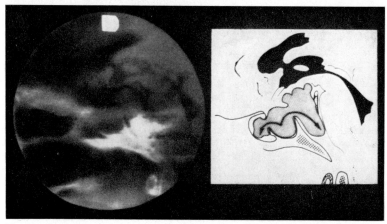

Fig. 11 Complicated case of both sphenoidal invasion and retrochiasmatic-retroclival extension of a pituitary adenoma. Necessity of 2 operative steps with (1) transsphenoidal and (2) subtemporal approaches.

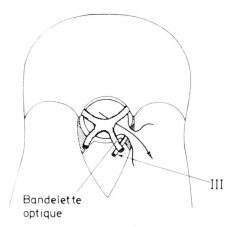

Bandelette
optique

Fig. 12a   Posteriolateral extension through a passage between the optic tract (homonymous hemi-anopsia) and the roof of the cavernous sinus (3rd nerve palsy).

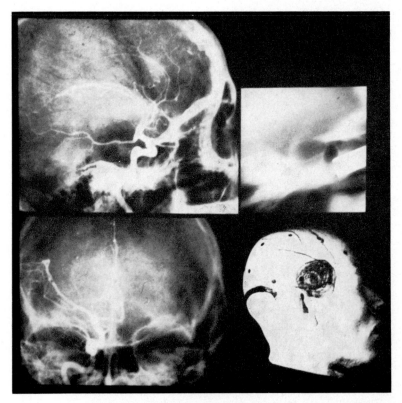

Fig. 12b   Tomography of the sella, angiography and isotope scanning in a case of temporal exten-sion. Again 2 operations were performed: (1) by transsphenoidal route in order to eva-cuate the intrasellar content of the adenoma, and (2) by 'transtemporal' route to remove the intratemporal extension.

		N. of Cases	%
LOGICAL	Downward intrasphenoidal "expansion" (without suprasellar expansion)..............................	5	1, 5
PREFEREN-TIAL	Age : 65-70................................. (or Bad condition)	15	4, 7
	Pituitary Apoplexy with adrenal insufficiency............	3	1
	Quasi blindness........................	6	2
ABSOLUTE INDICATIONS	Age : over 70.............................	7	2, 2
	Sphenoidal "invasion"..................	47	15
	Desperate cases of paninvasive Ad.	7	2, 2
		90	28, 6 %

Fig. 13   Indication for a transsphenoidal approach in a series of 317 cases of non-functioning pituitary adenomas.

P₀₀₀ Emma   79 ans

ADENOME CHROMOPHOBE

opéré le 3 juin 1966

	Preop.	Postop. (5 juillet 1966)
ACUITE v OD	1 / 20	2 / 10
v OG	1 / 10	4 / 10
CHAMP VISUEL	D G	D G
FOND D'ŒIL	ATROPHIE OPTIQUE BILATERALE	PAS DE CHANGEMENT

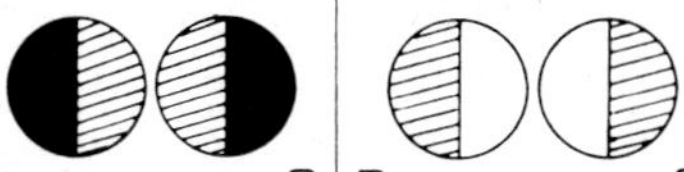

Fig. 14   Diagram of visual recovery after transsphenoidal removal of pituitary adenoma in a woman 79 years old.

in 4 of the 7) was removed and postoperative irradiation therapy was given. Two patients, blind before surgery, remained so. In 3, there was no further deterioration of vision. Two patients were improved. All of them are alive and in good general condition 3–10 years after the operation, and 4 are now working. These results indicate the value of both transsphenoidal surgery and radiotherapy (Figs. 15 and 16).

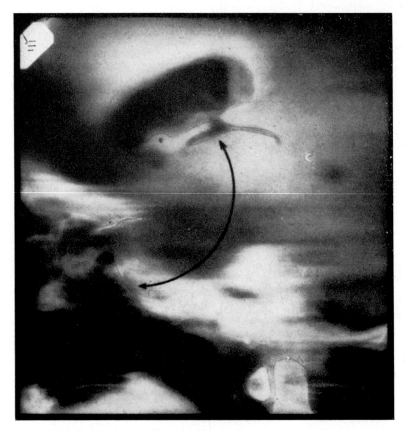

Fig. 15   Paninvasive adenoma (recurrence).

(b) *Downward tumor extension*. In addition to these clinicopathologic conditions, there is an anatomical basis which makes the transsphenoidal route logical or absolutely indicated for some adenomas. These are tumors which extend only in an inferior direction (Fig. 17) or tumors which have invaded the sphenoidal sinus (Figs. 18 and 19). This type of invasion has been observed in 15 % of cases.

In our series (see below) the transsphenoidal route was considered either as the preferable or as the only route of surgical approach in 28.6 % of cases. Although the estimate is somewhat subjective, we believe that in at least 20 % of patients with pituitary adenomas, the intracranial route is contraindicated.

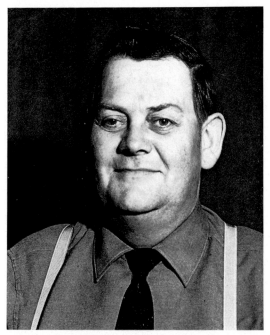

Fig. 16 The patient 6 years after paninvasive adenoma with destruction of the entire sphenoid. Intracranial multidirectional extension.

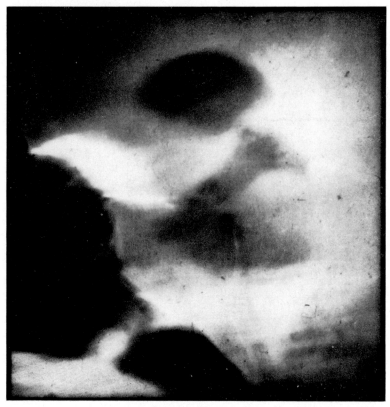

Fig. 17 Large intrasphenoidal extension without suprasellar extension.

Analysis of our series

As shown in Table I, 485 pituitary adenomas, 10 of which were recurrent, have been operated upon between 1957 and October 1972. Adenomas were non-functioning in 317 cases, secreting in 158 and not classified in 4 of these 485 patients. Results of treatment of these patients are summarized below.

Mortality

Eight patients died during the first 4 weeks after the operation (Table III). Four had chromophobe adenomas and 4 had acromegaly. Among patients with chromophobe adenomas, the fourth death was in patient No. 127 in the series. The causes of death were: (1) bronchial obstruction at the end of the operation in a patient with a recurrent adenoma, (2) rupture of the carotid artery during the course of biopsy of what was erroneously thought to be a malignant tumor of the base of the skull, (3) hemorrhagic syndrome in an elderly woman who recently had surgery for a gastrointestinal carcinoma, (4) endocrine disorders.

The other 4 deaths occurred in acromegalic patients: one patient (No. 50) had meningitis after cerebrospinal fluid rhinorrhea. During the last 2 years, 3 patients died with paninvasive eosinophilic adenoma.

In addition to patients expiring in the first 4 weeks postoperatively, 4 patients died within 6 months postoperatively – 2 cases of chromophobe adenoma with a picture of general and

Table III

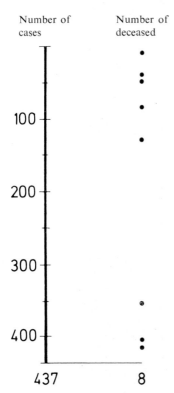

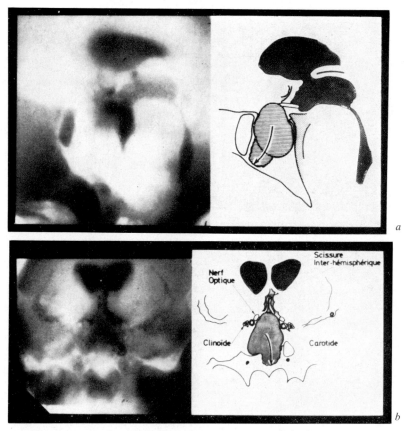

Fig. 18 Invasion of both (*a*) sphenoidal sinus and (*b*) clivus.

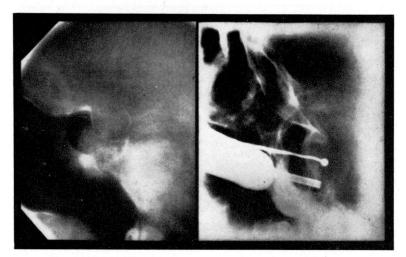

Fig. 19 Invasion of the sphenoidal sinus. On the right, intraoperative X-ray control showing that the sinus has been evacuated. A blunt instrument is introduced within the sella through the perforation made by the tumor in the anterior wall of the sella.

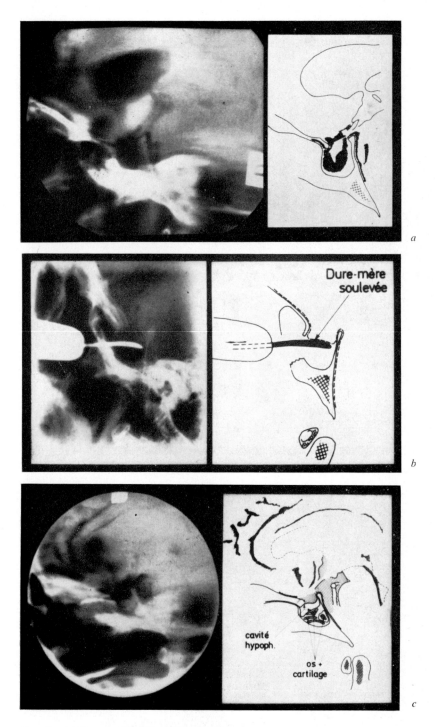

Fig. 20   (*a*) Empty sella with visual impairment.
(*b*) Elevation of the dural floor of the sella.
(*c*) Postoperative pneumoencephalography. Pieces of bone filling the inferior half of the sella can be seen.

mental deterioration, and 2 acromegalic patients with a Korsakoff's syndrome and endocrine disorders.

Complications in surviving patients

These are summarized in Table IV. Twelve patients required early reoperation for either a suspected hematoma or rhinorrhea.

Sudden worsening of vision and/or appearance of an oculomotor palsy postoperatively led us to suspect a hematoma in the operative site and to reoperate by the transsphenoidal route. Two of these patients had non-functioning (chromophobe) adenomas and one of them had a functioning adenoma with acromegaly. In one case, a small clot was found and the pieces of bone which had been put within the tumor cavity at operation in order to prevent descent of the optic nerves postoperatively were removed. The patient recovered vision immediately after removal of the clot. In the other 2 cases, the tumor cavity was empty. A previous invasion of the cavernous sinus by the tumor was suspected to be responsible for the ophthalmoplegia in one patient, who died later. Diplopia persisted for 2 years in the other patient, who survived.

Table IV   *Foch Hospital - Neurosurgical Department. Transsphenoidal operations for pituitary adenomas (from 1957 until 1972, Oct. 30)*

PRIMARY OPERATIONS	475
Reopening for - suspicion of hematoma	3
- rhinorrhea	9
2 chromophobe adenomas	
7 { small hypersecreting adenomas	
{ or functional hypophysectomy	
SECONDARY OPERATIONS for	
Rhinorrhea in the course of subsequent irradiation	3
Empty sella with visual disorders	5
Recurrence	10
7 after T. transsphenoidal route	
3 after intracranial route	

In an additional fourth case, the patient was reoperated by the subfrontal route the 10th day after an initial transsphenoidal operation. He had become blind on one side and almost blind on the other side. At reoperation, the optic nerves were found to have plunged down into the empty sella and the chiasm was stretched upon the right posterior clinoid process. Four years later, he had recovered 2/10 and 4/10 of visual acuity, with a persistent asymmetric field defect.

Nine patients were reoperated early for rhinorrhea. Two of them had non-secreting (chromophobe) adenomas and 4 had small intrahypophyseal eosinophilic adenomas. Postoperative rhinorrhea is apt to occur in the cases of small secreting adenoma or following functional hypophysectomy, because cerebrospinal fluid freely enters the hypophyseal chamber. On the other hand, it is an exceptional complication of transsphenoidal removal of a chromophobe adenoma. In most instances where the transsphenoidal route is selected, the tumor has chronically obliterated the foramen of the diaphragm, permitting the stalk with its arachnoidal sheath to enter the sella, but excluding cerebrospinal fluid from the operative cavity. Three cases of meningitis complicated the rhinorrhea.

Three cases of rhinorrhea occurred during the course of irradiation between 2 and 4 months postoperatively. These were cases in which an invasive adenoma had destroyed the sphenoid bone.

All these patients with rhinorrhea were reoperated in order to obliterate the tumor cavity with pieces of muscle, to close it with pieces of bone, and to plug the sphenoidal sinus. In addition, a lumbar drainage of CSF was maintained for a week. All patients were cured and there is no case of permanent fistula in the whole series. With an increasing experience of transsphenoidal surgery these complications have become rare.

Recurrences

Until now a second operation has been required for recurrence after transsphenoidal removal of a pituitary adenoma in 7 patients. In addition, 3 recurrences were observed after intracranial surgery and reoperated by transsphenoidal route.

The 3 patients who were operated on initially by the intracranial route, and 3 of the 7 patients operated on initially by transsphenoidal route, had not received postoperative irradiation. The first symptoms of recurrence were noted between 10 months and 9 years after the operation. Nine out of 10 cases were invasive adenomas at the time of the second operation and 7 had some radiological signs of invasion at the time of the original operation.

Empty sella and visual disorders

Five patients were reoperated on for visual disorders associated with an 'empty' sella, demonstrated by pneumoencephalography following transsphenoidal surgery for pituitary adenomas. Four had non-secreting (chromophobe) and one had a secreting (eosinophilic) adenoma. An extradural filling of the sella was performed, with pieces of bone, in order to elevate the optic nerves (Fig. 20). The results of these operations included 2 failures, one slight improvement and 2 gratifying recoveries.

All patients with the 'empty' sella had been operated on for the first time prior to 1966. Thereafter, in order to prevent this complication, the inferior half of the sellar cavity was systematically filled if it was particularly deep and if the pituitary adenoma was large. It is definitely easier to prevent than to cure a symptomatic empty sella.

Summary

Surgical problems posed by non-functioning and by secreting adenomas are quite different. The major reason is that external irradiation given after surgical ablation of non-functioning adenomas is effective in inhibiting further growth of the tumor, but relatively ineffective in inhibiting secretory processes of the adenoma. Therefore, the surgical goal for non-functioning adenomas consists essentially in reduction of the compressive effects and removal of all possible tumor mass without any risk to life or function. It is reasonable to expect that postoperative irradiation will impede or abolish the growth potential of residual fragments of most non-functioning adenomas.

Residual fragments of secreting adenomas, although unable to proliferate after irradiation, retain their secretory potential. The endocrine cure of a secreting adenoma is achieved only by radical removal or destruction of all the pathologic tissue. Depending upon the stage when surgery is performed for secreting adenomas, a surgical cure is possible, problematic or illusory. Normalization of hormonal secretion is possible in small intrahypophyseal adenomas removed by the transsphenoidal route. Again this is possible, but at the risk of pituitary insufficiency, in intrasellar enclosed adenomas. In secreting adenomas with suprasellar expansion, the dural capsule of the adenoma is often infiltrated and has to be removed.

Therefore the intracranial route gives a better chance for radical excision. Finally, when a secreting adenoma has become an 'invasive' adenoma, endocrine cure is unlikely, irrespective of the route of surgical removal.

In the case of non-functioning adenomas, both intracranial and transsphenoidal routes are equally suitable for 'global' and 'enclosed' adenomas (60 %). The choice between the 2 approaches depends not on the volume but on the shape and encapsulation of the tumor. The intracranial route is absolutely indicated in cases of transdiaphragmatic extension and of dumbbell-shaped tumors with a narrow neck between intracranial and intrasellar portions of tumor. On the contrary, invasion of sphenoidal sinus is an absolute indication for transsphenoidal route. Also, the transsphenoidal route is the route of choice for elderly patients, patients with acute intra-sellar hypertension and patients with extreme visual impairment. Finally, some desperate cases of paininvasive adenomas can be cured by a combination of transsphenoidal surgery and irradiation.

Both intracranial and transsphenoidal approaches have been required (in two steps) for 7 cases in our series.

References

(1) BAKAY, I. (1950): The results of 300 pituitary adenoma operations (Olivecrona's series). *J. Neurosurg.*, 7, 240.

(2) CUSHING, H. (1914): Surgical experiences with pituitary disorders. *J. Amer. med. Ass.*, 63, 1515.

(3) DEMAILLY, P., GUIOT, G. and OPROIU, A. (1967): Résultats visuels des exérèses d'adénomes hypophysaires par voie transsphenoïdale. *Arch. Ophtal. (Paris)*, 27, 5.

(4) DOTT, N. and BAILEY, P. (1925): A consideration of the hypophyseal adenomata. *Brit. J. Surg.*, 13, 314.

(5) ELKINGTON, S. G. and McKISSOCK, W. (1967): Pituitary adenomas: Results of combined surgical and radiotherapeutic treatment of 260 patients. *Brit. med. J.*, 1, 263.

(6) EMMANUEL, I. G. (1966): Symposium on pituitary tumors. Historical aspects of radiotherapy. Present treatment, technique and results. *Clin. Radiol. (Lond.)*, 17, 154.

(7) GUIOT, G., BOUCHE, J. and OPROIU, A. (1967): Les indications de l'abord transsphenoïdal des adénomes hypophysaires. *Presse méd.*, 75, 1563.

(8) GUIOT, G., ROUGERIE, J., FOURESTIER, M., VULMIERE, J. and COMOY, C. (1963): Explorations endoscopiques intracraniennes. *Presse méd.*, 71, 1225.

(9) GUIOT, G., ROUGERIE, J. and HERTZOG, E. (1958): L'utilisation de l'amplificateur de brillance en neurochirurgie. *Sem. Hôp. Paris*, 12, 689.

(10) HALSTEAD, A. E. (1910): Remarks on the operative treatment of tumors of hypophysis (two cases operated on by an oro-nasal route). *Trans. Amer. surg. Ass.*, 27, 75.

(11) HARDY, J. and CIRIC, I. (1968): Selective anterior hypophysectomy in the treatment of diabetic retinopathy. A transsphenoidal micro-surgical technic. *J. Amer. med. Ass.*, 203, 73.

(12) HARDY, J. and WIGSER, S. (1965): Transsphenoidal surgery of pituitary fossa tumors with televised radiofluoroscopic control. *J. Neurosurg.*, 23, 612.

(13) HEIMBACH, S. B. (1959): Etude suivie de 105 cas d'adénomes chromophobes et acidophiles de l'hypophyse, dûment vérifiés après traitement par opération transfrontale et radiothérapie (Krayenbuhl's series). *Acta neurochir. (Wien)*, 7, 101.

(14) HENDERSON, W. R. (1939): The pituitary adenomata. A follow-up study of the surgical results in 338 cases (Dr. Harvey Cushing's series). *Brit. J. Surg.*, 26, 811.

(15) HIRSCH, O. (1910): Endonasal method of removal of hypophyseal tumors, with a report of two cases. *J. Amer. med. Ass.*, 55, 772.

(16) JEFFERSON, G. (1940): Extrasellar extensions of pituitary adenomas. *Proc. roy. Soc. Med.*, 33, 433.

(17) JEFFERSON, G. (1955): *The Invasive Adenomas of the Anterior Pituitary*. University Press, Liverpool.

(18) KANAVEL, A. B. (1909): Removal of tumors of the pituitary body by an infra-nasal route. *J. Amer. med. Ass.*, 53, 1704.

(19)   NURNBERGER, J. I. and KOREY, S. R. (1953): *Pituitary Chromophobe Adenomas.* Springer-Verlag, New York, N.Y.
(20)   TÖNNIS, W., OBERDISSE, K. and WEBER, E. (1952): Bericht über 264 operierte Hypophysenadenome. *Acta neurochir. (Wien), III/2,* 113.

Transsphenoidal surgery of hypersecreting pituitary tumors

JULES HARDY

Service of Neurosurgery, Notre-Dame Hospital and University of Montreal, Montreal, Canada

Major progress has been made in the transsphenoidal open surgical approach to the pituitary by the introduction of the operating microscope and the development of microsurgical techniques of dissection. These have contributed to new therapeutic concepts and better knowledge about the pathophysiology of pituitary related disorders. In another chapter, Guiot has reviewed in detail the therapeutic problems of the non-secreting pituitary tumors with particular emphasis on the advantages of the transsphenoidal approach. This presentation will therefore be limited to the treatment of hypersecreting lesions of the pituitary.

434 transsphenoidal operations were carried out at the Notre-Dame Hospital and University of Montreal Neurosurgical Service over the last 10 years. These included 277 normal pituitary ablations for the treatment of advanced carcinoma of the breast and prostate (196 cases) and diabetic retinopathy (81 cases). There were 157 cases of pituitary fossa lesions of various kinds including craniopharyngioma, chordoma, meningioma, reticulosarcoma, chondrosarcoma and primary pituitary adenoma. Among the latter, there were 70 cases of pituitary adenoma associated with clinical syndromes of pituitary hypersecretion: 40 acromegalic patients, 20 patients with galactorrhea and 10 patients with Cushing's disease.

An extensive study from clinical, endocrinological, radiological and pathological points of view is in preparation. This paper is a preliminary summary with particular emphasis on the surgical therapeutic aspect by the transsphenoidal approach.

Endocrinological indications for transsphenoidal approach

For many years specific clinical syndromes of pituitary hypersecretory disorders have been attributed to diffuse hypertrophy and hyperplasia of the pituitary cells as a result of a primary hypothalamic disturbance of the releasing factors. This hypothesis was supported by patients who had no radiological evidence of enlargement of the sella turcica that might confirm the presence of a pituitary adenoma. In other cases with radiological signs of an expanding pituitary adenoma, the clinical syndrome was attributed to the adenoma.

However, on the basis of our experience in the exploration of the sella turcica in well documented cases of hypersecreting pituitary disorders with normal size sella, we have always found a well localized circumscribed nodule embedded within the pituitary parenchyma varying in sizes from 3 to 10 mm that we have given the appellation of 'microadenoma', as long as the lesion was smaller than 10 mm in diameter. As a consequence, the indications for transsphenoidal surgical exploration of the pituitary fossa have been extended to all cases of well documented pituitary disorders (both hypo- and hypersecreting) as a method of further diagnostic procedure as well as the first therapeutic approach.[1] The value of the early detection of these lesions in comparison with larger size tumors will be reflected in the clinical and biological results.

Surgical technique

Among the various extracranial transsphenoidal procedures so far described, the subnasal, midline, rhinoseptal transsphenoidal approach to the sella turcica has been adopted because it offers definite advantages and it is the most convenient and simple for neurosurgeons. Mainly, it respects a fundamental principle of surgical anatomy which obliges the surgeon to encounter the sella turcica in a strict medial sagittal plane. Adequate exposure and symmetrical visualization of the intrasellar contents allow the safest dissection in avoiding the risk of trauma to the surrounding neurovascular structures. This approach has already been described in detail elsewhere.[4] Thus, only the key steps in the procedure will be briefly illustrated in Figures 1, 2 and 3.

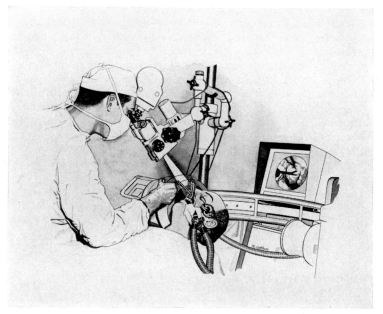

Fig. 1   Operating set-up for transsphenoidal surgery using the binocular surgical microscope and televised radiofluoroscopic control.

After the sphenoidal cavity is widely exposed, the operating microscope is positioned. The advantages of magnification are particularly evident since direct visualization allows the recognition and management of anatomical variations and anomalies about the sella such as the malposition of the circular and cavernous sinuses, the presence of carotid arteries in the sella, the finding of an arachnoidal diverticulum herniating through a large opening in the diaphragm and also the presence of unsuspected lesions such as extension of a carotid

a

b

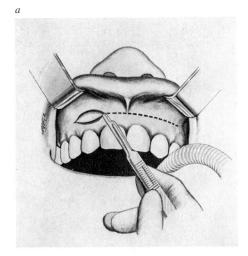
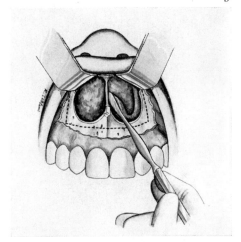
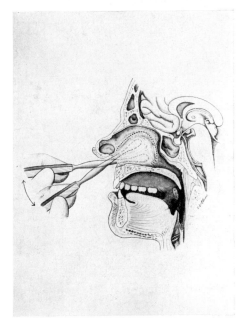
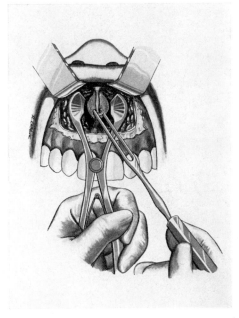

c

d

Fig. 2 Key steps of the oronasal, rhinoseptal, transsphenoidal approach to the sella turcica: (*a*) sublabial incision; (*b*) elevation of the nasal mucosa from the floor and submucosal dissection from the septum; (*c*) sagittal view of the submucosal dissection; (*d*) resection of the cartilaginous septum with a swivelled knife.

aneurysm into the sella turcica as found in 1 case. In large tumors herniating into or filling entirely the sphenoidal sinus, magnification is not indispensable, although it is useful at 10×. In smaller lesions magnification of 16× is used routinely, and in special cases of intrapituitary microadenoma magnification up to 25× will be necessary to distinguish the normal from the pathological tissues.

e 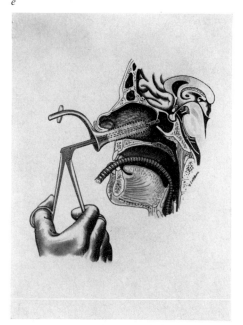 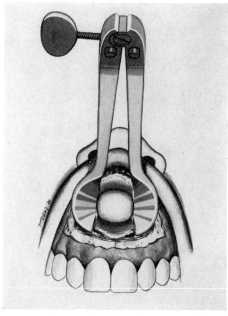 *f*

Fig. 2   (*e*) Position of the nasal bivalve speculum and opening of the sphenoid sinus; (*f*) final position of the bivalve speculum after removal of the floor of the sphenoid sinus producing a wide exposure of the cavity and of the sella turcica which is enlarged by a pituitary tumor.

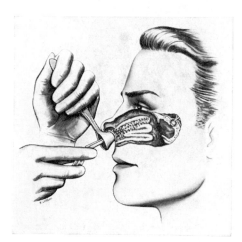 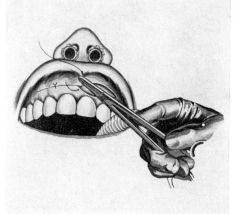

Fig. 3   (*a*) Simple closure by reapproximation of the nasal mucosa with vaseline gauze endonasal packing which is removed on the second postoperative day; (*b*) a few loose catgut sutures on the alveolar incision.

Our primary goal in the therapeutic management of hypersecreting pituitary adenoma is to achieve a complete excision of the lesion with all effort to identify and preserve the remnant of the normal hypophysis in order to avoid postoperative hypopituitarism. As a matter of fact, this has been possible in most patients who had had no previous operative manipulation or radiotherapy. In patients who had previous treatment and who already had hypopituitarism requiring substitution therapy before the operation, all the intrasellar content has been excised including the normal pituitary remnant. During the removal of the adenoma by fragments with blunt dissecting instruments and aspiration, grey reddish, soft tissue, white gelatinous or dark purple necrotic substances are easily distinguishable from the yellow orange, firm tissue of the normal anterior lobe. Usually, this normal adenohypophyseal tissue was found lying in the posterior and superior region of the sella above the tumor having the appearance of a thin layer, a tongue of tissue or even the anterior lobe having kept its nodular appearance. There is no point in further stressing the advantages of the extracranial transsphenoidal approach *since in hyperpituitarism most of the tumors expand downwards, herniating into the sphenoidal cavity.* Unless the tumor is extensively invasive, complete excison is possible in all cases. After the tumor has been removed, a biopsy with frozen section of the normal pituitary tissue is taken in order to obtain an immediate confirmation that this was in fact normal gland. If this biopsy is reported as pathological tissue, further removal is accomplished. In order to achieve complete eradication of tumor tissue within the sellar cavity, fixation with alcohol is also accomplished.

In patients with radiological evidence of suprasellar expansion as outlined by preoperative pneumographic study with tomography, the method is slightly modified. Prior to surgery, a catheter is inserted in the lumbar space to allow injection of a few ml of air to serve in outlining the suprasellar contour. At this time, televised radiofluoroscopy is mandatory to control the position of the curettes in the intracranial cavity. As the tumor collapses down into the sella turcica, further injection of air confirms immediately during surgery the re-filling of the chiasmatic cistern and the position of the anterior recess of the third ventricle.

Since a pituitary adenoma has no capsule of its own,[1] no attempt should be made to detach the 'capsule', which is the aponeural sheath of the sella and the diaphragm. Metallic clips are applied to the collapsed diaphragm to serve as opaque markers for follow-up radiological controls. Occasionally, when a cerebrospinal fluid leak occurs, it requires an immediate correction during surgery by the transplantation of a fascia lata graft with a piece of muscle taken from the patient's thigh. In rare instances of persisting oozing after tumor removal, it is recommended to leave a rubber catheter in the sphenoidal cavity to serve as drainage in the postoperative period. Systemic antibiotic therapy is given intramuscularly starting the day before surgery and during 5 days postoperatively; then it is continued orally for 10 days.

Criteria for the evaluation of the results

In reviewing our material, we found it was impossible to evaluate the clinical results in general in the treatment of hypersecreting pituitary adenoma since these results are dependent upon various factors – the most important of which are the type of lesion and the nature of surgical excision.

Classification of the types of lesion

From the radiological point of view, we have classified the pituitary adenoma in 2 major groups that have corresponding radiological changes on the sella turcica.

1. *The enclosed adenoma* The enclosed adenoma is described as a tumor which remains within the anatomical confines of the osteoaponeural sheath of the sella turcica. In these cases, the floor of the sella is always *intact*, although it may be enlarged. Thus, there are 2 grades:

Grade I: the sella turcica is normal in size (length <17 mm; height <14 mm; surface less than 208 mm² on the lateral view). However, careful study with tomo-

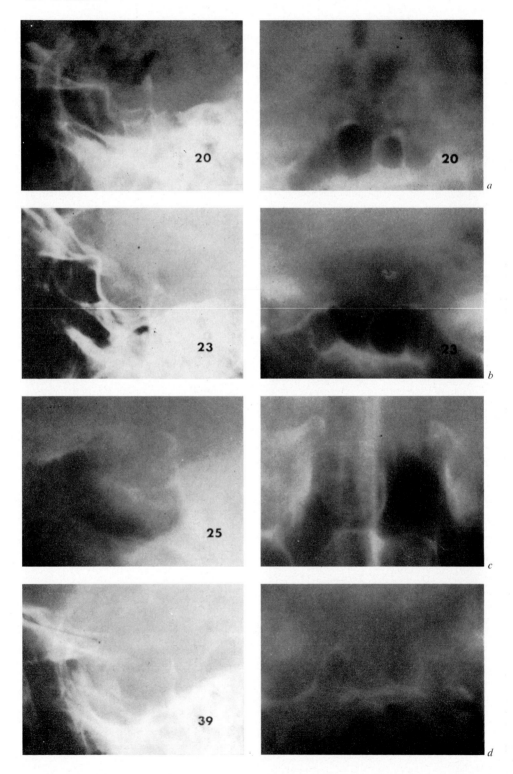

Fig. 4   Radiological classification of pituitary adenomas as illustrated from cases of acromegaly (on the left: lateral view; on the right: AP tomogram): (*a*) enclosed left-sided microadenoma in normal size sella (grade I); (*b*) enclosed right-sided adenoma in an enlarged sella (grade II); (*c*) local invasive adenoma with partial destruction of the floor and herniation of the tumor into the right sphenoid sinus (grade III); (*d*) diffuse invasive adenoma with 'phantom sella' (grade IV).

gram reveals an asymmetry of the floor of the sella characterized by the lowering on one or the other side in cases of acromegaly and galactorrhea. In these cases, the tumor is always less than 10 mm in diameter and is referred to as a 'microadenoma' (Fig. 4*a*).

Grade II: the sella turcica is enlarged to various degrees but the floor is always *intact* (Fig. 4*b*).
These may be associated with a suprasellar expansion as outlined by the pneumoencephalogram.

2. *The invasive adenomas*   In these cases, the tumor has eroded the floor of the sella with herniation of the pathological tissue into the sphenoidal sinus.

Grade III: when the erosion is well localized to one area of the floor of the sella (Fig. 4*c*).

Grade IV: when the entire floor of the sella is diffusely eroded or destroyed giving the aspect of a 'phantom sella' where all the boundaries are barely visible (Fig. 4*d*).

Again, in these last 2 grades, there might also be a suprasellar expansion of various degrees. Our present concept of the growth pattern of acidophilic adenomas is schematically illustrated in Figure 5.

We found that this classification was most important in order to obtain an adequate evaluation of the clinical results in the various clinical syndromes of hypersecreting pituitary adenoma.

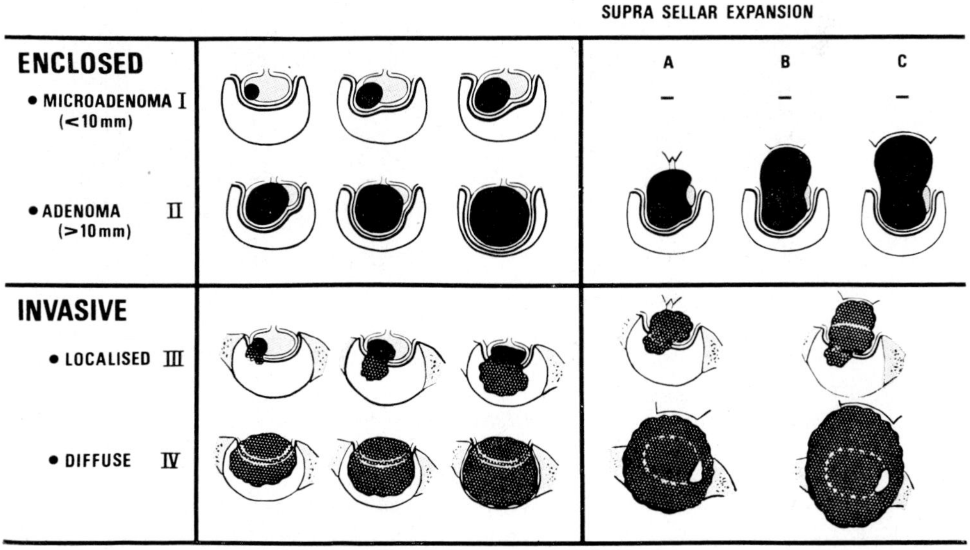

Fig. 5   Growth pattern of acidophilic adenomas.

Nature of surgical excision

Depending upon the various types of lesion that have been described above, it is obvious that the nature and the extent of the surgical excision have varied from one case to the other. Moreover, the ideal conditions were not always met to achieve the ideal goal of the selective radical excision of the lesion with preservation of the normal pituitary tissue since several patients already had previous treatment, either a first surgical approach not performed by the author or irradiation therapy. Because of these various factors, the nature of the surgical excision has been assessed from 4 different aspects:

1. *Non-selective total removal*:   in these cases, radical excision of all the intrasellar content was performed including the normal and pathological tissue.

2. *Non-selective subtotal removal*   is when there has been a partial removal of the pathological tissue and it is most likely that some residual tissue remains.

3. *Selective subtotal removal*   is when the normal pituitary gland has been identified with a biopsy but the surgeon has not been completely assured to have accomplished a complete excision of the pathological tissue. In this case, he will prefer to return in a second stage rather than producing panhypopituitarism by the removal of the remnant of the normal gland.

4. *Selective total removal*   is when the normal pituitary has been well identified and biopsied and the surgeon is sure to have excised all the pathological material. This latter method is schematically illustrated in Figures 6 and 7.

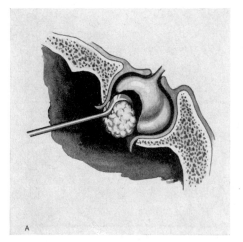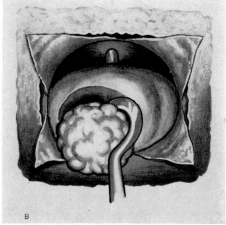

Fig. 6   (*a, b*) Illustration of a selective removal of an intrapituitary microadenoma located in the lateral wing of the gland as found in cases of acromegaly with normal size sella.

Clinical and biological evaluation of the results

At the present time, there are 3 clinical syndromes which are well documented as being caused by an oversecreting pituitary adenoma: *acromegaly* due to overproduction of growth hormone, *Cushing's disease* due to overproduction of ACTH resulting in an increase of cortisol secretion, and *galactorrhea* due to overproduction of lactogenic hormone; the latter disease is frequently associated with menstrual disorders or amenorrhea.

a   *b*

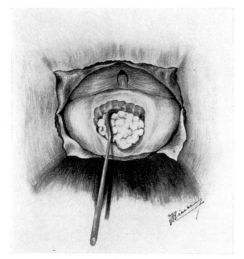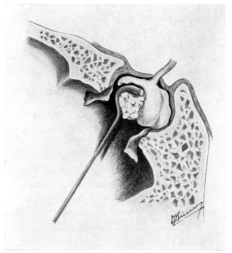

Fig. 7   (*a, b*) Illustration of the position of an intrapituitary basophilic microadenoma located in the median central part of the gland as found in cases of Cushing's disease with normal size sella.

From the clinical point of view, an adequate assessment of the therapeutic results varies considerably from one group to the other, and because of this the relative value of the different methods is not easy to compare. As a general principle, the ideal result would be the clinical arrest of the symptoms and signs of the disease with biological confirmation of the reduced pituitary oversecretion to normal level without inducing hypopituitarism requiring hormonal substitution therapy. The second best result would be the clinical improvement without hypopituitarism but with persistence of elevated hormone secretion. Partial success would be the clinical improvement with reduced oversecretion but with postoperative hypopituitarism of the other secretions. Finally, unsuccessful result would be the cases in whom no clinical improvement is observed and oversecretion persists. This general appraisal may provide an adequate method of evaluation so that postoperatively the patients may be classified as *cured, improved* or *unchanged*. More specifically, with each of the clinical syndromes, these are the criteria that we have used in the assessment of our patients.

In *acromegaly* we consider that the patient is cured when all symptoms and signs of pituitary hyperactivity have disappeared: disabling headache, perspiration and the soft tissue manifestations of the disease have shown significant regression as well as improvement of concomitant diabetes mellitus. But also, from the biological point of view, the previously elevated growth hormone should be reduced to *normal levels* as verified with the glucose tolerance test. Thus, a cure is assessed from both the clinical and biological point of view. Although a patient may be clinically cured according to the above mentioned criteria, if the previously elevated growth hormone levels are markedly reduced but still above the normal values, this patient will be classified as *improved*. Otherwise, the persistence of high levels of growth hormone despite some clinical improvement will be classified as unchanged or unsuccessful result.

In *Cushing's disease* well known clinical features: obesity, moon face, hypertension, etc., should be markedly reduced together with lowering of plasma cortisol to normal levels in order to classify this patient as cured. Otherwise, he is improved or unchanged.

In *galactorrhea* the arrest of lactation is the criterion for a successful result. Prolactin measurement has only been available recently but it is the biological assay that confirms the cure of pituitary oversecretion. In several patients the return of normal menstruation would be an additional factor to consider as a favorable result.

Acromegaly

Forty acromegalic patients with various types of lesion had a transsphenoidal surgical exploration and excision of the tumor. In this group of patients, 16 cases had previous radiotherapy which has been unsuccessful in reducing the growth hormone level. Three cases had previous surgical excision performed elsewhere.

In using the rigid criteria mentioned above, favorable results were obtained in 35 cases (87.5 %). These include 25 cases with clinical and biological cure and 10 cases with clinical and biological improvement. Correlations between the types of lesion, the extent of surgical excision and results are summarized in Tables I, II and III. It is important to notice that these favorable results were obtained mostly with the enclosed adenoma or with local invasive adenoma. Only one patient with a large suprasellar expansion remained unchanged. The operation was done because of severe visual loss which markedly improved. A second operation will be necessary on this patient to remove the residual pathological tissue. The other 4 unsuccessful cases with diffuse invasive lesions remained unchanged though a radical

Table I　*Results in acromegaly (40 cases)*

Type of lesion		No. of cases	Results		
			Cured	Improved	Unchanged
Enclosed adenoma					
Gr. I:	microadenoma	10	8	2	0
Gr. II:	adenoma				
	no s.s.	14	12	2	0
	with s.s.	5	1	3	1
Invasive adenoma					
Gr. III:	local invasion				
	no s.s.	3	2	1	0
	with s.s.	2	2	—	0
Gr. IV:	diffuse invasion				
	no s.s.	3	—	1	2
	with s.s.	3	—	1	2
Total		40	25	10	5

s.s. = suprasellar extension.

Table II　*Correlation between the results and the type of lesion in acromegaly*

Results	No. of cases	Enclosed adenoma		Invasive adenoma	
		Gr. I	II	III	IV
Cured	25	8	13	4	0
Improved	10	2	5	1	2
Unchanged	5	0	1	0	4
Total	40	10	19	5	6

Table III   *Correlation between the type of lesion, extent of surgical excision and results in acromegalics*

Extent of surgical excision	Grade of lesion	No. of cases	Results				
			Cured	Improved	Unchanged	F.R.	Hypo.
Selective total	I	10	8	2	—	4	0
	II	10	10	—	—	3	0
	III	3	2	1	—	—	0
	IV	2	—	1	1	—	0
Selective subtotal	II	1	—	1	—	—	0
	IV	1	—	—	1	—	0
Non-selective subtotal	II	5	1	3	1	—	0
	III	1	1	—	—	—	1
Non-selective total	II	3	2	1	—	—	3 (2)
(radical)	III	1	1	—	—	—	(1)
	IV	3	—	1	2	—	3 (2)
Total		40	25	10	5	7	9 (5)

F.R. = functional recovery of preoperative pituitary insufficiency; Hypo. = postoperative pituitary insufficiency; ( ) = preoperative pituitary insufficiency.

excision was performed. One of these cases had a surgical complication and died 4 months later. The autopsy showed that the lesion had extensively invaded the base of the skull, both cavernous sinuses, toward the temporal fossa and into the midline brain structures. The remaining 2 cases had a second operation with further removal of invasive tumor resulting in improvement with marked reduction of growth hormone but not to normal level. With regard to endocrine function, 5 patients were already suffering from panhypopituitarism due to previous treatment. Three patients were deliberately rendered panhypopituitaric as a result of the second operation with radical excision of all the intrasellar content. None of the patients who had selective excision of the lesion with preservation of the normal pituitary developed postoperative hypopituitarism requiring hormonal substitution therapy. On the other hand, 7 patients with preoperative partial pituitary insufficiency of gonadotrophin and/or thyrotrophin secretion had resumed normal function after surgery.

Galactorrhea

Twenty female patients with *galactorrhea* had a transsphenoidal exploration of the sella turcica. There were 14 cases below the age of 30, 4 cases between 30 and 40, and 2 patients between 45 and 50 years old.

In the youngest group, most of the patients were young females who had a history of menstrual disorders and infertility. Sixteen cases have taken oral contraceptive pills for a period of time during which galactorrhea appeared for most of the patients. After cessation of this medication, amenorrhea remained unchanged. Eighteen of the cases had amenorrhea which lasted from 6 months to 8 years with a mean of 3 years before surgery. Two patients had only galactorrhea without amenorrhea. Prolactin measurement by radioimmunoassay was obtained in 10 cases. In all of these cases, prolactin levels were markedly elevated above the normal value (30 ng/ml in our laboratory). In 4 cases, the sella turcica was radiologically enlarged, confirming the presence of a pituitary adenoma. Two of these patients had also visual difficulties. In the other cases, the sella was normal in size although a slight asymmetry of the floor could be detected on the tomographic study.

At operation, these 16 cases had an intrapituitary microadenoma that was found located *in the lateral wing of the gland.* The lesion was selectively removed under high magnification and microdissection whereas the normal pituitary glandular tissue was preserved. In the 4 other cases, 2 had an obvious expanding primary pituitary adenoma that was also selectively removed. In the other 2 cases, unsuspected cystic lesions were found and removed as well. These were a Rathke pouch cyst and a craniopharyngioma.

Results

There were no intraoperative complications. Postoperatively the patient with a craniopharyngioma developed panhypopituitarism with diabetes insipidus. Another patient had a transitory diabetes insipidus. Two patients with visual difficulties recovered completely. Two patients had preoperative thyroid insufficiency that remained unchanged. None of the 19 cases developed further hypopituitarism requiring substitution therapy as a consequence of surgery. Galactorrhea disappeared in all cases within a few days to a few months after surgery. Five patients resumed normal regular menstruations. High prolactin levels were reduced to normal in 4 cases. In 1 patient prolactin was reduced to 50 % of the preoperative levels in specimens collected postoperatively. In the other 5 cases, measurements were done but the results are not yet available.

The following case is an example of the ideal goal that can be obtained with the early detection of these intrapituitary microadenomas and selective removal with microsurgical dissection through the transsphenoidal approach. A 26-year-old married woman had a problem with irregular menstruation. She has been treated with contraceptive pills that restored the normal cycle. After cessation of this medication, she noticed the appearance of lactation and her menstruations stopped. The endocrinological study showed a selective pituitary insufficiency in gonadotrophins. Prolactin measurements were markedly elevated.

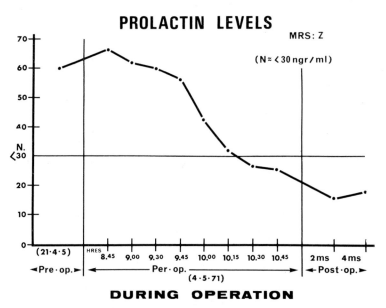

Fig. 8   Illustration of the immediate fall of high prolactin level at the time of surgery, during the removal of a prolactin-secreting microadenoma.

Skull X-ray showed a normal sella turcica. On the tomogram there was a suggestion of a very slight asymmetry with lowering of the floor on the right side. A transsphenoidal micro-surgical exploration was carried out on 4 June 1971, and permitted the detection and selective removal of a tiny intrasellar lesion located within the lateral wing of the gland measuring 5 mm in diameter. Galactorrhea stopped after 2 months. One month later she was found to be pregnant and on 4 June 1972 she delivered a normal child, the first since her marriage. Moreover, prolactin measurements done at the time of surgery show the early reversal of oversecretion immediately following surgical excision of the lesion (Fig. 8).

Cushing's disease

Ten patients with Cushing's disease were operated on transsphenoidally. There were 4 cases below the age of 20, 2 between 30 and 40, and 4 above 50 years old.

Three patients had been adrenalectomized before the pituitary surgery. Two of these had developed hyperpigmentation (Nelson's syndrome). In referring to the above mentioned classification, 6 patients had a small sella turcica grade I, 1 of grade II, 2 of grade III, 1 of grade IV. Results are summarized in Table IV.

Table IV   *Cushing's disease (10 cases)*

Results	No. of cases	Type of lesion			
		Enclosed		Invasive	
		Gr. I	II	III	IV
Cured	8	6		2	
Improved	1		1		
Unchanged	1				1

Eight patients were cured. Five of these have been cured without hypopituitarism after selective total removal of the tumor with preservation of the normal residual adenohypo-physeal tissue. Among these, 3 were intrapituitary microadenomas and 2 had an intra-sphenoidal expansion grade III. In the 3 other cases who had previous adrenalectomy removal of tumor tissue was successfully accomplished, but with resultant hypopituitarism. One patient was improved but the follow-up was lost and no biological confirmation could be obtained. An unsuccessful result occurred in 1 patient with a grade IV tumor despite 2 operations in an attempt to achieve a radical excision of the lesion with hypophysectomy after stalk section. She died later of hypertensive encephalopathy with intracerebral hemor-rhage. The postmortem study showed a malignant invasive lesion spreading in the base of the skull beyond any surgical anatomical feasibility. A 19-year-old boy was cured 6 years ago. He married, had normal sexual potency and fertility and became a father.

Because of the varieties of the cases in this small series, statistical results are not significant. However, it is worthwhile to notice that complete cure of Cushing's disease can be obtained in patients with selective excision of basophilic adenoma without producing hypopituitarism requiring substitution therapy. Clinical improvement is obvious early after surgery.

Malignant exophthalmos

We have only 1 case of a female patient who was suffering from malignant edematous exophthalmos. After total thyroidectomy, the exophthalmos got worse. The sella turcica was found to be slightly enlarged grade II. Hypophysectomy was recommended. At the surgical transsphenoidal exploration, a small cystic adenoma located in the median central part of the sella was found and selectively removed. The exophthalmos was markedly reduced shortly after surgery and she remained stable on a long-term follow-up.

Surgical mortality and morbidity

In this series of 70 cases, 1 patient died 4 months later as a consequence of surgical complication. She was an acromegalic patient who despite cobalt therapy did not have clinical improvement. At surgery, the tumor was extremely hard in consistency and fibrotic with adhesions to the cavernous sinus wall. Postoperatively, she developed hemiplegia due to left cerebral infarction, although a carotid angiogram did not show thrombosis of the artery. She died of pulmonary complications. The autopsy revealed that the tumor had a diffuse extension in the base of the skull, in both cavernous sinuses, towards the left temporal fossa with invasion of the midline cerebral structures.

One acromegalic patient had a transitory diplopia due to injury of the sixth nerve, obviously due to the fact that his small adenoma was far laterally placed in the corner of the sella turcica requiring manipulation towards the cavernous sinus. On the other hand, he was clinically and biologically cured without endocrinological deficit. There was no postoperative rhinorrhea or infection.

Comment

In reviewing our material, an interesting observation occurred to us concerning the localization of the various types of hypersecreting microadenomas within the pituitary gland. In acromegaly, the somatotropic microadenomas were located in the anterior inferior part of the

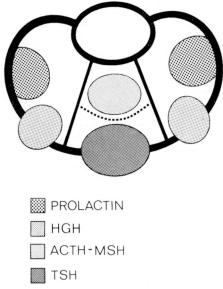

▓ PROLACTIN

▒ HGH

□ ACTH-MSH

▓ TSH

Fig. 9   This schematic drawing illustrates the localization of the various types of microadenomas as found under microsurgical exploration of the pituitary gland in cases of acromegaly, galactorrhea and Cushing's disease.

lateral wing of the gland. In galactorrhea, prolactin-producing microadenomas were also located in the lateral wings, although apparently more deeply or posteriorly in the gland. In Cushing's disease the microadenomas were located in the central core of the gland on the midline, as well as the microadenomas in Nelson's syndrome. In the single case of presumed TSH producing microadenoma, it was located also on the central area, near the surface of the gland. Therefore, it can be deduced that within the pituitary body there is a topographical distribution of hypersecreting microadenomas that might correspond to 'nuclei' or 'pools' of secreting cells in the normal gland (Fig. 9).

This clinical surgical observation has found a basic histological confirmation. Studies carried out by the late Robert Phifer (unpublished data) from the University of South Carolina using immunofluorescent staining methods has confirmed a histological distribution of these various cells in normal gland.

Summary

In more than 400 transsphenoidal operations, including 157 cases of pituitary fossa tumors, there were 70 patients who presented with hypersecreting pituitary disorders. With the operating microscope and techniques of microdissection, an attempt to perform a selective excision of the adenoma with identification of the normal pituitary gland was made in order to avoid postoperative hypopituitarism. Because of the various types of lesion that were encountered, the nature of the surgical excision and the pathological findings, we found it impossible to discuss in general the result of the therapeutic management of the various clinical diseases due to oversecreting pituitary adenomas. Thus, a classification of the various types of pituitary adenomas has been devised. There are 2 major groups: the enclosed adenomas and the invasive adenomas with a subdivision in 4 grades. Results are reported according to this classification.

In 40 cases of acromegaly, 5 patients remained unchanged after extensive surgical excision of the lesion. There were 4 cases of diffuse invading lesions extending beyond the confines of the sella turcica. One case had a large suprasellar extension and had a subtotal removal for visual difficulties which improved. She will require a second operation to remove further tissue in order to obtain a biological cure. 35 cases (87.5 %) had successful clinical improvement. In 25 of these, biological cure was confirmed as the growth hormone levels returned to normal values. In the other 10, it remained slightly above the normal value, although it was markedly reduced from the preoperative level and the patients are clinically restored. The best results were obtained in the series of microadenoma with a normal size sella and with a small adenoma in an enlarged sella.

In 10 cases of Cushing's disease, 8 patients were cured, 5 without hypopituitarism, 3 having had previous adrenalectomy. One case of invasive malignant lesion remained unchanged despite 2 radical surgical excisions of the lesion.

The major recent progress in the treatment of hypersecreting pituitary disorders is the early detection and selective excision of prolactin secreting adenoma producing galactorrhea often associated with amenorrhea. In 20 cases, 16 patients had a selective removal of an intra-pituitary microadenoma. Only 1 patient with an unsuspected concomitant craniopharyngioma developed postoperative hypopituitarism. Five patients resumed normal menstruation and one young female became pregnant 3 months after surgery and had a normal delivery 1 year after surgery. Galactorrhea was arrested in all of the cases within a few days to a few months after excision of the lesion.

Because of the benign, rapid and non-traumatic nature of the operation, the transsphenoidal open surgical approach is indicated as an additional method of diagnostic procedure in the exploration of the sella turcica in well documented cases of pituitary related disorders. The concept of microadenoma in early detected cases allows the achievement of a selective excision of the lesion with preservation of the normal pituitary tissue, thus producing clinical and biological cure without inducing postoperative hypopituitarism. The main advantage of surgical excision is the early reversal of pituitary oversecretion and rapid improvement of clinical signs in the immediate postoperative period. The ideal goal that can be achieved at the present time in the treatment of hyperpituitarism is to obtain a biological state of eupituitarism.

Acknowledgement

Figures are reproduced by kind permission of the editors of the *Journal of Neurosurgery*.

References

(1)   HARDY, J. (1969): Transsphenoidal microsurgery of the normal and pathological pituitary. *Clin. Neurosurg.*, *16*, 185.

(2)   HARDY, J. (1969): Microneurosurgery of the hypophysis: subnasal transsphenoidal approach with television magnification and televised radiofluoroscopic control. In: *Microneurosurgery*, *Chapter 8*, p. 224. Editor: R. W. Rand.   C.V. Mosby Co., St. Louis, Mo.

(3)   HARDY, J. (1969): Transnasal-transsphenoidal approach to the pituitary gland. In: *Microsurgery, applied to Neurosurgery*, p. 230. Editor: M. G. Yasargil.   George Thieme Verlag, Stuttgart; Academic Press, New York - London.

(4)   HARDY, J. (1971): Transsphenoidal hypophysectomy. *J. Neurosurg.*, *34*, 581.

(5)   HARDY, J. and PROVOST, J. (1969): Microneurochirurgie. *Un. méd. Can.*, *98*, 187.

(6)   HARDY, J. (1971): Microchirurgie des adénomes hypophysaires hypersécrétants. In: *Les Adénomes Hypophysaires Sécrétants*, pp. 195-196. Masson et Cie, Paris.

Discussion

DR. VAN BUREN: I am delighted to find in the current results that the incidence of rhinorrhea has not been important and likelihood of meningitis is very low. Five years ago, Bristol presented a series of some 350 transsphenoidal hypophysectomies for treatment of breast cancer. He had 51 instances of rhinorrhea with this group. He was doing a radical extracapsular removal with tearing through the stalk. His results included 11 cases of meningitis, 4 of which were fatal. This morbidity concerned me greatly.

DR. PEARSON: I would like to describe our first case of microadenoma which has been successfully removed. This was a prolactin secreting adenoma in a 25 year old male with galactorrhea and gynecomastia, which probably is the counterpart of the Forbes-Albright syndrome in women. The sella turcica was entirely normal on X-ray and there was no asymmetry. Air studies showed a convex upward air soft tissue interface within the confines of the sella turcica. Prolactin levels were elevated, failed to rise with a provocative test using chlorpromazine, and failed to suppress with the administration of L-DOPA. Thus, the endocrine data were strongly suggestive of an autonomous prolactin-secreting lesion, and we proceeded to look for a microadenoma. On entering and exploring the sella turcica, Dr. Brodkey found an adenoma, weighing about 200 mg, which secreted prolactin in vitro. We are impressed that we can cure the patient and leave normal endocrine functions behind. I am surprised at the number of cases Dr. Hardy has and wonder how he selects his patients for surgery.

DR. HARDY: These cases have been selected out of a large group of patients with galactorrhea. Dr. Henry Friesen can describe the endocrine tests we used for selection.

DR. FRIESEN: The prolactin levels have been quite high in all of Dr. Hardy's patients. In fact, it is impressive how high they can be. We have seen levels up to 12,000 ng/ml, and the frequency with which one sees elevations above the level of 500 ng/ml level is really quite high.

We have arbitrarily said that any patient with a level over 200 ng/ml probably has a primary tumor. The ones with concentrations between 30 and 200 could be on a functional basis, but again, some of them with a level of 60 ng/ml turned out to have a microadenoma, hence the arbitrary division is clearly not absolute.

Dr. Hardy, I think in some of your patients the levels of prolactin after operation still are not down to normal, and I wonder if you generally consider it appropriate to operate a second time in this circumstance, especially in the face of rather few clinical side effects in most patients with prolactin secreting tumors? Do you feel it is always justified to go back simply to try and reduce the prolactin levels to normal?

DR. HARDY: Since the clinical symptoms of galactorrhea are not life threatening, I think we have to follow such patients carefully to be sure they don't develop recurrent tumor. In such cases I do not think it would be wise to reopen on the basis of an arbitrary prolactin level alone.

DR. FRIESEN: Let me just add one comment with regard to prolactin secreting tumors. I think it is now widely appreciated that many, perhaps the majority, of patients with such tumors do not have galactorrhea. In our experience with studies on prolactin levels in all patients with pituitary tumors, prolactin-secreting tumors are the most common of all functional tumors of the pituitary.

DR. FRANTZ: I think it is important to emphasize that not all patients with galactorrhea will have elevated plasma prolactin, as Dr. Friesen mentioned, and some may have only minimally elevated levels.

I would like to ask Dr. Hardy if he or his associates have had any experience in irradiating patients with galactorrhea and high prolactin levels, because where tumors exist, they may be small, causing no pressure symptoms, little or no sellar enlargement, and no endocrine abnormalities except galactorrhea and possibly amenorrhea. In that case, might it not be possible they could be treated successfully by conventional radiotherapy?

DR. HARDY: I am a surgeon; I have no experience with irradiation in these cases. However, I think it would be difficult for the radiotherapist to focus on a target only 3 mm in diameter.

DR. ODELL: What is the incidence of increased prolactin concentrations in patients with galactorrhea? What per cent have normal prolactin concentrations?

DR. FRANTZ: We have looked at somewhat over 70 patients with galactorrhea at the Presbyterian Hospital in New York, and it depends to a considerable extent on how you select your patients. A considerable number of patients with galactorrhea do not have associated amenorrhea. These are frequently women who have had a child and simply continue to lactate, even though menses resume normally, and in some cases they go on to have further children.

In this rather large group with normal menses, you will find most have normal prolactin levels. If, however, you take only those patients who have galactorrhea with amenorrhea, you will find the vast majority of those do have hyperprolactinemia, although there are some who do have prolactin levels that fall within the normal range.

Patients with galactorrhea and proven pituitary tumors, with perhaps one exception, have all had at least minimally elevated plasma prolactin, in our experience. The higher the prolactin, the greater the likelihood of a tumor, and we would agree with Dr. Friesen that prolactin concentrations of greater than 200 ng/ml are very strongly suggestive of a tumor.

DR. ROBINSON: Do you think that patients with chromophobe adenomas treated with transsphenoidal surgery should have postoperative radiotherapy?

DR. GUIOT: Almost all of our patients have been radiated. In the case of a chromophobe adenoma, we have no tests to prove that the tumor has been completely removed, therefore we have irradiated patients in whom we were uncertain about total tumor removal.

DR. FAGER: If you look at the statistics from all of the larger series, Dr. Ray's, Dr. Randall's, our own, you will find, I am certain, that the rate of recurrence is far lower in those patients who have had radiation following surgery.

DR. DAUGHADAY: Dr. Hardy, have you ever recovered more than one microadenoma?

DR. HARDY: Multiple adenomata were reported by Costello. We have had two possible cases, but these have been the subject of some controversy with our pathologists.

DR. KRIEGER: If I understand Dr. Hardy correctly, the pituitary pathology in the patients with acromegaly has always been that of an adenoma, either a discrete encapsulated adenoma or what he has called invasive adenomas. Does the invasive adenoma correlate with what may be described as eosinophilic hyperplasia? Some of the transsphenoidally obtained pituitary specimens that our pathologists have reported have not been described as adenoma, but rather as eosinophilic hyperplasia.

DR. HARDY: I don't believe in eosinophilic hyperplasia. There is a tumor, an adenoma, that may be well localized or may grow rapidly towards the aponeural sheet, but it is an adenoma, not a hyperplasia.

DR. HORWITH: In Dr. Ray's absence, I would like to point out that in New York we don't feel that all patients with acromegaly have discrete lesions in the pituitary. Dr. Ray has gone on record to point out that frequently the tumor tissue is diffusely spread throughout the gland making it quite impossible to differentiate the adenomatous tissue from the rest of the pituitary.

DR. KRIEGER: Dr. Hardy, did you say that there has been some alteration in the floor of the sella as seen on tomography in all of your patients with microadenomas? Especially in the cases of Cushing's disease that you presented in whom normal sellas were reported, was the floor of the sella completely normal, or could you see some displacement of the sellar floor with tomography?

DR. HARDY: Not always, but we have to study the sella carefully with tomography to rule out abnormality.

DR. KAUFMAN: Minor degrees of asymmetry of the sella are not unusual. They have been well described by Di Chiro and by Rådberg. The problem is to correlate these changes with small adenomas of the pituitary. The ones Dr. Hardy illustrated do show minor degrees of asymmetry of the sella compatible with the size of the adenoma proven at surgery. The small adenoma will give sellar changes which may be localized or one-sided. Usually the adenomas which cause these changes are about 10 mm or more in size by the time they involve the sella floor and certainly that size or larger when they involve an anterior clinoid process.

The question essentially is one of evaluation of the size and configuration of the gland in a normal size sella. If the sella is 10×12 mm or slightly larger, one will usually have the normal gland in the bottom one-half of the sella and the upper surface will be concave upward. If there is an adenoma of about 10 mm or so, as in our case of galactorrhea in a male, then the gland literally will bow upward. In the case presented it had not gone beyond the confines of the sella, but the upper surface was convex upward. In the A-P projection of this case, no change in the floor occurred. The location of this particular adenoma could not be predicted from the studies. In essence, if you have a small sella, the gland fills the sella completely and in many cases bows slightly out of the sella. This would give a convex upward surface and radiographically one could not say whether an abnormality was present. If, however, the sella is larger than the usual size of the gland as described by Rasmussen and others, then one would not expect the pituitary gland to fill the entire sella and certainly not in those cases to give a convex upward surface even though it is within the confines of the sella as visualized on radiographs. One has to consider the size of the adenoma relative to the size of the sella and recognize that with certain combinations one cannot make the diagnosis.

DR. DI CHIRO: I would like to point out the necessity, indeed the indispensability, of studying the sella turcica in three dimensions. In my office I have a series of at least 12 cases of sella turcica radiograms, perfectly normal in the lateral views, but showing marked changes in the frontal projections. You are going to miss a lot of pathology if you do not study the sella in the three dimensions.

DR. KRIEGER: How successful is transsphenoidal surgery in cases of craniopharyngiomas, which may be so difficult to remove totally, even with transfrontal approaches?

DR. GUIOT: In our series a few cases of craniopharyngioma were operated on by the nasal route, but I must confess that half of those were not diagnosed correctly prior to surgery since the tumor was believed to be an adenoma. Occasionally craniopharyngiomas do appear as strictly intrasellar tumors, but they are extremely rare.

DR. HARDY: I have removed some microcraniopharyngiomas in children with excellent results. There are clearcut indications for intracranial approaches or transsphenoidal approaches. Indeed, it is possible to make a complete excision of the capsule of the craniopharyngioma transsphenoidally with preservation of the normal gland. In over 20 cases, I have done 12 craniopharyngiomas transsphenoidally. I think it is a problem of anatomy. To begin with, there are two types of craniopharyngiomas, which originate above the diaphragma sellae and those which arise underneath the diaphragm. The first should be approached intracranially. Some patients have a history of hypopituitarism first and later have visual problems.

In those children who have a very enlarged sella turcica, the craniopharyngioma has taken origin from the bottom of the sella, and growth has resulted in a cystic ballooning of the diaphragma sellae while the primary lesion remained below. I believe it is logical to take these out from below. As a matter of fact, it is logical and more convenient to make a radical excision of these lesions from below.

Sometimes a combined procedure is advisable in patients with acute increased intracranial pressure with a large cystic lesion in a large sella turcica. The first operation is just a puncture of the lesion to remove the fluid and obtain a mechanical decompression. Then we have time to complete endocrinological work-up and finally decide whether to go back from above or from below.

DR. GUIOT: In acromegaly, when there is a large sella, do you think it is because there is a large tumor? Why is the sella enlarged? Sometimes we see a large sella and the diaphragm is depressed into the sella. So I wonder why the sella is large.

DR. DI CHIRO: I think that the sellar enlargement in acromegaly is due to direct compression by the adenoma. I have taken part in a study sponsored by the National Pituitary Agency on the effects of growth hormone treatment in a very large group of dwarfs, mostly hypopituitary dwarfs. The body growth response of these patients to the growth hormone has been dramatic, but the sella turcica size has remained unchanged, even in patients followed for several years of treatment. In these patients the growth hormone supplementation has not, therefore, modified the sella turcica volume. From these observations I would infer that in acromegaly, the large sella is not due to an indirect hormonal effect, but rather to direct pressure.

V. Radiation treatment of pituitary tumors

A. Conventional radiation therapy
B. Heavy particle radiation therapy

Treatment of chromophobe adenomas of the pituitary gland and acromegaly

GLENN E. SHELINE

Section of Radiation Oncology, Department of Radiology, University of California, San Francisco, Calif., U.S.A.

This paper represents a review of our experience with chromophobe adenomas of the pituitary gland and with acromegaly. It includes data from approximately 300 patients who received their entire therapy at the University of California, San Francisco (UCSF). Some of these patients have been included in previous reports.[1-3] The discussion of chromophobe adenomas considers the course of the untreated adenoma, results of treatment of adenomas, and the results of retreatment of our own treatment failures. Both radiation therapy and treatment by transsphenoidal cryohypophysectomy for acromegaly will also be discussed. Since authors representing most points of view are included in this symposium, an exhaustive literature review will not be attempted.

Chromophobe adenomas

Untreated chromophobe adenomas

Between 1934 and 1968, a diagnosis of chromophobe adenoma was made for 64 patients who, at least initially, did not receive treatment for this disease.[1] Thirty-three of the adenomas were of microscopic size and diagnosed only by necropsy. Seven others, also diagnosed only upon postmortem examination, were large enough to cause erosion of the sella turcica but had been unsuspected clinically. Eight other patients with diagnosed chromophobe adenoma were seen only once.

This leaves 16 patients who had a presumptive diagnosis of chromophobe adenoma and who were observed for periods of 4-20 years (Table I). The diagnosis of chromophobe adenoma was based partly on the presence of a grossly enlarged sella with no evidence of acromegaly or of the type of calcification frequently associated with a craniopharyngioma. One-half of the patients had visual field defects, and most had hypopituitarism and pneumoencephalographic evidence of an intrasellar mass. Tending to confirm the diagnosis was the fact that during the subsequent period of observation in 13 of the 16 patients the sella turcica increased in size, visual field deficits appeared or increased, or both visual field deficit and size of the sella increased. For the 16 patients treatment was withheld either because the patient refused therapy or because the physician thought the disease inactive or the patient untreatable.

Table I *Initially untreated chromophobe adenomas (16 patients)*

	No. of patients	Interval (years)*
Normal visual fields		
Never treated	2	4,20
Ultimately treated because of		
larger sella	3 ⎫	5, 6, 15
appearance of visual field deficit	2 ⎬ 6	1, 5
progressive headaches	1 ⎭	4
Visual field deficit		
Never treated	0	—
Ultimately treated because of		
increased deficit	5 ⎫ 8	1/2, 2, 3, 5, 8
increased deficit and sella	3 ⎭	1, 4, 5

* Interval between observation and date of treatment or of last follow-up examination.

Of the 16 diagnosed but untreated adenomas, 2 showed neither clinical nor roentgeno-graphic evidence of growth. The other 14 displayed evidence of growth – some as early as 6 months, others as late as 15 years from the time of the initial diagnosis. In 13 patients the sella turcica increased in size, visual field defects appeared or increased, or both visual field deficit and size of sella increased. One patient developed progressive incapacitating headaches. All 14 patients with evidence of growth of the adenoma eventually required treatment. The post-treatment result in 7 was either an increase in the visual field defect as compared with that initially present or a visual field defect where none existed initially. Another patient developed a persistent cerebrospinal fluid rhinorrhea. This patient, 18 years of age when he was first seen, was observed periodically for 6 years, during which time the tumor grew from one that caused slight sellar enlargement and erosion to one that completely obliterated the sphenoid sinus. Thus, 14 of the 16 patients observed without treatment eventually required treatment and 8 had permanent damage that could have been prevented by earlier treatment.

Although these data do not permit numerical evaluation of the risk involved, they do indicate that, given time, many apparently inactive chromophobe adenomas will show growth.

Treated chromophobe adenomas

Between 1934 and 1968, 133 patients were given primary treatment at UCSF for chromo-phobe adenoma of the pituitary gland. The results of treatment in these 133 patients are presented here. An approximately equal number of patients, who received part of their primary treatment elsewhere or were referred to us only for recurrence of the tumor, are ex-cluded from this study. Also excluded are those patients who, during the earlier years, received radiation therapy with doses of less than 2000 rads; such exclusion seems reasonable in view of the reported dose-dependence for radiation control of chromophobe adenomas. [2,4]

During the period of study, 3 treatment regimens were used: radiation therapy alone (RT), surgical decompression with biopsy and partial removal of the adenoma (S), and partial surgical resection plus postoperative radiation therapy (S+RT). With the exception of 2 patients, in whom the surgical procedure was carried out via the transsphenoidal approach, all surgical patients underwent a craniotomy. Histologic proof of the diagnosis was obtained for all patients undergoing operation.

Only one of the 20 patients treated by radiation therapy alone had biopsy confirmation of the diagnosis. In this case biopsy material was obtained from the nasopharyngeal exten-sion of the adenoma. Among the 19 patients without a histologic diagnosis, all had enlarged eroded sellae, 15 had visual field defects consistent with a suprasellar mass, all 4 with normal visual fields had pneumoencephalographic evidence of a suprasellar mass, 15 had hypopituitarism, and none had the type of calcification characteristic of a craniopharyngioma. As will be seen, 73 % of those with visual field defects showed improvement following RT, indicating that the lesion present was radiosensitive and thus not an aneurysm. It seems reasonable to assume that the presumptive diagnosis of a chromophobe adenoma was correct in nearly all, if not all, of the 19 patients treated without biopsy.

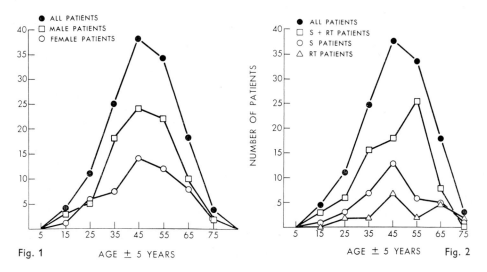

Fig. 1   AGE ± 5 YEARS

AGE ± 5 YEARS   Fig. 2

Fig. 1   Number of patients according to age at time of diagnosis.
Fig. 2   Number of patients according to age and type of treatment.

Composition of patient material.   Although the ratio of male to female patients was 1.7 to 1.0, little or no difference was found in their age distribution (Fig. 1). The age distribution of patients according to method of treatment is shown in Figure 2: 35 % (7/20) of the RT patients were older than 60 years of age, whereas only 12 % (14/133) of those undergoing surgical procedures (S and S+RT) were over 60 years.

Initial findings for the 3 groups of treated patients are presented in Table II. The various treatment groups appear comparable with respect to incidence of enlarged sellae and locally invasive adenomas. Since some surgical patients did not have complete endocrine studies before operation, comparison of the incidence of hypopituitarism for the various treatment

Table II   *Initial findings for patients subsequently treated for chromophobe adenoma (133 patients)*

Abnormality	No. of patients			
	RT (20 patients)	S (36 patients)	S+RT (77 patients)	Total (133 patients)
Visual field defect	15	35	72	122
Enlarged sella	20	34	74	128
Hypopituitarism	15	17	39	71
Nasopharyngeal extension	1	0	1	2
Other invasion	—	6	5	11
Cystic lesions	—	14	19	33

groups is probably not meaningful. A disproportionately high percentage (25 %) of RT patients had normal visual fields as opposed to the low percentage (5 %) of those patients who underwent surgery. A total of 11 patients had normal visual fields. In one of these patients there was massive invasion of the brain and in 2 others the adenoma extended into the nasopharynx. Both patients with nasopharyngeal extension subsequently developed cerebrospinal fluid rhinorrhea. In one it occurred subsequent to nasopharyngeal biopsy and RT, and in the other it occurred after transsphenoidal hypophysectomy.

The 33 patients with cystic adenomas represent 29 % of all the operated patients (Table III). Cystic lesions were found in 14 or 34 % of the female and in 19 or 26 % of the male operated

Table III   *Age distribution of patients with cystic chromophobe adenomas compared with that of all patients receiving surgical treatment*

Age	No. of patients with cystic adenomas			Total No. of patients
(years)	Male	Female	Total	operated on
11–20	2	1	3	4
21–30	2	2	4	9
31–40	5	2	7	23
41–50	4	3	7	31
51–60	4	5	9	32
61–70	2	1	3	13
> 70	0	0	0	1
Total	19	14	33	113

patients. Of all the operated patients 30 years of age or younger, 54 % had cystic adenomas. This suggests that the younger patient may have a greater tendency toward cystic lesions. The numbers, however, are small.

The duration of visual symptoms for the 3 treatment groups and for those with cystic adenomas is shown in Table IV. The only clear difference between treatment groups is in the large fraction (8 of 20) of the RT patients who had no visual symptoms. About one-third of all patients had visual symptoms for longer than one year; the average duration was 13.5 months. The percentage of adenomas found to be cystic did not correlate with duration of symptoms.

Table IV   *Duration of visual symptoms in patients with cystic chromophobe adenomas as related to that in the 3 treatment groups*

Duration of symptoms	No. of patients			No. of patients with
(months)	RT	S	S+RT	cystic adenomas*
None	8	1	11	4 (33 %)
< 1–2	2	3	11	4 (28 %)
> 2–6	2	8	10	6 (33 %)
> 6–12	0	10	18	8 (28 %)
> 12–24	1	5	14	6 (32 %)
> 24–36	1	4	4	2 (25 %)
> 36	4	3	5	1 (13 %)
No data	2	2	4	2 (33 %)
Total	20	36	77	33 (29 %)

* Percentage is based on total number of patients who underwent surgical procedures (S and S+RT).

Selection of therapy. Selection factors which played a role in determining which patients were to receive radiation therapy without surgical decompression are given in Table V. As stated above, the RT group contained a disproportionately high number of older patients as well as of those who had no visual symptoms or visual field defects. The older group accounts for most of the patients considered to be poor surgical risks.

Table V *Reason for selection of radiation therapy only (RT) as treatment for chromophobe adenomas*

Reason	No. of patients
Patient refused surgery	5
Poor surgical risk	6
Normal visual fields	5*
Minimal field deficit	2
Unknown	2
Total	20

* One patient had biopsy-proved chromophobe adenoma, the other 4 had suprasellar tumors verified by pneumoencephalogram.

Primary surgical decompression was usually selected for those patients who had large lesions or evidence of recent change in visual fields. Patients whose visual fields failed to improve after surgical decompression tended to be referred for postoperative radiation therapy.

Radiation therapy. In general, radiation therapy was given via bilateral opposed fields using 1 MeV or higher energy photon beams with radiation doses to the pituitary of 4000–5000 rads. The overall treatment time was usually 5–6 weeks with 5 fractions per week. Several exceptions to this treatment policy occurred during the early period of this study. Twelve patients were treated with 250 kVp or 400 kVp X-rays, and 13 received doses between 2000 and 4000 rads.

Results. A tumor was considered to be controlled as long as there was no evidence of further growth and any improvement in symptoms or signs was maintained. Although all available data were used in the evaluation of results, primary reliance was placed on serial visual field determinations performed by a neuro-ophthalmologist.

The changes in visual fields which occurred within the first 12 months after treatment are shown in Tables VI and VII. Each eye is considered separately and the visual deficits are

Table VI *Visual field response to treatment of chromophobe adenomas*

Deficit before therapy*	Visual field after therapy											
	Normal			Improved, not normal			No change			Worsened		
	RT	S	S+RT	RT	S	S+RT	RT	S	S+RT	RT	S	S+RT
None	11	5	12	0	0	0	0	0	0	0	1	0
≦ 1/4	11	7	21	2	2	1	4	0	7	0	0	4
> 1/4 to ≦ 1/2	0	8	27	6	11	19	4	1	31	0	4	8
> 1/2 to > HM**	0	0	1	0	4	1	0	2	8	0	0	1
HM to blind	0	1	0	2***	2	0	0	2	5	0	3	0
Total	22	21	61	10	19	21	8	5	51	0	8	13

* There were insufficient data for 3 eyes of the S series and 8 eyes of the S+RT series.
** HM = vision limited to perception of hand motion.
*** Minimal improvement.

Table VII   *Results of treatment of chromophobe adenomas for eyes with deficit involving one-half or less of visual field*

Visual field after therapy	Treatment group			
	RT	S	S+RT	S and S+RT
Normal	40 %	46 %	41 %	42 %
Improved	30 %	39 %	17 %	22 %
No change	30 %	3 %	32 %	26 %
Worse	0	12 %	10 %	11 %

tabulated according to the fraction of the field which showed reduced vision. Classification of a visual field deficit as '> ½ to ≤ ½' means that the deficit involved more than a quarter but not more than one-half of the field. 'HM' means that vision was limited to perception of hand motion. The designation '> ½ to > HM' includes eyes in which the defect involved more than one-half of the field but in which there was useful vision.

If patients with normal pretreatment visual fields are excluded from the analysis, treatment resulted in some degree of improvement in 73 % of the RT, 75 % of the S, and 52 % of the S+RT patients. The average for the 2 surgical series was 58 %. The difference between 73 % improved visual fields for the RT and 58 % for the combined surgical series (S and S+RT) is probably because the surgical patients tended to have more extensive visual defects. The pretreatment defect involved more than a quarter of a field in 70 % of the combined surgical groups but only 30 % of the RT patients had such defects.

Table VII represents an attempt to get around the bias introduced by the treatment selection factors. In this table, consideration is limited to patients with eyes having relatively early and approximately comparable deficits, i.e. deficits present but involving one-half or less of the visual field. In these patients, normal fields followed therapy in 40 % of those patients treated by radiation alone, 46 % by surgery alone, and 41 % by surgery plus radiation therapy. Improvement, but without return to completely normal fields, followed treatment by RT, S, and S+RT in an additional 30 %, 39 %, and 17 % of the patients, respectively. The low incidence, namely 3 %, of eyes showing no change after surgery alone (S) indicates that patients in whom improvement did not follow decompression were almost invariably referred for postoperative irradiation. Because the initial improvement in visual fields of S+RT patients is largely due to the decompression, it was thought valid to combine the 2 surgical series (S and S+RT) for the purpose of comparison with the radiation series (RT). When this was done (right-hand column of Table VII), the only difference between those treated with irradiation alone and those treated with surgery, with or without irradiation, is that 11 % of the surgery patients experienced a permanent increase in visual field defect. With this exception, the percentage of visual fields improved or remaining unchanged

Table VIII   *Current status of all patients treated for chromophobe adenomas*

Status	No. of patients		
	RT	S	S+RT
No known recurrence			
Under observation	11	3	55
D.I.D.*	8	1	14
Lost to follow-up study	1	5	0
Known recurrence	0	19	7
Unassessable (brain damage)	0	0	1
Surgical death	—	8	—
Total	20	36	77

* D.I.D. = Dead from intercurrent disease without evidence of recurrence.

during the first year after treatment is virtually the same whether the initial procedure was with irradiation or surgery.

The current status of all treated patients is summarized in Table VIII. In the RT series, 11 of 20 patients remain under observation and there has been no known recurrence. Eight patients have died of intercurrent disease without recurrence and 1 refuses to return for study. The high intercurrent disease death rate in this group was because many of the elderly patients selected for RT had other non-related medical problems. Patients treated by surgery alone have shown a high recurrence rate. Of the 28 patients who survived the surgical procedure but did not receive postoperative irradiation therapy, 19 (68 %) have had a definite recurrence, one has died of intercurrent disease, and 5 have been lost to follow-up study. Only 3 of this group are under observation and their disease known to be controlled. Of the 77 patients treated by S+RT, 55 are living and the disease currently under control, 14 have died of intercurrent disease without evidence of recurrence, and only 7 (9 %) have adenomas which have recurred.

Absolute and determinate control rates, as a function of time after treatment, for the various treatment groups are presented in Table IX. The *absolute rate* includes all patients.

Table IX   *Control rates for treated chromophobe adenomas*

Post-treatment interval (years)	Absolute control rate			Determinate control rate		
	RT	S	S+RT	RT	S	S+RT
2	$\frac{17}{20}$ (85 %)	$\frac{18}{36}$ (50 %)	$\frac{74}{77}$ (96 %)	$\frac{17}{17}$ (100%)	$\frac{18}{23}$ (75 %)	$\frac{74}{74}$ (100%)
5	$\frac{13}{14}$ (93 %)	$\frac{9}{32}$ (28 %)	$\frac{54}{62}$ (87 %)	$\frac{13}{13}$ (100%)	$\frac{9}{21}$ (43 %)	$\frac{54}{57}$ (95 %)
10	$\frac{4}{6}$	$\frac{2}{29}$ (7 %)	$\frac{27}{36}$ (75 %)	$\frac{4}{4}$	$\frac{2}{18}$ (11 %)	$\frac{27}{33}$ (82 %)
15	$\frac{1}{2}$	$\frac{0}{24}$	$\frac{14}{22}$ (64 %)	$\frac{1}{1}$	$\frac{0}{15}$	$\frac{14}{19}$ (74 %)
20	$\frac{0}{2}$	$\frac{0}{21}$	$\frac{6}{13}$ (46 %)	—	$\frac{0}{13}$	$\frac{6}{9}$ (67 %)

The *determinate rate* was calculated by excluding the patients who died as a result of the surgical procedure as well as those dead of intercurrent disease or lost to follow-up study. These exclusions were made because: (1) many patients who were selected for RT had severe non-related medical problems which resulted in a high intercurrent disease death rate independent of the form of therapy; (2) the number of postoperative deaths may have been influenced by the fact that the larger and more aggressive adenomas were selected for initial decompression; and (3) intercomparison between the 2 surgical series would certainly require elimination of the postoperative deaths. Disregarding patients who died of intercurrent disease biases the results in favor of RT, but removal of patients dying postoperatively or lost to follow-up provides a bias in favor of surgery. As will be discussed below, the conclusions to be reached are the same whether the absolute or the determinate rate is used.

For periods up to 10 years, there was no evident difference in the absolute control rates for those patients treated with RT as compared with those treated with S+RT. The determinate control rates are also similar for the 2 series in which radiation therapy was used. There are too few RT patients observed longer than 10 years to permit comparison at later times.

Results for both the RT and S+RT groups are clearly better than those for the S group at all intervals after treatment, regardless of whether comparison is based on the absolute or the determinate rates. For example, at 5 years the absolute control rates for the RT and the S+RT series are 93 % and 87 % respectively, but only 28 % for the S series. At 10 years the absolute and determinate control rates for the S+RT series were 75 % and 82 %, whereas they were only 7 % and 11 % for the S group. By 15 years all patients treated only by a surgical procedure had had a recurrence, but one-half to two-thirds of those patients treated with S+RT were without recurrence even at 20 years. Furthermore, it is probable that the late control rates in the S+RT patients would be even higher if some of the patients treated during the early phase of the study period had received larger doses of irradiation.

Recurrence as related to radiation dose. Earlier reports[2, 4] have suggested that a direct relationship exists between control rate and radiation dose. The data presented in Table X, although containing too few low-dose cases to permit a definitive conclusion, are consistent

Table X *Recurrence of chromophobe adenomas as related to radiation dose*

Dose	Number treated		Known recurrences (years)*	
(rads)	RT	S+RT	RT	S+RT
2000 to < 3000	0	5	0	2 (0.5 and 6.0)
3000 to < 4000	1	7	0	1 (2.5)
≥ 4000	19	65	0	4 (1.0 to 9.6)

* Time of recurrence in years.

with such a relationship. With doses between 2000 and 3000 rads, 2 of 5 lesions have recurred. On the other hand, only 4 lesions in 84 patients receiving doses of 4000 or greater have recurred. Since 1959, 34 patients have been treated with doses greater than 4000 rads and observed at least 5 years; there has been only one recurrence (Table XI)*.

Complications. In the S and the S+RT groups, the visual field deficit was permanently greater after treatment in 21 of the 200 eyes for which data were available (Table XII). In each case the change was noted immediately following and was directly attributable to the surgical procedure. Seven patients, about 5 % of those operated, experienced major damage

Table XI *Recurrence of chromophobe adenomas in patients irradiated since 1959**

Time at risk	Number treated		Known recurrences	
(years)	RT	S+RT	RT	S+RT
5	9	25	0	1
10	1	5	0	0

* All doses were greater than 4000 rads.

---

* This single recurrence was not evident from clinical examination, visual field change, or plain skull roentgenograms; it was found as a small suprasellar tumor on repeat pneumoencephalograms. The pneumoencephalograms were done one year post-irradiation as part of a re-evaluation of a carotid aneurysm which had been discovered at the time of the original treatment.

Table XII   *Analysis of visual fields made worse by surgical treatment of chromophobe adenomas*

A. Minor increase in deficit: 11 eyes (9 patients)

B. Major increase in deficit: 10 eyes (7 patients)

Before surgery	After surgery
3 patients: bilateral hemianopsia	bilateral blindness
1 patient: blind+hemianopsia	bilateral blindness
3 patients: unilateral hemianopsia (i.e. contralateral eye normal in 1 and hemianopic in 2)	unilateral blindness (i.e. contralateral eye unchanged)

to vision. In 4 patients with one-half of one or both visual fields intact preoperatively, the end result was total blindness. Three patients with a hemianopic deficit in one eye became blind in that eye but had useful vision remaining in the second eye.

The major complications of treatment, other than damage to optic nerves, are shown in Table XIII. There were 8 deaths due to the surgical procedure, 7% of all patients operated.

Table XIII   *Complications other than visual in treatment of chromophobe adenomas*

Complication	Treatment group		
	RT	S	S+RT
Operative deaths	—	8	—
Cerebrospinal fluid rhinorrhea			
transient	0	0	2
permanent	1	0	0
Wound infection	—	2	0
Severe brain damage	0	1	2
Permanent cranial nerve damage	0	1	1

In the 90 patients operated since 1945 there have been 4 postoperative deaths: one due to a cerebral infarct and the other 3 involved adenomas which had extensive local invasion. This represents a 30% postoperative death rate in lesions described at the time of surgery as locally invasive.

Cerebrospinal fluid (CSF) rhinorrhea occurred in 2 patients in whom the tumor had extended into the nasopharynx and in one in whom there was erosion through the floor of the sphenoid sinus. There were 3 instances of severe brain damage resulting in epilepsy and mental deterioration. The 2 instances in patients treated by S+RT involved lesions that extensively infiltrated the brain and it was not possible to determine whether the brain damage was due to the adenoma, the treatment, or a combination of both*. Many patients had transient postoperative electrolyte problems, cranial nerve palsies, diabetes insipidus, or increased steroid requirements.

Other than epilation, usually transient, no complication has definitely been attributable to radiation therapy. One of the patients with CSF rhinorrhea was in the RT group but his adenoma extended into the nasopharynx where it had been biopsied.

Summary.   The initial response of the visual fields was the same whether treatment was by surgical decompression alone or by surgical decompression followed by radiation therapy. The control rates – both absolute and determinate – showing freedom from recurrence

---

* One had received excessive irradiation (7200 rads in 32 days via 10 × 10 cm bilateral opposed fields) and the other has had 2 craniotomies and 2 courses of radiation therapy.

were, however, much greater at all intervals from 2 to 20 years when postoperative irradiation was given. In fact after 10 years, no patient without irradiation was free of recurrence. With respect to both visual field improvement and lack of recurrence, patients treated by radiation therapy alone did as well as those given combined therapy (S+RT).

In terms of mortality and morbidity, radiation therapy alone yielded the best result. No major complication could be attributed to irradiation. Surgical procedures, on the other hand, yielded a 7 % mortality rate, and about 5 % of the patients experienced major damage to the optic nerves or chiasm.

Because of differences in selection factors used to determine the form of therapy for each patient, direct comparison of the results of primary irradiation with surgical decompression is open to question. It is the author's opinion, however, that selected cases of presumed chromophobe adenomas may properly be treated by radiation therapy alone. However, whenever a reasonable doubt of the diagnosis or a severe or recently changed visual field deficit exists, primary surgical decompression is necessary. If the primary therapy is irradiation, surgery should be reserved for irradiation failure. On the other hand, irradiation should be given postoperatively for all patients initially treated by surgery.

Treatment of recurrent chromophobe adenomas

Twenty-two of our 26 known treatment failures have been retreated. Table XIV shows the secondary treatment used and the results thereof. Of those adenomas initially treated by surgery alone, 10 were retreated by means of radiation therapy. Eight of the 10 showed improvement of their visual fields and had no complication attributable to treatment. Four, however, subsequently recurred again.

Table XIV   *Visual field improvement in patients with retreated chromophobe adenomas*

Secondary treatment	Improved by secondary treatment*	
	Initially treated by S	Initially treated by S+RT
RT	8 of 10 (4)	1 of 1 (1)
S	1 of 2 (1)	2 of 2 (1)
S+RT	2 of 3 (1)	1 of 3 (0)

* Number in parentheses indicates number that recurred again.

Eleven patients had a secondary craniotomy, with or without RT; 6 showed improvement which, to date, has been maintained in 3. Following secondary craniotomy there were, however, 3 significant complications. These consisted of postoperative death in one patient and an acute brain syndrome with incapacitating frontal lobe seizures in another. Neither of these patients had had radiation therapy. The third patient, initially treated by S+RT, became totally incapacitated (deaf, dumb and blind) after retreatment 5 years later by S+RT. Since this patient received only 2600 rads initially and the retreatment was limited to 3000 rads, it seems unlikely that the damage was due to radiation therapy but rather that it was surgically induced.

In summary, of 22 patients retreated 15 showed a positive response but there were major complications in 3 and 8 have already recurred again. Such results of retreatment emphasize the importance of the primary treatment. It is thought that many of the recurrences could have been prevented with adequate initial radiation therapy. As indicated previously, most of our failures occurred in patients not irradiated or irradiated with less than optimal doses.

Acromegaly

Between 1942 and 1959, 65 patients with acromegaly were studied at UCSF. Approximately one-half (37 patients) had convincing clinical and laboratory evidence of active acromegaly and were treated with conventional radiation therapy. Surgery was, at that time, usually reserved for irradiation failures.

Results, presented in part in an earlier report[3], were judged on the basis of change in endocrine activity and pressure effects. The growth hormone assay was not available at the time these patients were treated; it was necessary, therefore, to base the evaluation of endocrine activity on evidence of hypermetabolism, decreased carbohydrate tolerance, increased serum phosphorus levels, adrenal hyperactivity (as measured by 17-ketosteroid and 17-hydroxysteroid excretion), and growth of skeletal and soft tissues. Reversal of chemical abnormalities and arrest or reversal of soft tissue changes were considered to represent a successful result. Pressure effects were evaluated separately on the basis of visual field deficits, expansion of the sella, and persistent unusual headaches. Pressure effects were considered to be controlled if there was improvement in visual fields, cessation of headaches, and no further expansion of the sella.

In evaluating the results of treatment, it should be noted that 41 % (15 patients) of this group, treated by conventional radiation therapy, had initial extrasellar extension of the pituitary tumor sufficient to produce a visual field deficit. On the other hand, cryohypophysectomy and heavy-particle irradiation have usually been limited to tumors without significant suprasellar extension[5, 6].

The control rate for patients treated with relatively low doses of irradiation (3500 rads or less) was about 25 % (Table XV). Seven of the low-dose failures were salvaged by retreat-

Table XV   *Results of conventional radiation therapy for acromegaly*

	Fraction (%) of patients controlled	
	Initial dose $\leq$ 3500 rads	Initial dose $>$ 3500 rads
Controlled by Initial treatment		
endocrine hyperactivity	5/19 (26 %)	13/17 (77 %)
increased pressure	5/17 (29 %)	14/18 (78 %)
Retreatment (irradiation)	7/19	None
Total controlled	12/19 (63 %)	14/18 (78 %)

ment using additional irradiation. When the dose was greater than 3500 rads the control rate was 78 %. Within each dose range, the control rates for endocrine hyperactivity and for the pressure effects were the same. Fourteen of the 15 patients with abnormal visual fields had posttreatment visual field evaluations. In 10 the fields became normal. Induction of hypopituitarism by irradiation was not seen in any patient. Complications occurred in 2 patients, both of whom were initially treated with a relatively low dose of irradiation and both eventually received multiple courses of radiation therapy. These complications consisted of transient superficial ulceration in the ear canal of one patient and a pituitary sarcoma in the other. Pituitary sarcomas have been described in non-irradiated patients and whether or not this sarcoma was radiation-induced is conjectural.

It is concluded from these results in patients treated before 1960 that about 75 % of acromegalic patients can be controlled by conventional radiation therapy and that the control rate is higher and the complication rate negligible for those receiving a single course of therapy with a dose in excess of 3500 rads.

Soon after the growth hormone assay became available[7], it was reported that the fasting serum growth hormone (FHG) level does not respond satisfactorily to conventional radiation therapy[8]. For example, at the NIH symposium in 1966, Glick reported on the results for 30 patients who had received conventional X-ray therapy with doses of at least 4000 rads. Only 7 of his 30 patients (about 25 %) had achieved FGH levels of less than 7.5 ng/ml at the time of reporting[8]. The initial studies implying the inadequacy of RT for treatment of acromegaly appeared about the time that techniques of transsphenoidal cryohypophysectomy (TCH) were being developed.

At UCSF since the mid-1960s, as a result of these reports, all active acromegalic patients in whom there was little or no suprasellar extension of the pituitary tumor have been treated by TCH. Before proceeding to the limited new information available for our patients treated by means of conventional radiation therapy, the results for our first 50 consecutive patients treated by TCH will be briefly reviewed. These results have been partially described in preliminary reports by Smith and Levin[5] and by Levin and his co-workers[9]. A more complete report by Levin is in preparation[10].

Before receiving cryohypophysectomy, 90 % of the patients had FGH levels greater than 10 ng/ml, 36 % had greater than 40 and the mean was 52 ± 11 ng/ml (Table XVI). After

Table XVI   *Results of transsphenoidal cryohypophysectomy in 50 acromegalic patients having no suprasellar extension**

	FGH level (ng/ml)
Pre-TCH	
90 % of patients	> 10
36 % of patients	> 40
Mean for all patients	52 ± 11
Post-TCH	
76 % of patients	< 10
Mean for all patients	17 ± 5

* Levin[11] and Levin et al. [5,6]

surgery, 76 % of these patients had levels less than 10 ng/ml and the mean was 17 ± 5 ng/ml. Improvement in other chemical and clinical parameters paralleled the decrease in growth hormone. When improvement occurred it became evident within 6 weeks and continued throughout the duration of observation. At the time of review 82 % of the TCH patients had been observed more than one year, some for 4 years. Decrease of the FGH level to 10 ng/ml or less occurred in 90 % of those patients who had a preoperative value of <40 ng/ml but in only 50 % of those patients with a preoperative value of > 40 ng/ml. In view of this 50 % failure rate of TCH in patients with FGH levels above 40 ng/ml, it is interesting that Lawrence et al.[11] found that one-half of their patients with pretreatment growth hormone levels greater than 40 ng/ml failed to respond to conventional external radiation therapy, but all their patients with initial levels less than 40 ng/ml responded favorably to radiation therapy.

Although a substantial number of transitory complications followed TCH in the UCSF series, permanent complications were limited to diabetes insipidus (4%), adrenal insufficiency (12 %), and hypothyroidism (10 %) (Table XVII). Thus, based on the UCSF surgical experience, TCH carries an acceptable morbidity rate and, to date, no mortality.

Table XVII *Complications of transsphenoidal cryohypophysectomy in 50 acromegalic patients having no suprasellar extension**

Complication	Frequency (%)
Transitory	
Diabetes insipidus	20
Extraocular muscle paralysis	14
Visual field defect	4
CSF rhinorrhea	6
Meningitis	4
Permanent	
Diabetes insipidus**	4
Adrenal insufficiency	12
Hypothyroidism	10

* Levin et al. [6]
** Remitted after 4–6 months.

Because patients with significant suprasellar extension are not suitable for cryohypophysectomy and about one-fourth of those so treated respond inadequately, interest in the possibilities of conventional external radiation therapy has reappeared. Conventional radiation therapy, if effective, would have the advantages of being applicable to all acromegalic patients regardless of extrasellar extension, of wide availability and associated with a minimum of complications. In this regard conventional radiation therapy is defined as megavoltage radiation given in a single fractionated course of about 5 treatments per week to a total dose of approximately 5000 rads in 5–6 weeks.

Because of the renewed interest in conventional radiation therapy for acromegaly, we have restudied our patients treated prior to 1965. All these patients had laboratory and clinical evidence of active acromegaly and it is assumed that the growth hormone levels were elevated at the time of treatment. Of 24 living patients treated prior to 1965, 17 have been re-examined. The other 7 are reportedly asymptomatic but unable to return for evaluation (for 6 this was because of excessive distances).

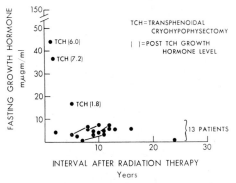

Fig. 3 FGH levels of 17 patients treated with conventional radiation therapy. 'TCH' means that a transsphenoidal cryohypophysectomy was performed at the time indicated by the black circle.

Figure 3 shows the FGH levels plotted as a function of time after radiation therapy for these 17 pre-1965 patients. Where more than one value is available for a particular patient, the points are connected with a line. At the time of restudy, 13 of the 17 patients had FGH levels of 7.5 ng/ml or less (considered in our laboratory to be values within the normal range). In 10 of these patients the level was ≤5 ng/ml. All 13 patients with normal FGH levels are free of clinical evidence of the disease.

At posttreatment intervals of 13 months to 9 years, the other 4 of the 17 patients were found to have elevated FGH levels and clinical evidence of hyperactivity. Three* of these 4 patients considered as radiation failures have now had TCH and are clinically controlled with normal growth hormone levels. In Figure 3 the postoperative growth hormone levels are shown in parentheses. The number of patients is small but the fact that all 3 radiation failures responded to TCH suggests that patients who do not respond to irradiation are not necessarily the ones who would have failed with TCH. Perhaps the 2 procedures complement each other.

Only 2 patients have been referred to us for radiation therapy since the growth hormone assay became available. The pretreatment and posttreatment FGH levels for these patients are shown in Figure 4. In one patient the FGH level dropped slowly until it reached the

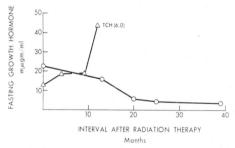

Fig. 4   Pretreatment and posttreatment FGH levels for 2 patients treated with conventional radiation therapy. 'TCH' means that a transsphenoidal cryohypophysectomy was performed; the past TCH FGH level is given in parentheses.

normal range in about 18 months. The second patient failed to respond to irradiation and 12 months later (too soon to evaluate the radiation therapy) was treated by TCH; this patient's FGH level subsequently decreased to the normal range.

These data, along with the results of Lawrence and co-workers, tend to refute the contention[8] that the FGH level does not respond satisfactorily to conventional radiation therapy, and are evidence that in many instances RT is effective in reducing FGH levels of the acromegalic patient to normal values.

Lawrence et al. reported in 1971 that 13 of 16 patients treated with conventional radiotherapy prior to 1965 had clinically inactive disease and growth hormone levels within the normal range (4 ± 4 ng/ml for adult men and 6 ± 4 ng/ml for women)[11]. They also reported that, 6 months to 4 years after treatment, 9 of 12 patients with preirradiation FGH levels of 20–332 ng/ml had posttreatment values within the normal range. From their report, the time required for the FGH levels to reach normal is not clear.

We are currently treating by means of conventional radiation therapy a group of patients considered TCH failures. These patients, however, may or may not respond to irradiation in the same way as would those with the type of acromegaly responsive to TCH. We would like to promote a study of the response to conventional radiation therapy of a randomly selected group of patients who are suitable for TCH. To be eligible for such a study a patient would be one in whom there is no urgency about reducing the growth hormone level but who, in all other respects, is qualified for transsphenoidal cryohypophysectomy. Failures

---

* Two of these 3 were operated at 13 months after radiation therapy; this interval is now known to be too short to permit evaluation of irradiation.

among either the irradiated or surgically treated patients would be reassigned to the alternate form of therapy.

Summary

(1.) Of 16 untreated patients with a presumptive diagnosis of chromophobe adenoma of the pituitary gland, 14 eventually required treatment. Growth of the adenoma during the period of observation (6 months to 15 years) resulted in additional and permanent damage for 8 patients.

(2.) A total of 133 patients with chromophobe adenomas were treated during the study period (1934–1968). Twenty received radiation therapy alone (RT), 36 had surgical decompression (S), and 77 had a surgical decompression followed by radiation therapy (S+RT). The improvement rate, judged primarily by change in visual fields, was approximately the same for all 3 modes of treatment. Patients who did not receive radiation therapy, however, showed a much higher recurrence rate than did those irradiated. At 10 years, the RT and S+RT patients had a control rate of about 75 % whereas that for the S patients was about 10 %. No patient treated without irradiation was controlled for 15 years. No significant complication could be definitely attributed to irradiation. The operative mortality rate was 7 %, and 5 % of the patients who underwent a surgical procedure experienced major damage of the optic nerves or chiasm.

It is concluded that radiation therapy alone is suitable treatment for selected patients with chromophobe adenomas and that whenever primary operative decompression is used radiation therapy should always follow.

(3.) At UCSF between 1966 and 1970, transsphenoidal cryohypophysectomy (TCH) was performed on 50 acromegalic patients, all of whom had elevated fasting growth hormone (FGH) levels. Approximately 75 % of these patients responded with clinical improvement and return of FGH levels to the normal range within 6 weeks. Measurement of FGH levels in 17 surviving patients treated with conventional radiation therapy before 1965 suggests a comparable control rate. Thirteen of the 17 pre-1965 patients are clinically free of evidence of active acromegaly and have FGH levels of ≤ 7.5 ng/ml. Three of the other 4 patients have been salvaged by secondary transsphenoidal cryohypophysectomy.

References

(1) SHELINE, G. E. (1971): Untreated and recurrent chromophobe adenomas of the pituitary. *Amer. J. Roentgenol.*, *112*, 768.

(2) SHELINE, G. E., BOLDREY, E. B. and PHILLIPS, T. L. (1964): Chromophobe adenomas of the pituitary gland. *Amer. J. Roentgenol.*, *92*, 160.

(3) SHELINE, G. E., GOLDBERG, M. B. and FELDMAN, P. (1961): Pituitary irradiation for acromegaly. *Radiology 76*, 70.

(4) KERR, H. D. (1948): Irradiation of pituitary tumors: results in 50 cases. *Amer. J. Roentgenol.*, *60*, 348.

(5) SMITH JR, L. J. and LEVIN, S. R. (1972): Manifestations and treatment of acromegaly. *Calif. Med.*, *116*, 57.

(6) LAWRENCE, J. H., TOBIAS, C. A., LINFOOT, J. A., BORN, J. L., LYMAN, J. T., CHONG, C. Y., MANOUGIAN, E. and WEL, W. C. (1970): Successful treatment of acromegaly: metabolic and clinical studies in 145 patients. *J. clin. Endocr.*, *31*, 180.

(7) GLICK, S. M., ROTH, J., YALOW, R. S. and BERSON S. A. (1963): Immunoassay of human growth hormone in plasma. *Nature (Lond.)*, *199*, 784.

(8) ROTH, J., GLICK, S. M., CUATRECASAS, P. and HOLLANDER, C. F. (1967): Acromegaly and other disorders of growth hormone secretion: combined Clinical Staff Conference at the National Institutes of Health. *Ann. intern. Med.*, *66*, 760.

(9)   LEVIN, S., SCHNEIDER, V., RUBIN, A., HOFELDT, F., BECKER, N., ADAMS, J., SEYMOUR, R. and FORSHAM, P. (1973): Rapid metabolic responses and lasting effects of cryohypophysectomy for acromegaly. In: *Abstracts, IV International Congress of Endocrinology, Washington, DC., 1972*, p. 133. Excerpta Medica, Amsterdam.
(10) LEVIN, S.: In preparation.
(11) LAWRENCE, A. M., PINSKY, S. M. and GOLDFINE, I. D. (1971): Conventional radiation therapy in acromegaly: a review and reassessment. *Arch. intern. Med.*, 128, 369.

Indications for, and results of, treatment of pituitary tumors by external radiation

SIMON KRAMER

Department of Radiation Therapy, Thomas Jefferson University Hospital, Philadelphia, Pa., U.S.A.

The pituitary adenomas have long been of particular interest to the radiation therapist. These benign tumors have been treated by radiation for many years; and since survival is usually prolonged, it has been possible to assess the effectiveness of radiation therapy, as well as any possible damage that may be caused by such treatment.

In judging the value of one form of therapy against another, it is essential to evaluate the quality of life which the patient will lead after his tumor has been cured. Ideally all abnormal pituitary function should be arrested, while the normal functions of the gland are preserved

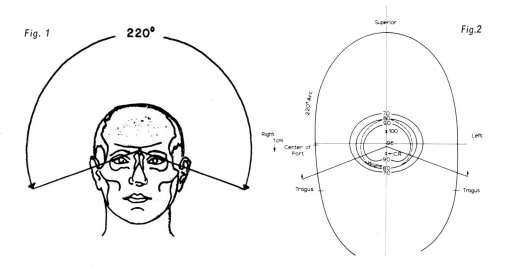

Fig. 1 Method of treatment with a 220° arc situated in the coronal plane.

Fig. 2 A typical isodose distribution for a 220° rotational field.

so that there will be a minimum need for endocrine replacement therapy. Supervoltage radiation therapy can achieve these goals in a high proportion of patients without causing appreciable morbidity. In patients in whom radiation therapy has failed to arrest excessive hormone production, or where the tumor has recurred, ablative procedures can be instituted without increased risk.

Because of the position of the pituitary gland, tumors in this region can be particularly well treated by beam-directed multiple fields or by rotational techniques. The advent of supervoltage therapy has made it possible to use small well-defined beams and to limit the high dose to the chosen target volume.

The technique most frequently employed by us is that of cobalt beam radiation with an arc rotation in the coronal plane. This technique is illustrated in Figures 1 and 2. The rotational arc most commonly chosen is 220°, but this arc can be increased or decreased to change the volume obtained. The positioning of the treatment arc is always carefully checked by means of the radiation therapy simulator, since the small size of the volume makes accurate positioning of the beams most important.

An alternative method presents itself where a large target volume is to be chosen because of the size of the tumor. Under these circumstances we use 2 lateral wedge fields and a central superior open field, as demonstrated in Figure 3. This gives an excellent homogenous dose within the target volume; it has the disadvantage of giving somewhat higher doses to the temporal lobes of the brain than does the rotational technique.

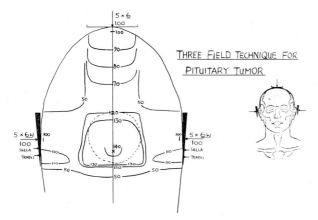

Fig. 3   Three-field treatment technique using 2 lateral wedges and a superior open field.

The management of pituitary tumors will be described separately for eosinophilic adenomas (acromegaly) and chromophobe tumors. We will mention our past experience with basophilic tumors only briefly.

Acromegaly

It has long been recognized that relatively small doses of radiation therapy will rapidly arrest the common symptoms of acromegaly, such as the acral, visual field and acuity changes, and the headaches so commonly found in this disease. Thus, until 25 years ago it was common practice to give perhaps 1000 rads and to repeat this course on many occasions as symptoms recurred. Since that time it has come to be recognized that a single course of radiation to a higher dose is considerably more successful in arresting the disease permanently and a great deal less likely to produce deleterious changes. Today, most radiation therapists give a single course of radiation therapy extending over 4–5 weeks. Until approximately 2 years ago it was our practice to deliver 4500 rads in $4\frac{1}{2}$ weeks, in daily fractions of 200 rads 5 times per week, for this disease. In the last 2–3 years, however, having found this dose to be entirely safe, and in the attempt to bring about a more rapid decrease in the growth hormone level, we have increased our tumor dose to 5000 rads in 5 weeks.

One of the most important developments in the management of acromegaly in recent years has been the radioimmunoassay of serum human growth hormone (HGH) levels. It has been suggested that these levels, which are invariably elevated in patients with acromegaly, are not reduced to normal by conventional radiation therapy[1]. Thus, although clinically the patient's disease is arrested, as evidenced by the disappearance of symptoms and the arrest of the progression of the acral changes, such a patient is supposed to run the risk of a persistently elevated HGH level. Our results, as well as the published data of Lawrence et al.[2] and Roth et al.[3], have shown that following conventional irradiation with 4000–5000 rads, the HGH serum levels do indeed return to normal or near-normal values, but that the decrease in such levels takes several months to become evident and may take as long as 1–2 years to return to normal. We therefore continue to believe that conventional radiation therapy is the treatment of choice for most patients with acromegaly because serious side effects are rare and the treatment is effective. Pretherapy surgery should be limited to those patients in whom there is an acute embarrassment of visual acuity or evidence of hemorrhage in a pituitary tumor. Of course, if the HGH level is extremely high in a patient, making it impossible to wait for the reduction in HGH level over a period of 6 months to 2 years, it may be necessary to resort to some form of pituitary destruction which is reported to bring about a more rapid decrease in HGH.

At the Thomas Jefferson University Hospital we have treated 29 patients with acromegaly between 1957 and 1971. Twenty-eight patients were treated on the basis of clinical diagnosis, and one patient was treated after craniotomy for what was thought to be a chromophobe adenoma, but was shown histologically to be an eosinophilic tumor. Radiation therapy was given as described; 2 patients received 4000 rads or less, while most of our patients treated in 1970–1971 received approximately 5000 rads or slightly more. Of our total group, 25 patients have shown no clinical evidence of recurrence, whereas 4 patients have had recurrences, a failure rate of 14 % (Table I).

Table I   *Acromegaly*

Total number of patients		29
Treated on clinical diagnosis	28	
Treated postcraniotomy	1	

Treatment		
Tumor doses (rads)	No. of patients	
≤ 4000	2	
4400–4600	20	
> 5000	7	

Factors: ^{60}Co   SA distance, 80 cm
160–220° arc rotation
Field size, 4.5×4.5–6.5×6.5 cm
1000 rads per week, five 200-rad fractions

Results		
No clinical evidence of recurrence	25	
Clinical evidence of recurrence	4	
Failure rate	4/29 or 14 %	

Table II   *Cases of acromegaly with no clinical evidence of recurrence*

Total number	25
Alive with no evidence of disease	21
< 10 yr	5/7
< 5 yr	12/16 (75 %)
< 3 yr	17/21 (81 %)
> 3 yr	4
Dead	
1 hypopituitarism (?) at 66 months	
1 coronary occlusion at 41 months	
1 ruptured splenic artery at 1 yr	
1 myocardial infarct at 2 yr	

Of the 25 patients who showed no evidence of recurrence (Table II), 21 are alive without evidence of progressive disease. Five of 7 have been alive for 10–15 years; 75 % of those treated more than 5 years ago are alive; 81 % have been alive for 3 years or more; and 4 patients have been alive for less than 3 years. Of the 4 patients who died without evidence of recurrence, one died of suspected hypopituitarism 5 years after treatment. This was a patient who refused to return for further management of any kind and slowly faded away at home. One patient had a coronary occlusion at 3 years and 5 months, one died of a ruptured splenic artery 1 year after treatment, and one died of myocardial infarct at 2 years.

Of the 4 patients who showed clinical evidence of recurrence (Table III), 3 were treated by craniotomy and hypophysectomy, and one was treated by a stereotaxic hypophysectomy. None of these 4 patients had any postoperative complications. Two patients are alive without evidence of disease, 5 and 11 years respectively, after their operations. In the first of these 2 patients, recurrence took place 3 years after his radiation; in the second one, within 4 months of the radiation. One patient died 15 months after his hypophysectomy, which took place 4 years and 7 months after his radiation treatment. One patient was lost to follow-up; he had a recurrence 3 years after his radiation therapy and we followed him for an additional 2 years after his operation.

Table III   *Cases of acromegaly with clinical evidence of recurrence*

Number of cases	4
Treated by craniotomy and hypophysectomy 3	
Treated by stereotaxic hypophysectomy 1	
Alive with no evidence of disease	
at 5 yr postop., 8 yr postradiation	1
at 11 yr postop., 11 yr 4 months postradiation	1
Dead (cause unknown)	
at 15 months postop., 6 yr postradiation	1
Lost to follow-up	
at 2 yr postop., 5 yr postradiation	1

Of considerable interest are the growth hormone studies which we have been able to perform on some of our patients. Nine patients were not studied; all these had been seen and treated prior to the availability of serum HGH tests. Eight patients were studied both pre- and postoperatively (Table IV). For the pretherapy levels found in these 8 patients, the fasting levels were 13–37 ng and the maximum levels, as measured during a glucose tolerance curve, ranged between 22 and 73 ng. The posttherapy levels of 7 of these patients have returned to normal in time intervals of 9 months to 2 years, with a fasting level of 4–10 ng

Table IV *Acromegaly: human growth hormone studies*

Not studied (1957–1966)		9
Studied pre- and posttherapy		8
Pretherapy HGH levels (ng)		
Fasting	13–37	
Maximum (glucose tolerance)	22–73	
Posttherapy HGH levels (ng)		
Return to normal (9 months–2 yr)		7/8
Fasting	4–10	
Maximum	8–9.9	
Still elevated (13 months)		1/8
Fasting	17.8	
	(pretherapy: 37)	
Maximum	20	
	(pretherapy: 60)	

and a maximum level of 8–9.9 ng*. One patient still has an elevated finding 13 months after treatment but even this shows marked reduction from the pretherapy levels. Details of these patients are given in Table IVa.

Eight patients were studied posttherapy only (Table V); all these patients have returned to normal levels, both at the fasting level and at the maximum level, as determined during a glucose tolerance curve.

One patient was studied pretherapy only; he died, without any further HGH level having been obtained, of heart failure 2 years later. Historically, he had had acromegaly for 27 years prior to therapy. Table Va gives the details of these patients.

Of the 4 patients who showed clinical evidence of recurrence of acromegaly, the HGH levels were studied in 3 patients (Table VI). In one patient, these were studied posthypophysectomy only and they were normal at 6 and 10 years postoperatively; this patient is well. Two patients were studied at the time of their recurrence, as well as posthypophysectomy. These studies show that even after hypophysectomy, at 3 and 5 months respectively, the postoperative HGH levels were still elevated; but in the one patient for whom data are available, it had returned to normal at 4 years postoperatively.

Thus, we conclude that of 19 patients who were studied post- or pre- and post-radiation therapy, 16 have shown no clinical evidence of recurrence; of these, 15 have returned to normal HGH values, and one patient has shown marked reduction of HGH levels 13 months posttherapy. Two of the 4 patients who showed clinical evidence of recurrence showed essentially elevated HGH levels. All 4 were submitted to surgery. It is reasonable, therefore, to conclude that the HGH levels by and large parallel the clinical condition of the patient and that, unless there is some overriding emergency, it would seem appropriate to treat acromegalic patients with a course of conventional radiation therapy and to withhold any surgical attack for a year or two, at least as long as their clinical condition is satisfactory.

It is of interest to note the need for endocrine replacement therapy in this group of patients (Table VII). Of 22 patients treated by radiation alone, 17 required no replacement therapy, 5 required some replacement therapy, including cortisone in only one patient. Of 7 patients who underwent craniotomy, hypophysectomy or both (one as a means of diagnosis,

---

* Normal levels in our laboratory are: Male resting, 0-2.5 ng/ml; after mild exercise, 0-4.5 ng/ml; Female resting, 0.15-20.5 ng/ml; after mild exercise, 3.5-20.0 ng/ml.

Table IVa *Details of 8 cases of acromegaly: growth hormone levels studied pre- and posttherapy*

Patient	Present status		HGH levels					Replacement	Complications
	Condition	Years posttherapy	Pretherapy		Years posttherapy	Posttherapy		therapy	
			Fasting (ng)	Maximum (ng)		Fasting (ng)	Maximum (ng)		
D.G.	Alive and well	5	23	31.5	$1\frac{1}{2}$ $1\frac{3}{4}$	13 4	19 8	Thyroid, Diabinese, cortisone	None
C.W.	Alive and well	$3\frac{1}{2}$	37	60	2	17.8	20.0	None	None
B.L.	Alive with partial vision	3	45	73	1 $1\frac{3}{4}$	25 3.5	25	Thyroid, cortisone	Very poor vision bilaterally. Craniotomy – no tumor; optic nerve vasculitis
M.C.	Alive and well	3	27	46	$\frac{2}{3}$ 1 2	28 16 5		None; cortisone for asthma	None
M.C.	Alive and well	$2\frac{1}{2}$	24	31	$2\frac{1}{4}$	9.5		None	Central scotoma right eye
L.P.	Alive with memory loss	$2\frac{1}{3}$	13	40	1 $1\frac{5}{6}$	9 4.2		None	Marked memory loss
I.T.	Alive and well	$1\frac{1}{2}$		22	$1\frac{1}{2}$	5.5		None	None
V.D.	Alive and well	1	40	40	$\frac{3}{4}$	10	9.9	Oricon	None

Table V   *Cases of acromegaly: human growth hormone studies*

Studied posttherapy only (1959–1970)	8
Posttherapy HGH levels (ng)	
Normal levels (31 months–13 yr)	8
Fasting 1.2–14	
Maximum 4–12.5	
Studied pretherapy only (1967)*	1
Pretherapy HGH levels (ng)	
Fasting 33	
Maximum 33.2	

* Died 2 yr later.

Table Va   *Details of 8 cases of acromegaly: growth hormone levels studied posttherapy only*

Patient	Present status		HGH levels			Replacement therapy
	Condition	Years post-therapy	Years post-therapy	Fasting (ng)	Maximum (ng)	
D.B.	Alive and well	13⅓	11	9.5	12.5	None
			13	4.5		
Q.F.	Alive and well	12	12	4	7	None; empty sella syndrome
M.J.G.	Alive and well	9	9	3	4	Clomiphene
M.K.	Alive and well	8¾	6	3	4	None
			8	3.4		
E.F.	Alive and well	7	7	1.2		None
H.F.	Alive, no vision left eye, post-craniotomy	5	5	1.2		Cortisone, thyroid postcraniotomy
C.C.	Alive and well	3¾	3¾	6		None
I.B.	Alive and well	3	3	14		None (insulin)

Table VI   *Acromegaly: human growth hormone studies in patients with recurrent tumors*

Patients with clinical evidence of recurrent acromegaly						3*
Studied posthypophysectomy only						1
HGH levels (ng):	6 yr postop.		10 yr postop.			
Fasting	5		2			
Maximum	9					
Studied at time of recurrence and posthypophysectomy						2
HGH levels (ng):	Patient E.S.			Patient J.S.		
	Pre-hyp.	3 months postop.	4 yr postop.	Pre-hyp.	5 months postop.	
Fasting	92	32	10	49	27.5	
Maximum	132	80	—	—	30.0	

* Three out of 4 such patients were studied.

2 in whom recurrences were suspected but not confirmed and 4 in whom recurrences were found), only one patient in whom no tumor was found at craniotomy is without replacement therapy; the other 6 require replacement with cortisone and thyroid hormone.

Table VII   *Cases of acromegaly: endocrine replacement therapy*

Patients treated by radiation alone	22
No replacement therapy	17
Replacement therapy	5
1 thyroid	
2 clomiphene, Oricon	
1 cortisone, thyroid, Diabinese pre- and posttradiation	
1 insulin	
Patients who underwent craniotomy/hypophysectomy	7
(1 diagnosis, 2 suspected recurrences, 4 recurrences)	
No replacement therapy	1
(no tumor found at craniotomy)	
Replacement therapy	6
(all on cortisone and thyroid)	

Morbidity, presumed due to irradiation, has occurred in 4 patients. One patient has suffered severe impairment of vision, occurring 6 months after irradiation. He was subsequently explored, but no cause for his visual deficit was found, nor was there recurrence of his pituitary tumor. A diagnosis of optic nerve vasculitis has been made by exclusion. Another patient developed a central scotoma in her right eye 9 months posttherapy. This has remained unchanged for the last 2 years. She, as well as a third patient, suffers from recurrent headaches due to an empty sella syndrome. The fourth patient has developed a marked memory loss 1 year after therapy. He shows no other neurological abnormality, but is unable to work.

Chromophobe adenomas

It has been well established that radiation therapy plays a major part in the management of chromophobe adenomas of the pituitary. It seems well founded that recurrence is high after conventional surgical management alone, and that adequate radiation therapy, either as an adjunct to surgery or as the sole treatment, offers the best results. Indeed many of my colleagues in radiotherapy believe that, once a clinical diagnosis has been established, the best management is by radiation therapy without surgical intervention.

I do not entirely share this belief, but think that in most patients the best approach lies in obtaining a biopsy prior to radiation. This can nowadays be obtained with minimum morbidity in skilled hands by the transsphenoidal route. Thus the histological nature of the tumor can be established and, since cystic lesions are frequently encountered in chromophobe adenomas (up to perhaps one-third of all tumors), it becomes possible to evacuate such a cyst before radiation; cystic tumors have been shown to be less amenable to radiation (probably because the pressure of the cyst causes the cells to be hypoxic and therefore less responsive to irradiation). It must also be remembered that craniopharyngiomas, although rare in adults, show calcification in less than 50 % of the cases in this category and may be clinically indistinguishable from chromophobe adenomas. It is, however, most important to make the distinction, since craniopharyngiomas require a considerably higher dosage of radiation for a cure to be obtained.

Most would agree, I believe, that patients with rapidly progressive visual impairment require surgical decompression. There are, however, 3 categories of patients in whom surgical intervention is probably not warranted. The first, obviously, are elderly patients in poor general medical condition which renders them unsuitable for surgical intervention.

The second is a group of young women with anovulatory amenorrhea and galactorrhea associated with an enlarging pituitary fossa, but without visual disturbances. In these patients we have been able to arrest the progression of the disease, as shown by radiographic evidence and the fact that galactorrhea ceased after radiation therapy. Menstruation, however, has not been re-established in this group.

The third group of patients to be treated by radiation only is fortunately rather uncommon. It is a group of patients with exceptionally large tumors and long histories of impairment of visual acuity and visual fields. Although our experience is limited in this group, we have found that surgical decompression carries an extremely high risk of mortality and morbidity, and little chance for improvement of the visual defects. In these patients it is often wisest to accept the loss of vision present and hope that radiation therapy will prevent further deterioration.

Even in these large tumors, radiation therapy will sometimes bring about marked improvement in acuity and visual field defects. This is well shown in a patient treated 12 months ago who had a huge tumor both extending suprasellarly and destroying the pituitary fossa and sphenoid sinus. Pretherapy, she had light perception only in the right eye and a dense hemianopic defect in the left eye, her vision being 6/60; vision in the left eye began to improve within 2 weeks after initiation of radiotherapy, and she is alive and well now, with a full visual field and excellent vision in the left eye, although the right eye remains practically useless (Figs. 4a, b, c).

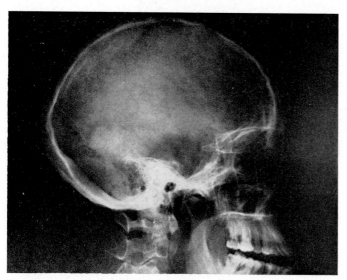

Fig. 4a Lateral view of skull showing destruction of sella and sphenoid sinus.

Our technique for treating chromophobe adenoma is the same as that for tumors in acromegalics. It is, however, essential in this group of tumors that both carotid angiograms and pneumoencephalograms be obtained prior to therapy, so that the extrasellar component of these tumors is defined. The dose given in these patients is 4500 rads in 4½ weeks to the target volume, given in 5 daily fractions per week of 200 rads each. We do not modify this

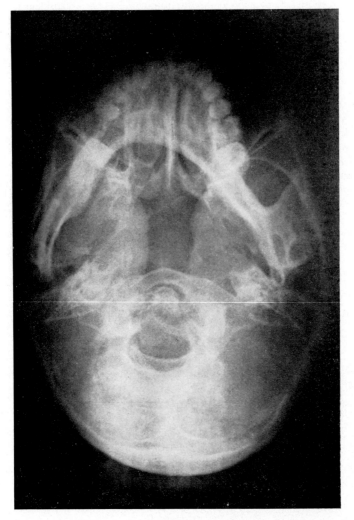

Fig. 4b   Submento-vertical view showing destruction of midline structure.

dose, whether the patient is treated by radiation alone or adjunctively with radiation after surgery.

Since 1956 we have treated 140 patients with chromophobe adenomas at the Thomas Jefferson University Hospital. My analysis, however, is based on the 98 patients treated up to 1969 (Table VIII); the 42 cases since then have been very similar in terms of distribution of management. Tables IX, X and XI give details of our management in these 98 patients. Twenty-four were treated on the basis of clinical diagnosis, without biopsy (Table IX); 63 were treated postoperatively, after either a craniotomy or a transsphenoidal stereotaxic biopsy (Table X); and 11 patients were treated for recurrence of their disease (Table XI). As mentioned, those treated on clinical diagnosis were often old and feeble or had endocrinological disturbances without compressive symptomatology. Twelve patients are alive and well, with at most minimal residual defects; 6 of these have been alive for over 5 years,

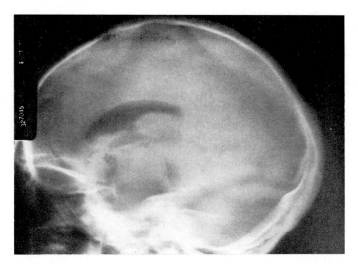

Fig. 4c   Pneumoencephalogram showing large suprasellar extension of tumor.

and 6 for less than 5 years. There have been 2 recurrences treated surgically who have fared badly: one died postoperatively, the other is alive but is totally blind. One patient was lost to follow-up and 9 have died of causes unrelated to their pituitary disease. Of these, 5 were over 65 years of age at the time they received treatment.

Table VIII   *Chromophobe adenoma cases*

Clinical diagnosis (no biopsy)		24
Treated postoperatively		63
Craniotomy	46	
Transsphenoid stereotaxic biopsy	17	
Treated for recurrence		11
Total		98

About two-thirds of our patients were treated postoperatively; of those treated more than 5 years ago, 75 % are alive and well. If those who were treated more recently are included, the crude survival figure becomes 82 %. Two patients either had a recurrence or were thought to have died with evidence of persistent disease, giving a failure rate of just over 6 %. The quality of life of those surviving is excellent, with only minimal visual field impairments in some.

The treatment of recurrent chromophobe adenoma is difficult indeed. In establishing the diagnosis of recurrence, some form of biopsy is almost always necessary. Where previous radiation therapy has been given, the dose delivered on the first occasion will determine subsequent management. If less than 3000 rads has been given, I would not hesitate to re-treat the patient with a dose of 3500–4000 rads. It is desirable under these circumstances for reoperation to be as complete as possible, so that the lowest possible dose can be employed to destroy the remaining cells. When an adequate course of radiation therapy has already been administered, I believe that a second full course of radiation therapy is too dangerous and we should place our reliance on the surgical effort alone. Of 11 patients referred to our

Table IX   *Chromophobe adenoma cases treated on clinical diagnosis*

Number of cases of clinical diagnosis (no exploration)		24
Treatment: 4500 rads in $4\frac{1}{2}$ weeks		
Results		
Alive and well with minimum residual visual defects		12
5–13 years	6	
< 5 years	6	
Recurrence treated surgically		2
at $1\frac{1}{2}$ years, died postoperatively	1	
at 9 months, blind postoperatively	1	
Lost to follow-up		1
D.O.C.		9
> 5 years	2	
< 5 years	7	
Amenorrhea and galactorrhea		6
Over 65 years of age when first seen		5 (4 D.O.C.)

Table X   *Chromophobe adenoma cases treated postoperatively*

	< 5 years	5–13 years
Number of postoperative cases	63	
Craniotomy	46	
Transsphenoid stereotaxic biopsy	17	
Treatment: 4500 rads in $4\frac{1}{2}$ weeks		
Results		
Alive and well	52/63	24/32
Lost to follow-up	4	3
D.O.C.	3	1
Recurrences	2	2
Dead with disease	2	2
Crude survival	82.5 %	75 %
Determinate survival	87 %	83 %

Table XI   *Chromophobe adenoma cases treated for recurrence (total number of cases: 11)*

Diagnosed by craniotomy			9
Had been treated without radiation therapy		8	
(Recurred at 3, 3, 4, 4, 5, 6, 9, 10 yrs)			
Had been treated with radiation therapy		1	
(3000 rads: recurred at 9 yrs)			
Treatment: approximately 4500 rads			
Two exceptions: 4000 rads (previously irradiated)			
3000 rads (died during treatment)			
Results			
Alive and well		6	
< 2 yrs	4		
$3\frac{1}{2}$ yrs	1		
$5\frac{3}{4}$ yrs	1		
Lost to follow-up		2	
Died during treatment		1	
Diagnosed clinically			2
Had been treated with radiation therapy			
(repeat courses; recurred at 2 yrs)			
Deteriorated at 1 yr		1	
Died at 1 yr		1	

department prior to 1969 for recurrent tumors, 9 were referred after a second craniotomy (Table XI). Eight of these had received no postoperative radiation therapy and recurred between 3 and 10 years after surgery. One patient had received 3000 rads postoperatively, and he recurred 9 years later. Those patients who had not received radiation therapy were given 4500 rads in $4\frac{1}{2}$ weeks, except for one patient who deteriorated and died during the course of radiation therapy; the previously irradiated patient received 4000 rads in 4 weeks. Six of these patients are alive and well between 2 and $5\frac{3}{4}$ years after treatment, 2 patients were lost to follow-up and one died during his treatment. In 2 additional patients, recurrence was diagnosed on clinical grounds and neither of these patients was deemed fit for reoperation; they both did badly, deteriorated and died within a year of their reirradiation. Thus, unlike the acromegalic patients, salvage in patients with recurrent tumors has been relatively poor in our hands.

Cushing's disease

Finally, in patients with Cushing's disease, our experience with irradiation of the pituitary has been quite limited. It has been restricted to a handful of patients in whom there was evidence of an enlarged pituitary and in whom an adrenal tumor could be excluded. We believe such patients should receive conventional radiation therapy to the pituitary and that a dose such as that given for chromophobe adenomas is adequate. Very satisfactory results can be obtained, with complete loss of the stigmata of Cushing's disease and return of normal menstruation.

Summary

There is now considerable evidence that early reports of supervoltage radiation therapy failing to control excessive human growth hormone levels in patients with acromegaly are erroneous. Data are now accumulating that the growth hormone levels parallel the clinical response, but that growth hormone levels after conventional radiation therapy require from 6 months to 2 years to return to normal levels. Since over 80 % of patients with acromegaly respond to conventional radiation therapy and continue well, without need for substitution therapy, and since morbidity from such treatment is minimal, this would seem to be the first treatment of choice in patients with acromegaly, except for those with high, life-threatening growth hormone levels or compressive symptomatology. Those who fail to respond to radiation therapy stand an excellent chance of being well managed by some operative surgical procedure.

Patients with chromophobe adenomas should all receive radiation therapy, either as the primary treatment or as adjunctive therapy to surgical intervention. A recurrence-free rate in excess of 80 % can be confidently expected. Our experiences with Cushing's disease are too limited to more than suggest that in suitable cases, conventional radiation therapy to a dose of 4500 rads in $4\frac{1}{2}$ weeks may well be the treatment of choice.

References

(1) ROTH, J., GLICK, S. M., CUATRECASAS, P. and HOLLANDER, C. S. (1967): Acromegaly and other disorders of growth hormone secretion: Combined Clinical Staff Conference at the National Institutes of Health. *Ann. intern. Med.*, *66*, 760.

(2) LAWRENCE, A. M., PINSKY, S. M. and GOLDFINE, I. D. (1971): Conventional radiation therapy in acromegaly: a review and reassessment. *Arch. intern. Med.*, *128*, 369.

(3) ROTH, J., GORDON, P. and BRACE, K. (1970): The efficacy of conventiona pituitary irradiation in acromegaly. *New Engl. J. Med.*, *282*, 1385.

The treatment of acromegaly by conventional pituitary irradiation

PHILLIP GORDEN and JESSE ROTH

Diabetes Section, Clinical Endocrinology Branch, National Institute of Arthritis, Metabolic and Digestive Diseases, National Institutes of Health, Bethesda, Md.,U.S.A.

It is now clear that conventional supervoltage irradiation is an effective way to reduce growth hormone (GH) concentration in acromegaly.[1, 2] We have demonstrated that nearly all irradiated patients show some fall in GH with time, while untreated patients show either no change or a rise in plasma GH concentration. It was concluded from our study that, while the rate of decrease in plasma GH may be slower than with other therapies, the overall efficacy was clearly in the same range as other more aggressive forms of therapy.[1] The crucial point is whether these conclusions remain valid or whether one mode of therapy has clearly emerged as superior. To help answer this question, we have expanded our series and had the opportunity to follow our patients for a longer period of time.

Since the hypersecretion of GH is the culprit in acromegaly, the measurement of GH concentration by radioimmunoassay before and after treatment is the most direct means of evaluating the effects of therapy. These determinations should be made in the basal state on several occasions; determinations made during stimulation or suppression tests, while possibly useful in making the diagnosis of acromegaly, have not been validated as yardsticks of therapy. Other clinical and metabolic parameters, which may be influenced by a variety of factors, are useful in individual patients but are less valuable for comparisons between groups of patients.

Patients with acromegaly were treated by irradiation regardless of the degree of elevation of the plasma GH concentration, the sella size, or the presence of supersellar extension (except when supersellar extension had resulted in significant loss of vision). Thirty previously untreated acromegalic patients have been treated with 4000–4500 R by conventional supervoltage irradiation and followed for 1–6 yr. All patients were restudied at the end of 1–2 yr and 16 of 30 were studied again at the end of 3–6 yr. Three additional patients were first treated by transfrontal hypophysectomy followed by irradiation.

The pretreatment mean GH concentration for the 30 patients was 58 ng/ml, median 29 and range 7–200 ng/ml (Fig. 1). By 1–2 yr after irradiation there was a 62% reduction in plasma GH for the 30 patients (mean GH = 22 ng/ml, median 14 and range 3–85 ng/ml) (Fig. 2). Further reduction in plasma GH occurred with time and by 3–6 yr postirradiation there was a 78% reduction in plasma GH for 16 patients (mean GH = 13 ng/ml, median 7 and range 3–50 ng/ml). The most recent GH determinations in this group of 16 patients indicate that almost 3/4 of the group have GH concentrations of 10 ng/ml or less and that almost 1/2 of the group have GH concentrations of 5 ng/ml or less.

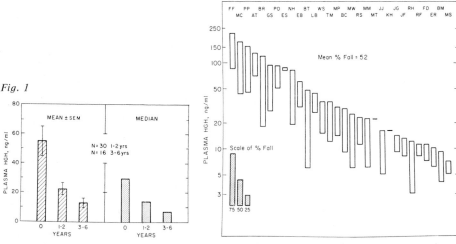

Fig. 1 Mean and median growth hormone concentrations for untreated acromegalic patients and for patients treated by supervoltage irradiation as a function of time.

Fig. 2 Plasma GH concentrations in acromegalic patients before and 1–2 yr after irradiation. Each bar represents a single patient; the top of the bar represents the mean pretreatment value and the bottom the mean posttreatment value. Since the verticle scale is logarithmic, the height of each bar is proportional to the % change in plasma GH.

The response of an individual patient to irradiation appears to be independent of whether the patient was first treated by surgery. Thus in 3 patients studied, there was a 46 % mean reduction in GH concentration following transfrontal hypophysectomy which was followed by a further 50 % mean reduction in plasma GH by 1–2 yr post conventional irradiation. By 3–5 yr postirradiation 2 of the 3 patients had GH concentrations of less than 5 ng/ml (Table I).

Table I *Comparison of hypophysectomy and irradiation*

Patient	Growth hormone (ng/ml)			
	Untreated	Post-hypophysectomy	Postirradiation (1–2 yr)	(3–5 yr)
J.M.	161	69	42	21
J.B.	62	15	6	3
H.T.	34	35	10	4

Transfrontal hypophysectomy was performed for large tumors in J.M. and J.B. with compromise of vision and for a small tumor in H.T. who had congestive heart failure, making a rapid GH reduction desirable.

The usefulness of any therapy is determined by the ratio of the benefits to risks. Benefits of irradiation are judged primarily by reductions in plasma GH. Risks are of 2 types: deficiencies of pituitary trophic hormones, and structural damage to the brain or cranial nerves. Single or multiple pituitary hormone deficits are common with pituitary tumors in the absence of therapy. Pituitary irradiation did not noticeably increase the incidence of hypopituitarism nor did it improve deficits that were already present. If we exclude hormone deficiencies that antedated the irradiation, then 1 of our patients required thyroid replacement and 1 adrenal corticoid replacement.

When conventional supervoltage irradiation is given with proper care in a single 4 to 5 week course and in doses that do not exceed 4500 R, structural damage to the brain or cranial nerves is rare. We have seen no such complication in the 30 patients reported in the present study. Since the potential benefits from a second course of treatment are slight and the risks considerable, we do not further irradiate patients who have been given up to 4000 R as initial treatment. The benefit to risk ratio of doses that exceed 4500 R is unclear. While doses of up to 6000 R have been given safely [2], it is possible that some patients will not tolerate these high doses. More recently we have modestly increased our therapy dose to 5000 R given over a 5 week period; one patient treated in this way developed a transient visual field cut 3 months post treatment unassociated with suprasellar extension of the tumor. The defect cleared spontaneously in one week and there was no further difficulty. A second patient with systemic sarcoidosis and acromegaly was treated with 5600 R over a 6 week period. Approximately 18 months post-treatment the patient developed a progressive visual field abnormalityunassociated with suprasellar extension. In this case, we could not specifically implicate irradiation but neither could we exclude the possibility of radiation-induced damage. Since the benefit of irradiation in excess of 4500–5000 R is unclear and the risk potentially significant, we now limit our therapeutic dose to a maximum of 5000 R given in 4–5 weeks.

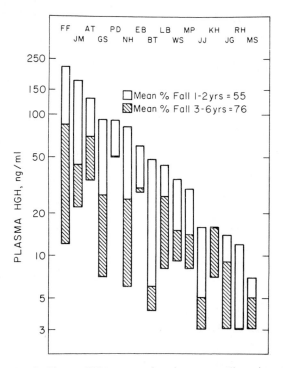

Fig. 3   Plasma GH concentrations in acromegalic patients before, 1–2 yr and 3–6 yr postirradiation. The bars are the same as in Figure 2. The % fall at 3–6 yr refers to the change from the untreated state.

At the present time patients are treated largely on the basis of regional expertise or preference. No single mode of therapy has emerged as ideal or clearly preferable. All therapeutic modalities to date leave some patients with distinctly elevated growth hormone concentrations. Finally, in individual patients we must frequently decide whether the treatment or the disease is preferable. Patient E.B. (Fig. 3) is a good example of the enigma. He was irradiated at age 23 and has been followed for almost 10 yr. During this period he has been gainfully employed, sired 2 children, has normal libido and generally has few complaints. Although he had a fall in GH following therapy, his values remain between 20–30 ng/ml. In our opinion the uncertain risks of his elevated plasma GH offset the real hazard of rendering him hypopituitary by a more aggressive ablative technique.

In summary, in an extensive prospective series conventional supervoltage irradiation by 5 yr after treatment reduces the plasma GH to the same extent as all other modalities of therapy reported thus far and is remarkably low in side effects. Presumably the benefits (and side effects) of newly introduced modalities of therapy should be compared with these data.

References

(1) ROTH, J., GORDEN, P. and BRACE, K. (1970): Efficacy of conventional pituitary irradiation in acromegaly. *New Engl. J. Med.*, *282*, 1385.
(2) LAWRENCE, A. M., PINSKY, S. M. and GOLDFINE, I. D. (1971): Conventional radiation therapy in acromegaly. *Arch. intern. Med.*, *128*, 369.

A system for therapy of pituitary tumors*

RAYMOND N. KJELLBERG and BERNARD KLIMAN

Massachusetts General Hospital, Boston, Mass., U.S.A.

New technology of the past decade has reduced the risk of operative mortality in patients with pituitary tumors to 0.3 %, while satisfactory results range from ca. 80 to 90 % for the various conditions treated. We have developed a system in which appropriate patients are selected for stereotactic Bragg peak proton ablation or microsurgical excision by the transsphenoidal or transfrontal routes. In the authors' experience with over 350 patients harboring various pituitary tumors (Table I), the sole procedure-related mortality occurred in 1962, due to pulmonary embolus on the twelfth postoperative day in a patient prepared for discharge. Because the assets of a single technical procedure under a given clinical circumstance may become liabilities under a different set of clinical conditions, we have devised a system for the choice of appropriate and effective relief of illness.

Table I *Surgical procedures for pituitary tumors (R.N.K.)*

Tumors	Open		Stereotactic		Total
	Frontal craniotomy	Trans-sphenoidal	Radio-frequency Hypophysectomy	Bragg peak proton beam	
Chromophobe adenoma	10	4	1	36	51
Acromegaly	3	5		233	241
Cushing's disease	2	1		52	55
Suprasellar meningioma	1				1
Craniopharyngioma	1				1
Other		2		2	4
Total	17	12	1	323	353

This discussion will review problems associated with surgery of the pituitary, experience with solutions of such problems, descriptions of the methods employed and other considerations, including the attitudes of patients involved and influences of non-medical third parties and government on the development of treatment programs.

---

* This project was supported by USPHS grants CA 07368 and AM 04501.

Problems

1. *Mortality*

By 1910, only 17 operations had been done on the pituitary.[1] In the ensuing generation, Harvey Cushing became considered the founding father of pituitary surgery and endocrinology. In 338 patients, his operative mortality was 5.5% and his patient mortality was 6.3%.[2] In his acromegalic patients, operation by the transsphenoidal route was associated with a mortality one-third that of the transfrontal route, but there was little difference in the routes of operation for chromophobe adenoma. The generation of neurosurgeons who followed Cushing devoted themselves largely to the transfrontal route. In recent years, the technical expertise of Bronson Ray has reduced the operative mortality of transfrontal craniotomy in patients with chromophobe adenoma and acromegaly to 1.2% and 0% respectively, or about 1% for both groups in his hands.[3, 4]

In our own experience, undesirable effects or complications of surgery with the potential risk of death tend to be higher in transfrontally operated patients than in transsphenoidally operated patients (Table II). Several of the complications are attributable to the fact that general anesthesia was required. In fact, our only mortality directly attributable to the procedure, namely pulmonary embolus, is attributable to the anesthetized state rather than the cranial procedure per se.

Table II   *All pituitary procedures (R.N.K.): undesirable effects*

	Open		Stereotactic
	Frontal craniotomy	Transsphenoidal	Bragg peak proton beam
Numbers of procedures	19	12	323
Wound infection	0	0	0
CSF leak	0	1	0
Coma	0	0	0
Seizures			
Major	0	0	0
Minor	0	0	4
Dilantin intoxication	1	0	0
Pituitary insufficiency			
Anterior partial	0	0	7
Anterior total	8	2	22
Posterior permanent	0	0	0
Posterior temporary	10	2	4
Pulmonary embolism	1 (died)	0	0
Hepatitis	2	0	0
Further treatment	7	3	21

2. *Morbidity*

a. Vision.   Deterioration of visual acuity or fields is an outstanding risk associated with untreated pituitary tumors or with virtually all the methods by which pituitary tumors are treated. Progressive visual loss is often the specific reason for undertaking therapy, as is the case with chromophobe adenoma. On the other hand, the risk to vision during frontal craniotomy makes this a less desirable approach. In our experience, the risk to vision by transsphenoidal microsurgical excision or proton hypophysectomy appears to have been reduced to very low levels.

During the first year (1963) of our clinical trial with the proton beam, we treated 3 cases of chromophobe adenoma with suprasellar extension of the tumor. In our inexperienced state, we attempted radiation of the whole mass. Two of these patients had previously received substantial amounts of X-radiation. All 3 experienced significant visual loss from 4 to 14 months following proton treatment. In addition, one died following craniotomy elsewhere. The operating surgeon thought optic nerve tissue was damaged by radiation, but we have no histologic confirmation. We have been additionally informed[5] that the lesion was apparently malignant.

Also in that year, we irradiated a girl with an unusual invasive pituitary lesion, considered to be a connective tissue neoplasm, possibly a meningiosarcoma. The beam diameter was large (51 mm), as was the dose (8000 rads). She lost all vision 15 months later and at craniotomy, when no clear basis was found, we attributed the blindness to proton radiation. This risk was to a degree anticipated in what we regarded as a life-preserving effort.

These cases demonstrated problems associated with the application of proton radiation to cases which we came to realize were not suitable for the Bragg peak method: (1) Patients with suprasellar extension of tumor are at risk; the paths of the optic nerves usually cannot be separated from the tumor by means of a pneumoencephalogram. (2) Prior X-radiation contributes a hazard to proton therapy. (3) Large diameter beams in a single horizontal plane develop a wedge of overlap as they converge on the pituitary, such that the cumulative dose may be above tolerance for neural tissue.

Other than the above 4 early cases, none of the patients subsequently treated for pituitary adenoma in our group has developed a visual handicap as the result of any of the therapeutic maneuvers employed. However, transfrontal craniotomy has produced many more partial alterations of visual function than transsphenoidal excision, where we have witnessed no decrease in visual acuity or fields in any instance. In 13 transfrontally operated patients, 4 experienced improvement in acuity and visual fields bilaterally. Three patients experienced improvement in visual function attributable to the improvement in one eye but the other eye was worse. Both fields improved in one patient, but acuity remained the same, and in 3 patients, both fields and acuity remained the same. Two patients have measurable decrements in either field or acuity but function at their preoperative levels of physical activity. We continue to regard risk to vision as an irreducible problem when the transfrontal route is employed.

By all forms of therapy – surgery, X-ray or proton beam – patients are subject to visual loss due to the development of the so-called 'empty sella syndrome'.[6] This phenomenon appears to limit the ultimate success of intervention, but it also occurs without treatment and it is fortunately rare.

b. *Mental status.*   Alteration of mental status may be related to massive tumors, malignant invasions or major endocrine disorders, and it represents another important risk of the transfrontal route of excision. We have not encountered complications of brain function related to transsphenoidal procedures. The only instance of temporary memory alteration was reported[7] in our first proton-treated acromegalic patient and has not been observed again with the improved dosimetry of radiation.

In our hospital, following a frontal craniotomy, a few instances have been seen of delayed alteration of mental status. Patients have been noted to be bright and alert following transfrontal excision, then, 2 to 5 days later, rather abruptly change and become poorly responsive. Angiography may reveal spasm of cerebral arteries. The hypothesis has been advanced that degenerating blood products in the subarachnoid space may be responsible.

c. *Endocrine.*   Total surgical excision of a pituitary tumor inevitably obligates a patient to lifelong dependence on replacement medication. While this is normally satisfactorily managed as a modest inconvenience, the occasional inadvertent catastrophe in a stressed cortisone-dependent patient should be reckoned in the overall risk. Diabetes insipidus and its management are significant sources of disability to the patients. Deliberate subtotal excision may often avoid this inconvenience and risk. However, the patient frequently requires retreatment with X-ray or later reoperation to control persistent hyperfunction or recurrent mass. Microadenomas, tumors that are 10 mm or less in diameter, may be excised by the trans-sphenoidal microsurgical route, preserving the remainder of the gland. Such small tumors, however, represent a very small proportion of all adenomas, and the operative separation of larger tumors from normal pituitary cannot be reliably performed. Either total hypophysectomy or secondary therapy is normally required. Optimally, both hypopituitarism and high prospect of retreatment should and can be avoided.

Conventional X-ray is being less frequently performed as a therapy for pituitary hyperfunction (acromegaly, Cushing's disease). The principal instrument leading to this reappraisal and redirection has been the development of radioimmunoassay techniques for measuring human growth hormone (HGH), adrenocorticotrophic hormone (ACTH) and other primary pituitary trophic hormones.

Thus, Glick found the values of HGH in acromegalic patients nearly identical before and after X-ray therapy.[8] We would not interpret his data to show that X-ray had no effect. We think it is proper to credit the X-ray therapy with arresting the tendency for HGH levels to increase as they normally do. They did not, however, fall. The data of Roth et al. on 20 cases require greater care in interpretation.[9] In none of their 5 patients with postirradiation HGH values below 5 ng/ml (R.H., B.M., M.S., J.G. and J.J.) was any acral change observed. The value of one of these (J.G.) appears to have been 5 ng/ml before treatment, and the HGH values of 3 of the others appear to have been 6.5, 8 and 11 ng/ml. The degree of 'activity' in these cases we would consider in doubt pending further information. Furthermore, in 2 of their 3 patients in whom acral regression was observed (G.S. and L.B.), the HGH levels were 39 and 28 ng/ml respectively after treatment. These very few patients (3 of 20 or 15 %) demonstrating acral improvement have done so only between 2 and 4 years after treatment. However, as for the prospects for improvement beyond the second year after X-ray therapy, their Figure 2 shows 7 patients, 2 with no growth hormone decrease after one year (B.T. and W.S.), 3 with no 2-year measurement (G.S., A.T. and M.S.), one tested only at 12 and 30 months (M.M.) and only one (J.J.) with a decrease between 24 and 48 months. The 'benefit' in that case is calculated by us to be another 10 % of control or only 2 ng/ml.

There is a substantial body of evidence from Ray,[4] Adams,[10] Rand,[11] ourselves and others that reduction of HGH below 5 ng/ml can be induced with substantially greater frequency, ranging from 50 % to 75 % of cases by the variety of means used by these authors. Furthermore, their experience and ours substantiates a strong correlation between levels of HGH in the normal range and remission of acral changes. We have observed acral regression when patients with 'active' acromegaly have their HGH reduced to or below 5 ng/ml. Furthermore, in such patients (with HGH of 5 ng/ml or less) the oral glucose tolerance test is likewise restored to normal, except in some patients with a family history of diabetes mellitus. In addition, the patient's experience with X-ray therapy deserves mention. The time for a course of X-ray therapy is normally 4–6 weeks, with a direct cost of $600–1000. If a patient is hospitalized for this treatment, the hospital bill may be in the range of $2800–4200. If the patient is an average earner and unable to work, his lost earnings may be $600–1000.

d. Seizures. The classic monograph on acromegaly by Davidoff[12] listed seizures in 7 of his 100 patients. Presumably, most cases represented parasellar extensions of tumor into the temporal lobe. This complication is much less frequently encountered in current practice because patients now seek medical evaluation at an earlier stage of their disease, and the prospect that the physician will correctly appraise the problem and set the course of therapy is quite high. Following frontal craniotomy, anticonvulsants are routinely employed. We have had one instance of Dilantin intoxication as a result of this practice. We have had no instance of a major (grand mal) seizure by any of the methods employed, but 4 instances of mild minor seizures have been noted in acromegalic patients following proton hypophysectomy.

3. *Therapeutic goals*

A proposal to restate the therapeutic goals in patients harboring pituitary tumors may seem superfluous. However, amidst the profusion of clinical expressions of pituitary lesions, the exquisite panoply of laboratory tests to define the biochemical status and the rich technology available for the therapy of pituitary tumors, the relatively simple goals of the patient may be obscured. Each patient desires safe, simple and reliable restoration to normal health at minimal expense of personal and financial resources. The differing clinical conditions associated with pituitary tumors have different requirements.

Most patients with acromegaly simply require a reduction in circulating HGH. In addition to improvement of glucose metabolism and cessation of acral growth, it is probably more important that the eventual metabolic disabilities of acromegaly be avoided. Crippling osteoarthritis and life-threatening hypertension or cardiomyopathy are often irreversible. Since the hyperfunctioning adenoma causes the visual disturbance relatively infrequently, it is undesirable to invoke a therapy which carries such a risk. When visual impairment is the presenting feature, early decompression of the optic nerves is essential. Pituitary overproduction should be curtailed, preferably without inducing hypofunction. Surgical resection by either the transfrontal or transsphenoidal routes can reduce HGH to less than 5 ng/ml. However, this normally requires total hypophysectomy and the lifelong obligations of replacement medication.

The needs in patients with Cushing's disease are similar to those in acromegaly, namely, correction of the hormone excess due to hyperfunction of the pituitary. The Vanderbilt study[13] indicates a cure of 10 of 51 patients and improvement in 13 patients by conventional X-ray alone. Other therapies were applied in many of the remainder. Total adrenalectomy is probably the most widely used therapy for Cushing's disease, but it uniformly requires lifelong dependence upon corticosteroid replacement. The number of these patients who go on to develop Nelson's syndrome seems to be increasing.[14-16] This fact, together with Cushing's early demonstration of 'microadenomas' in his cases[17] and the Columbia series on pathology findings in the pituitary,[18] is in our view an adequate basis for including Cushing's disease of pituitary origin under the rubric of pituitary tumors. Subtotal adrenalectomy often fails to provide adequate corticosteroid reserve, and the adrenal remnant may hypertrophy to allow recurrence of Cushing's disease. Open surgical hypophysectomy has been applied with surprising rarity.

Non-functioning chromophobe adenomas need to be appraised in a somewhat different context. The usual symptom associated with these is visual field defect. We learned early in our experience with the proton beam (above) that excess hazard accrues when this therapy is applied to chiasmal syndromes. Our present view is that chiasmal compression requires open surgery, preferably by the transsphenoidal route. Frontal craniotomy is followed by recurrence in 22 % of patients unless X-ray is given, in which case the recurrence rate is reduced to 8 %.[3] We are unaware of any patient exhibiting a requirement for full maintenance of cortisone and thyroid who was restored to normal function by any method of therapy. Consequently, we do not consider restoration of normal function a feasible clinical goal in these patients.

More recently, we have treated a group of patients exhibiting an enlarged sella, no suprasellar extension of the tumor, and normal visual and endocrine functions. We have conducted

Bragg peak proton radiation in them at about one-half of the dose we use in hyperfunction, since our therapeutic objective is to produce only growth arrest but not necrosis. No complications have occurred since 1964. The problems in these patients are twofold: (1) is therapy of any sort indicated and for what goals? and (2) how is the effectiveness of therapy to be measured? In addition, we have given proton radiation to the sella in several patients following an open surgical operation on a pituitary tumor.

The problem of malignant change in pituitary adenomas is particularly difficult. We understand that the histologic criteria are remarkably unreliable.[19] The cellular character of malignant pituitary tumors is often indistinguishable from the usual benign tumor. Jefferson[20] and others have considered tumors malignant when they invade surrounding structures independent of their cytoarchitecture. Implants near the pituitary may be observed. Invasion and rapid growth can occur in tumors of long duration, suggesting that the change to malignancy may have occurred late in the course of a previously benign lesion.

One problem is to develop a diagnostic method for identifying malignant growth potential independent of histologic character. It would then be more readily possible to state whether a 'cure' of a malignant tumor had been achieved. Under the present circumstances, we can only be certain of our failures.

Craniopharyngiomas, meningiomas and various other neoplasms occur with sufficiently low frequency to require management on an individual basis. We advocate microsurgical technique in dealing with such lesions.

Solutions

1. *Case selection*

Our method of case selection is rather simple. We always use the Bragg peak proton method in any instance without suprasellar extension and without excessive prior radiation exposure. If a candidate for therapy has been radiated within the previous 2 years, we allow 24 months to elapse, or we perform transsphenoidal hypophysectomy. If a patient has had more than 6000 rads of X-ray at any time in the past, we do not use protons. If he has had a full course of radiation less than 6000 rads, more than 24 months previously, we use protons and reduce our dose by 1000 to 2000 rads.

If a patient has suprasellar extension, we draw a line in the pneumoencephalogram from the nasal spine to the tuberculum of the sphenoid. If the dome of the tumor is below the line, we do a transsphenoidal hypophysectomy. If the dome of the tumor is above the line, we perform frontal craniotomy. In marginal cases, if the distance between the tuberculum and the posterior clinoids is long, we do transsphenoidal hypophysectomy and allow the dome to descend as the sella is evacuated. When the distance between the tuberculum and posterior clinoids is short, the tumor is impacted and will not descend and thus necessitates a frontal craniotomy.

2. *Acromegaly*

A program for pituitary therapy has been developed on the basis of personal experience with over 230 acromegalic patients. Our initial intention was to induce focal radionecrosis of a large proportion of the adenoma. The newly developed radioimmunoassay of HGH provided a precise documentation of this procedure. Thus, in ideal instances, an acromegalic with elevated HGH and abnormal metabolism of glucose can be cured of his metabolic abnormality and experience a cessation of bone growth, accompanied by soft tissue regression. This is accomplished with local anesthesia and with less than 2 hours on an operating table. Convalescence is uneventful. The hospital bill may be one-third to one-half of the amount of that for open intracranial procedures. He retains normal pituitary function.

The effect of Bragg peak proton hypophysectomy on the HGH levels and clinical features of acromegaly is shown in Figure 1. The postoperative HGH is listed in relation to pre-operative HGH. The data points themselves are recorded as 4 grades of results on clinical criteria normally supplied by the referring physician. The solid black dots are graded 'Remission' and represent reversal of all clinical indications of acromegly – digits and facial features reduce in size, glucose intolerance improves toward normal, and various individual manifestations such as fatigability, joint pain or carpal tunnel syndrome subside. Nearly all the cases falling to or below 5 ng/ml are in this grade, and this accounts for 53 % of all the patients on whom we have data. Furthermore, many of these patients have values 10 % or less than their preoperative HGH values.

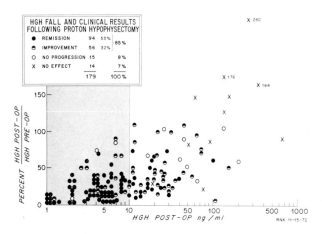

Fig. 1   Posttreatment values of HGH are shown in relation to the percentage of fall from pre-operative values in 151 patients. The data points indicate the degree of clinical response to therapy as shown in the box at the top of the figure (clinical follow-up is on 179 patients). The values represent those available at the time of the most recent follow-up without respect to the interval following treatment. (See text for discussion of time course of response to therapy.)

There are several instances of patients we graded clinically as 'Remission' with HGH levels above 5 ng/ml, in fact above 10 ng/ml, but these usually developed a fall to 30 % or less of their preoperative values. In reviewing reports of therapy for acromegaly, a variety of values for HGH appear to be accepted as 'normal'. For the present, rather than debate the merit of one value or another for 'normal', we would prefer to emphasize careful ap-praisal of the clinical findings and their correlation with HGH values. In Figure 1 we have recorded the most recent values we have for each patient without respect to the interval following therapy. Many of the values are less than 2 years postoperative and further lowering of the HGH is anticipated. We are inclined to regard the value of HGH at 2 years postoperative as the final effect, but we are aware of further decrease in HGH in some cases.

Patients who exhibit reversal of some, but not all, of the features of active acromegaly are graded as 'Improved' and are represented on the figure as half-black and half-white circles. These two grades, 'Remission' and 'Improved', represent 85 % of the patients.

The third grade, 'Arrested', is represented as open circles. Six per cent of the patients fall in this group and are considered as failures in the sense that clinical signs of acromegaly persist. This degree of response is comparable to that reported following conventional X-ray therapy.[8, 9]

Seven per cent of our patients, noted by x's, were frank 'Failures'. They persisted in having clinical signs of active disease and, as might be expected, their growth hormones remained high in absolute value and increased in comparison to preoperative levels. Further treatment was indicated in these patients and was provided by surgery when circumstances allowed. In general, our failures have reduced with added experience (Table III).

Table III   *Proton hypophysectomy: acromegaly. Results of therapy*

Case numbers	Remission	Improvement	No progression	Failure	No follow-up
1–50	26	16	2	6	0
51–100	27	10	3	4	6
101–150	22	14	3	2	9
151–200	17	13	5	3	12
Total	92	53	13	15	27
	145				

Mortality risk in acromegalic patients is zero. Morbidity has been generally low and further reduced in recent years as technical resources and experience with a new method improved (Table IV). As is the case with most forms of pituitary ablations, it can be anticipated that the morbidity is related to structures in the immediate vicinity of the pituitary.

Table IV   *Proton hypophysectomy: acromegaly. Undesirable effects*

Case numbers	Temporary EOM disturbance	Visual	Hypopituitary			Seizures	Retreatment
			Partial anterior	Total anterior	Transient D.I.		
1–50	16	3	1	7	0	0	4
51–100	14	0	0	6	1	2	4
101–150	9	1	2	3	1	1	2
151–200	3	1	1	3	2	1	3
Total	42	5	5	19	4	4	13

Two factors contribute to successful application of the Bragg peak proton beam. The exact spatial distribution of the radiation must be known and controllable. Secondly, the exact spatial distribution of the pituitary and surrounding structures must be established without direct invasion of the region by the operator. Precise definition of the spatial distribution of the proton radiation was achieved by a member of the Harvard Physics Department, Mr. Andreas Koehler. Using a silicon diode radiation detector of 0.25 mm² cross-section sensitive area, the single beam of protons is carefully mapped in 3 dimensions. A computer program was designed to assemble a family of isodose curves of various dimensions, such that predictably high doses (up to 15,000 rads) may be developed while allowing low doses a few millimeters away. In general, the dose falls off from the central high intensity region at the rate of 1000–2000 rads per mm (Fig. 2).

It is mandatory to secure radiographically precise measurements of the pituitary area in each individual patient. Several necessary studies have evolved with the aid of our neuroradiological colleagues, Drs. Taveras, New and Roberson. Since all X-ray films are secured

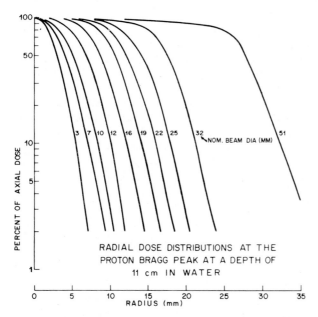

Fig. 2   Our convention is to state the total dose in terms of the axial dose. This dose falls along radii from the axis depending upon the beam diameter. Note that although the rate of fall of the dose below about 70 % of the axial dose is linear on the graph, the vertical scale is logarithmic.

with more or less enlargement of the skeletal or contrast images, it is necessary to correct for such magnification. We secure marker films taken with leadshot markers at intervals of 10 mm placed in the three planes of the pituitary – midline, coronal and horizontal (to Reed's line). Pneumoencephalography is used to evaluate regions above the clinoids. It is imperative to determine whether suprasellar extension of the tumor exists, for such cases are ordinarily excluded from proton beam therapy. In addition, the course of the optic nerves can be established from the recesses of the third ventricle and the details of the optic cistern, in part with the aid of tomography. Coronal polytomes of the floor of the sella are very helpful. During the past year, cavernous sinography has been routinely employed to provide additional precise measurement of the internal limits of the tumor.

We have had 2 optic nerve complications (one hemianopsia and one quadrantanopsia) since a new dosimetry has been employed (after case No. 100). In 2 other patients in whom X-radiation had been done prior to proton radiation, field defects developed. The risk to optic nerves in patients who have previously received X-ray therapy is about twice as great as in those without prior radiation exposure. Visual loss in association with the 'empty sella syndrome' is, in part, associated with whatever therapy is employed, and it accrued in 2 of these patients. Two patients developed visual loss postoperatively due to diabetic retinopathy, and another patient had a visual defect due to an arachnoid cyst of the middle fossa and chiasmatic cistern.

a. Temporary oculomotor disturbance.   This has been the most persistent problem. Many patients are aware of the problem only intermittently upon waking, turning, changing gaze or when fatigued. In others, the eye casts out or ptosis may occur. The disturbance recovers in a variable number of months. In one patient, a second course of radiation was followed by diplopia which has persisted for 55 months and is evidently permanent. Another patient has worn an eye-patch continuously and her diplopia has persisted. The frequency of this problem has decreased with the technical maneuvers described below.

In our early experience, instances of transient oculomotor disturbance occurred with a significant frequency (Table IV). This table shows a substantial reduction with improved dosimetry and other technical refinements. The high dose radiation was moved 1 mm medial to the perimeter of pituitary tissue in the anticipation that the outermost zone should be normal gland rather than adenoma. In addition, by moving the center of rotation of the radiation pattern 5 mm beyond the midline, the beams passing through the cavernous sinus are more divergent, and the radiation attributable to overlap is reduced.

The decrement in frequency of oculomotor complications in case Nos. 101–200 does not include the anticipated advantage from cavernous sinography. The oculomotor nerves range between 2 and 7 mm lateral to the pituitary. Thus, nerves which are closest to the pituitary are at greater risk than those further laterally. In the sinograms, the lateral walls of the pituitary are evident, but the individual oculomotor nerves cannot be identified.

b. Hypopituitarism.   We consider hypofunction of the pituitary an undesirable effect. The majority of patients treated by the Bragg peak proton method retain normal pituitary function. We have hypofunction in 28 cases of the 231 acromegalics treated to date (Table IV) by the proton beam. The requirement for cortisone and thyroid was present in 19 patients. An additional 5 patients required either thyroid or cortisone but not both. In addition, we have identified HGH deficiency in 5 patients with HGH values below 1 ng/ml who fail to respond to insulin or arginine stimulation and develop reactive hypoglycemia late in a glucose tolerance test. Four patients had transient diabetes insipidus.

c. Seizures.   We have been concerned from our beginning with Bragg peak proton therapy that the dose of radiation to the medial temporal lobe may be significant. In collaboration with pathologists, we studied 8 brains of patients who had received proton radiation by our original technique.[21] These patients had all been irradiated with the beam portals in a single horizontal plane (since at that time we did not have the resources to compute isodose curves in a three-dimensional system). Although none of these patients exhibited appropriate clinical symptoms, several of the medial temporal regions show changes regarded as consistent with radiation effects a few millimeters in size. Our concern over this matter had induced us to modify the arrangement of portals prior to the time this study was completed, so that the portals diverged vertically as well as horizontally. No instance of histologic change has been seen since.

In the clinical cases, no grand mal convulsions have occurred. Four patients have had brief episodes of aura, smells, sensations, etc. which stopped when anticonvulsants were instituted.

3. *Cushing's disease*

The principles evolved in the treatment of acromegaly are all directly applicable to Cushing's disease due to pituitary ACTH excess. A radiographically normal sella is found in fewer cases of acromegaly (about 5 %) than in Cushing's disease. (This figure is not well established for Cushing's disease, but in our experience at least 30 % ultimately develop abnormal sellae.)

Nevertheless, the principles and techniques of hypophysectomy by the Bragg peak proton method are identical. The results are quite similar (Table V). To date we have treated 52 patients. We can report follow-up on 45 of them. Eighty-nine per cent are improved, including 58 % with complete remission. Patients with sustained high levels of cortisol or who required additional therapy were rated as failures (11 %). Whether or not the patient has had prior adrenal surgery has little influence on the prospect or interval to achieve a remission. However, in a few instances of early or mild Cushing's disease, a good response has been evident in only one month following therapy. The ideal result is superior to that experienced in acromegalic patients since all the stigmata of the condition may be obliterated.

Complications have been mild and infrequent, and they follow the pattern of those seen in the acromegalic patients (Table VI). They are: one unilateral quadrantanopsia, 4 instances of temporary oculomotor disturbance, and 4 cases of hypopituitarism. One patient underwent, at approximately 2-year intervals, X-ray, proton beam, transsphenoidal hypophysectomy, and bilateral total adrenalectomy. Her adrenals showed multinodularity with one large hyperplastic nodule thought to be autonomous. She did poorly after her adrenalectomy and died of a stroke, but was not autopsied.

Table V   *Proton hypophysectomy: Cushing's disease. Results of therapy*

	Hypercorticism	Nelson's syndrome	Total	Percent of followed cases
Remission	23	3	26	58 % } 89 %
Improved	10	4	14	31 % }
Failed	5	0	5	11 %
No follow-up	6	1	7	
Total	44	8	52	

Table VI   *Proton hypophysectomy: Cushing's disease. Undesirable effects*

	Hypercorticism	Nelson's syndrome	Total
No. of patients	44	8	52
Temporary oculomotor disturbance	3	1	4
Visual loss	1	0	1
Hypopituitary			
Anterior partial	1	1	2
Anterior total	2	0	2
Posterior temporary	0	0	0
Posterior permanent	0	0	0
Retreatment	5	0	5

4. Chromophobe adenoma

Risk to the optic nerves is avoided by identifying in a pneumoencephalogram the absence of tumor above the clinoids and tracing the course of the optic nerves from the chiasm between the suprachiasmatic and suprapituitary recesses to their entrance into the optic foramina just below the level of the tuberculum of the sphenoid. When significant suprasellar extension exists, one cannot define in a pneumoencephalogram the separation between the dome of the tumor and the optic nerves. The solution is simply not to treat such patients with the proton beam.

Patients with suprasellar extension require open surgical hypophysectomy, for which we prefer the transsphenoidal route. Our reason is that none of our patients treated in this manner have experienced a fatality, nor have they experienced the emergence or aggravation of a field defect. Subtotal excision is probably adequate. We line the cavity with gold foil and can then follow the patients with periodic X-rays to detect shifts of the gold foil and with visual field examinations.

Retreatment can be done by any of several methods. We do not know the reoperation rate for the transsphenoidal operation in the larger series, but this may soon be documented. In some centers, conventional X-ray is given routinely immediately postoperatively. Ray et al. had a recurrence rate of 8 % in transfrontally operated patients who received postoperative X-ray. We consider it to be a liability if it is necessary to X-irradiate all patients for the limited gain of reducing the recurrence rate from 22 % to 8 %. Thus, only 14 % are really benefitted, while 100 % are subject to the expense, inconvenience and income loss that is associated with a course of X-ray therapy.

Of 33 patients treated since 1964 by the proton beam for benign chromophobe adenoma, one has been known to develop a recurrence of solid tumor and transsphenoidal hypophysectomy was done. Two other patients with developing field defects were operated on by the transsphenoidal route and we found fluid-filled cysts, one with a tan layer on the walls and the other with glistening white fibrous tissue on its walls. Pathologic examination confirmed no recurrence in the cyst walls.

It is considered that therapy of asymptomatic non-functioning adenomas will prevent the progress of these lesions to chiasmal compression. It is probably better to employ the minimal risk of limited dose radiation therapy than to deal with the chiasmal syndrome by craniotomy at a later date. The custom of serial plain skull X-rays and visual field examinations does little to protect the patient from the development of a suprasellar extension of the tumor.

Authors' methods

1. Stereotactic Bragg peak proton hypophysectomy

The accelerated protons are extracted from the cyclotron by bending magnets and are concentrated into a beam by focusing magnets. Figure 3 diagrammatically portrays the sequence of manipulations of the proton beam. Detailed point by point measurement of the beam is made possible by a silicon diode detector which was developed by one of our physics staff.[22] The tiny dosimeter with a cross-section sensitive area of 0.25 mm has been used to map the beams of various diameters.

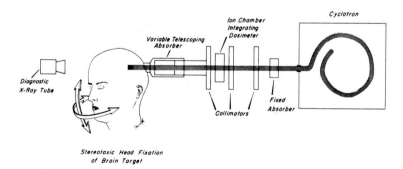

Fig. 3 Diagram of the sequence in the course of a proton beam from acceleration to cranial target. The diagram indicates the basic relation between the principal components of the system.

Figure 4 shows the isodose contours of such a beam, 7 mm in diameter. The radiation to the pituitary gland is delivered through 12 portals of entry. The computations of the three-dimensional isodose curve for one central coronal plane is done by a computer, as shown in Figure 5.

DOSE IN PERCENT OF PEAK DOSE
7mm DIAM. BEAM WITH ~12.5 cm RANGE

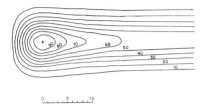

Fig. 4   Isodose curve of a single proton beam. The cross-section of the beam through its central axis is mapped in three dimensions by a silicon diode radiation detector with a sensitive area of 0.25 mm².

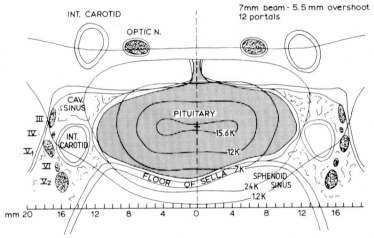

Fig. 5   Computer-produced isodose curve of 12 converging beams superimposed on a diagram of the pituitary region. Isodose curves are a three-dimension composite determined by a computer for beams of various diameters and for various widths of the pituitary fossa.

To induce frank radionecrosis in most pituitary targets (except chromophobe adenoma), large doses of 6000–10,000 rads at the Bragg peak are used. When the object of therapy is to induce growth arrest of chromophobe adenoma, the dose is 2000–4000 rads. The dose at the site of entrance and along the path of a single beam is about one-tenth to one-twentieth that of the central target dose. Figure 6 is an example in which 7000 rads are delivered to the pituitary with a 12 mm beam. In this example, the dose to the temporal lobe along the beam path is 300 rads and the remaining temporal lobe and cerebrum receive essentially no radiation (less than 1 rad).

In our method, the entire course of radiation is completed in normally 30–40 minutes. The stereotactic instrument as shown in Figure 7 is a modification of our general purpose stereotactic instrument.[23] To illustrate the method, Figure 8 shows radiographic confirmation of this superimposition of the proton beam upon the pituitary (a small circle and a central dot on the radiograph marked by a beam spot in the pituitary fossa). Depth of penetration of the Bragg peak is controlled by the variable water absorber (Fig. 3). Computed corrections in length of the path are introduced to account for variations in radiation absorption by the bone and tissues.

PITUITARY TARGET DOSE: 7000 RADS
(12 mm BEAM)

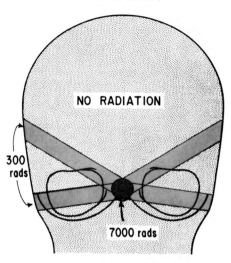

NO RADIATION

300 rads

7000 rads

Fig. 6   Example of proton radiation dose and distribution in the coronal plane. The diagram represents an approximately coronal plane of the head through the pituitary target, taken from the protocol of a typical patient with acromegaly. Four of the 12 entering beams are shown; the remainder are anterior or posterior to this plane. It illustrates the small dose of radiation along the beam path and the absence of radiation throughout most of the brain. The pituitary target dose is ample to induce radionecrosis confined to the pituitary.

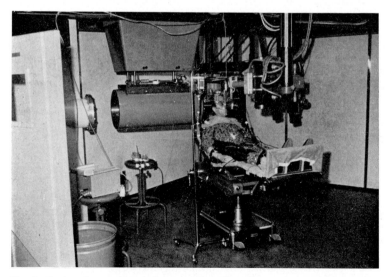

Fig. 7   Patient in stereotactic instrument undergoing proton radiation. The patient's head, fixed to the stereotaxic instrument, is seen in the center. To the left, the system of collimators and the ion chamber is housed in a large cylinder. To the far left is the source of the beam from the cyclotron. To the right is the diagnostic X-ray equipment for centering the pituitary target.

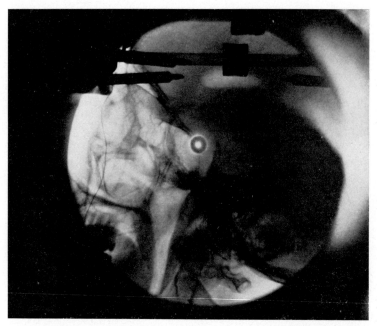

Fig. 8   Beam spot: exposure of protons on a radiograph of sella turcica. A skull X-ray taken during
the alignment of the proton beam with the pituitary target shows the brief exposure of the
proton beam exposed on the X-ray film – the 'beam spot'.

From the pneumoencephalogram, we determine the course of the optic nerve. The center
of the beam is brought to lie a distance below the plane of the optic nerves so that they receive not more than 1000 rads. Figure 2 displays the radial dose distribution for beams of
several sizes, from which we establish the radiation dose at any particular point. The beam
center is placed 2 mm anteriorly to the midpoint of the sella to spare the posterior lobe from
high doses of radiation. In patients with acromegaly and Cushing's disease, the beam diameter
is selected to leave a 1 mm shell around the margins of the sella, since this usually is the remnant of normal pituitary gland, and normal pituitary function may thus be preserved.

The entire therapeutic procedure is done in a single stage or sitting under local anesthesia,
usually in 1½ hours. The patient walks to and from the procedure, leaving the hospital in
2 days, and can immediately return to his occupation.

2. *Microsurgical, transsphenoidal*

Our technique is similar to that developed and described by Professor Guiot and Dr. Hardy.
We normally line the cavity with multiple-folded segments of gold foil placed against the
diaphragm, cavernous sinus and bony boundaries. The gold foil markers have proved to be
useful in follow-up evaluation for the question of recurrence. We have adopted the policy
of not conducting postoperative radiation on a routine basis. Instead, the patients are followed with periodic radiographic examinations wherein we compare the gold foil contour
and position with that obtained shortly after the operation. We anticipate that shifts in the
foil would be evidence of recurrence and radiation would then be performed.

3. *Microsurgical, transfrontal*

We began using the operating microscope for pituitary surgery in 1963 and later included the image amplifier in much the same manner as for transsphenoidal surgery. We seek scrupulously to preserve the blood vessels on the superior surface. Bergland and Ray[24] drew attention to the importance of this blood supply nourishing the optic chiasm. Occasionally, a tiny mirror is useful in visualizing the depths of the sella. Gold foil is placed on the floor and the lateral walls. The image amplifier confirms that the foil is applied closely to the bony outlines and that no gaps representing tumor are remaining. Gold foil is also placed against the diaphragm, and the postoperative X-rays are as shown in Figure 9.

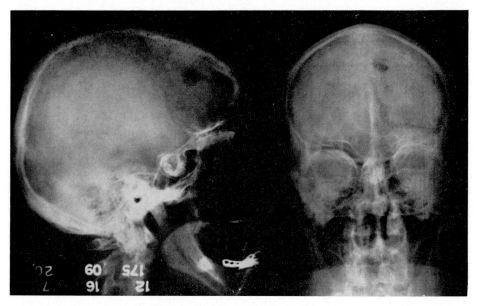

Fig. 9 X-rays showing folded layers of gold foil lining the sella turcica. Gold foil is folded in several layers and matted against the inner boundaries of the pituitary tumor after it has been excised. Follow-up X-ray examinations can be compared to detect shifts in the foil, which would be early evidence of tumor recurrence.

Discussion

The system of surgery described herein for pituitary tumors appears to have virtually eliminated the risk of mortality associated with therapeutic procedures, except for those risks associated with the use of general anesthesia, such as pulmonary embolism and hepatitis. The overall morbidity is low, largely attributable to the preponderance of proton-treated cases.

The patients' acceptance of the proton procedure under only local anesthesia is quite good. Their attitude and emotional preparation is largely attributable to the fact that all the members of the clinical team – endocrinologist, surgeon, nurse and anesthetist – spend ample amounts of time explaining the procedure and answering their questions. They are, in general, comfortable and reassured during the 1.5–2-hour period of the stereotactic procedure.

The hospital costs associated with proton therapy compare well with the other methods in these patients, as shown in Table VII. The expense of frontal craniotomy is about 3 times greater than proton hypophysectomy, and transsphenoidal hypophysectomy is midway between these. This is largely attributable to the difference in length of hospital stay following

Table VII   *Surgical treatment methods: comparison of hospital costs*

	Open		Bragg peak
	Frontal craniotomy	Transsphenoidal hypophysectomy	proton beam hypophysectomy
Average	$ 5,005	$ 2,713	$ 1,569
Minimum	$ 4,227	$ 2,338	$ 855
Maximum	$ 6,501	$ 3,154	$ 2,391

Table VIII   *Hospital days: procedure to discharge*

Diagnosis	Open		Bragg peak
	Frontal craniotomy	Transsphenoidal hypophysectomy	proton beam hypophysectomy
Acromegaly	18	10	2
Cushing's disease	17	16	2
Chromophobe adenoma	16	18	2
Other	14	20	3

a procedure, as shown in Table VIII. In addition to the short in-hospital convalescence, there is no home convalescence or work disability.

We presume it to be the intention of this symposium to allow comparisons to be made between the many alternatives available in diagnosis and management of pituitary tumors. Because of the difficulty in making worthwhile comparisons between non-standardized format and definitions employed by various workers, we recommend that uniform standards for evaluation of methods and results be formulated for systems of pituitary therapy. This is an instance in which physicians should exercise initiative before they find others doing it for them.

This symposium also gives testimony to the fact that the management of pituitary tumors tends to be more or less a function of 'centers'. An epidemiologist tells us[25] that there are about 2500 newly diagnosed pituitary tumors each year in the United States or a little over one per year per neurosurgeon. Inevitably, most of the pituitary surgery will be performed by a limited number of neurosurgeons. The epidemiologist further reports that only about 300 new cases of acromegaly emerge each year. On this basis, between the Berkeley cyclotron[26] and ourselves, about half the new cases of acromegaly are being treated by particle radiation beams.

We are grateful to referring endocrinologists who have permitted us to work in this fascinating area. In many instances the referral is accompanied by a pneumoencephalogram and test results for the major pituitary functions. A detailed endocrine and physiologic survey is completed during the same time required for the further radiodiagnostic procedures. Visual acuity and perimetry are obtained immediately prior to the treatment procedure. Patients return to their referring physicians, who have been extraordinarily helpful in providing follow-up evaluation and data. We have recommended extensive follow-up at 6, 12 and 24 months with an annual follow-up thereafter. This approach has provided the most useful information as to the reliability of treatment techniques and secures a high degree of medical observation and care for every patient.

Acknowledgments

The authors gratefully acknowledge the theoretical and technical services of the cyclotron crew of the Harvard Physics Department, particularly Mr. Andreas M. Koehler and Dr. William M. Preston. We thank the nurses and technicians of the Endocrine Unit and Laboratory. We especially thank Dr. William H. Sweet, Chief of Neurosurgery, and Dr. Alexander Leaf, Chief of Medicine, of the Massachusetts General Hospital, for counsel and support. We particularly thank Miss Rita Thompson and Mrs. Billie Swisher for the compilation of data and editorial work.

References

(1) WALKER, A. E. (1951) (Ed.): *A History of Neurological Surgery*, p. 166. Williams and Wilkins, Baltimore.

(2) HENDERSON, W. R. (1939): The pituitary adenomata. A follow-up study of the surgical results in 338 cases (Dr. Harvey Cushing's series). *Brit. J. Surg.*, 26, 811.

(3) RAY, B. S. and PATTERSON, R. H. (1971): Surgical experience with chromophobe adenomas of the pituitary gland. *J. Neurosurg.*, 34, 726.

(4) RAY, B. S., HORWITH, M. and MAUTALEN, C. (1968): Surgical hypophysectomy as a treatment for acromegaly. In: *Clinical Endocrinology, II*, pp. 93–102. Editors: E. B. Astwood and C. E. Cassidy. Grune and Stratton, New York.

(5) HAMLIN, H.: Personal communication.

(6) LEE, W. M. and ADAMS, J. E. (1968): The empty sella syndrome. *J. Neurosurg.*, 28, 351.

(7) KJELLBERG, R. N., SHINTANI, A., FRANTZ, A. G. and KLIMAN, B. (1968): Proton beam therapy in acromegaly. *New Engl. J. Med.*, 278, 689.

(8) GLICK, S. M. (1967): Acromegaly and other disorders of growth hormone secretion: combined Clinical Staff Conference at National Institutes of Health. *Ann. intern. Med.*, 66, 760.

(9) ROTH, J., GORDEN, P. and BRACE, K. (1970): Efficacy of conventional pituitary irradiation in acromegaly. *New Engl. J. Med.*, 282, 1385.

(10) ADAMS, J. E., SEYMOUR, R. J., EARL, J. M., TUCK, M., SPARKS, L. L. and FORSHAM, P. H. (1968): Transsphenoidal cryohypophysectomy in acromegaly, clinical and endocrinological evaluation. *J. Neurosurg.*, 28, 100.

(11) RAND, R. W. (1966): Cryosurgery of the pituitary in acromegaly: reduced growth hormone levels following hypophysectomy in 13 cases. *Ann. Surg.*, 164, 587.

(12) DAVIDOFF, L. M. (1926): Studies in acromegaly. III. The anamnesis and symptomatology in one hundred cases. *Endocrinology*, 10, 461.

(13) ORTH, D. N. and LIDDLE, G. W. (1971): Results of treatment in 108 patients with Cushing's syndrome. *New Engl. J. Med.*, 285, 243.

(14) SPRAGUE, R. G., WEEKS, R. E., PRIESTLEY, J. T. and SALASSA, R. M. (1961): Treatment of Cushing's syndrome by adrenalectomy. In: *Modern Trends in Endocrinology*, pp. 84–99. Editors: H. Gardiner-Hill. Paul B. Hoeber Inc., New York.

(15) SALASSA, R. M., KEARNS, T. P., KERNOHAN, J. W., SPRAGUE, R. G. and MacCARTY, C. S. (1959): Pituitary tumors in patients with Cushing's syndrome. *J. clin. Endocr.*, 19, 1523.

(16) RANDALL, R. V.: Personal communication.

(17) CUSHING, H. (1932): The basophil adenomas of the pituitary body and their clinical manifestations (pituitary basophilism). *Bull. Johns Hopk. Hosp.*, 50, 137.

(18) PLOTZ, C. M., KNOWLTON, A. I. and RAGAN, C. (1952): Natural history of Cushing's syndrome. *Amer. J. Med.*, 13, 597.

(19) RUSSFIELD, A. B. (1968): Diseases of the pituitary. In: *Pathology of the Nervous System. I.*, pp. 619–638. Editor: J. Minckler. Mc-Graw Hill, New York.

(20) JEFFERSON, G. (1960): Extrasellar extensions of pituitary adenomas. In: *Sir Geoffrey Jefferson: Selected Papers*, p. 375. Charles C. Thomas, Springfield, Ill.

(21) NIELSEN, S. L., KJELLBERG, R. N., ASBURY, A. K. and KOEHLER, A. M. (1972): Neuropathologic effects of proton-beam irradiation in man. II. Evaluation after pituitary irradiation. *Acta Neuropath.*, 21, 76.

(22) KOEHLER, A. M. (1967): Dosimetry of proton beams using small silicon diodes. *Radiat. Res., Suppl.*, 7, 53.

(23) KJELBERG, R. N., KOEHLER, A. M., PRESTON, W. M. and SWEET, W. H. (1962): Stereotaxic instrument for use with the Bragg peak of a proton beam. *Confin. neurol. (Basel)*, *22*, 183.

(24) BERGLAND, R. and RAY, B. S. (1969): The arterial supply of the human optic chiasm. *J. Neurosurg.*, *31*, 327.

(25) POSKANZER, D. C.: Personal communication.

(26) LAWRENCE, J. H., TOBIAS, C. A., LINFOOT, J. A., BORN, J. L., LYMAN, J. T., CHONG, C. Y., MANOUGIAN, E. and WEI, W. C. (1970): Successful treatment of acromegaly: metabolic and clinical studies in 145 patients. *J. clin. Endocr.*, *31*, 180.

Treatment of pituitary tumors with heavy particles

JOHN H. LAWRENCE, CLAUDE Y. CHONG, JOHN T. LYMAN, CORNELIUS
A. TOBIAS, JAMES L. BORN, JOSEPH F. GARCIA, EDWARD MANOUGIAN,
JOHN A. LINFOOT and GERALD M. CONNELL

Donner Laboratory, Lawrence Berkeley Laboratory, University of California,
Berkeley, Calif., U.S.A.

The treatment of pituitary disorders with externally delivered radiation posed a problem for radiotherapists because of the relative radioresistance of the normal pituitary gland[1] as well as of the hyperplastic or adenomatous glands such as we find in acromegaly, Cushing's disease and Nelson's syndrome. Metabolic effects from conventional pituitary irradiation procedures have not usually been seen[5-7] because of the limitation placed on the pituitary dose in order to avoid possibly damaging doses to surrounding vital structures such as cranial nerves, hypothalamus, and the temporal lobes. However, the availability of high energy, charged, heavy-particle beams provides a safe and effective method for intense irradiation of small volumes deep within the body.[5] When studies demonstrated that it is possible to suppress pituitary function safely in animals with heavy particles,[6] we began investigating their use in treating human disease.

In 1954, 340-MeV protons were first used to suppress pituitary function in patients with far advanced metastatic breast cancer.[7, 8] Since 1957, higher energy 910-MeV alpha particles have been used, and their therapeutic applications were soon extended to include the treatment of patients with disorders of the pituitary gland, including acromegaly, Cushing's disease, Nelson's syndrome, and chromophobe adenoma.[9-12] With these high energy, charged, heavy particles, it is possible to overcome the relative insensitivity of the pituitary gland to externally delivered radiation and to deliver safely to the pituitary area sufficiently large doses of energy to treat these pituitary disorders successfully. In addition, the patient is ambulatory during the treatment period, the procedure is painless, and there is no need to enter the cranium either surgically or by needle.

Acromegaly

Acromegaly is a disorder usually caused by an eosinophilic tumor of the pituitary gland, with resultant hypersecretion of growth hormone leading to the development of its many signs and symptoms. The life expectancy of these patients is reduced. One study reports that in 100 cases of acromegaly, 50 % had died before the age of 50 years and 89 % by age 60 years;[13] another study reports that the number of deaths in 194 patients was almost twice that expected from a matched general population.[14] In addition, both these studies indicate an increased incidence of deaths due to cardiovascular and cerebrovascular causes.

Until recently, surgical partial hypophysectomy or limited doses of X-ray had been the usual therapeutic methods. With the availability of cortisone for replacement therapy, surgical hypophysectomy has been used with considerable success[15, 16] as have pituitary implants of gold-198 or of yttrium-90,[17-20] and more recently cryosurgery,[21] thermocautery,[22] and transsphenoidal hypophysectomy as developed by Jules Hardy.[23] However, using an externally delivered high energy alpha particle beam from a cyclotron, it is possible to deliver sufficiently large doses to the pituitary area to control the excessive growth hormone secretion and thereby to treat acromegaly successfully.

Since 1958, we have used 910-MeV alpha particles to treat 191 patients with acromegaly. Following therapy, the relief of signs and symptoms is gradually achieved. Headache, the most frequent and troublesome symptom encountered, has either markedly improved or disappeared in most of the patients within one year. Lethargy and weakness improve following treatment. The acral enlargement has not progressed, and has decreased in one-third of the patients within 4 years after completing therapy. The typical coarse heavy facial appearance of these patients has undergone satisfying changes in one-third of the group followed for at least 4 years. This was evident in a refinement and decrease in mass of the supraorbital ridges, the malar prominences, the jaw and the nose. Primarily the changes occur in the soft tissue mass, but there is also evidence of change in the bones as demonstrated by comparative head casts, X-ray examinations of the hands and feet, and studies of calcium metabolism. The paresthesias, which were present in about 50 % of the patients, had improved in 54 % within one year and in 81 % within 3 years.

The plasma growth hormone levels, as determined by radioimmunoassay[25] were lower following treatment. The level had dropped to within normal limits (≤ 5 mμg/ml) in 37 % of the patients within 2 years, and 94 % of those followed for 9 or more years. When the growth hormone level has dropped to 10 mμg/ml or less, significant metabolic improvement is usually seen: this level was achieved in 71 % of the patients within 2 years. Other abnormalities in carbohydrate metabolism, including insulin resistance, diabetic-type glucose tolerance curves, and the presence of diabetes mellitus, usually disappear following treatment.

Although some degree of hypopituitarism has occurred in about one-third of the patients as a result of achieving adequate control of their disease, this develops slowly in most patients. Cortisone replacement therapy has been required in only one-third of those patients whom we have followed for at least 2 years, with replacement therapy being initiated usually between 2 and 4 years after completion of heavy-particle therapy (range 1–12 years). About 35 % of the patients required thyroid replacement at some time following treatment, but this was more difficult to assess because many patients had been placed on thyroid prior to treatment without clear documentation of the need for such therapy. Androgen therapy was subsequently given to about 10 % of the men and estrogen therapy to slightly more than 10 % of the women. We have no clinical evidence of sterility occurring in any of these patients. Nevertheless, we encourage young couples to initiate their families promptly after treatment. Three patients have become pregnant following therapy, and the wives of 5 other patients have also become pregnant, with subsequent normal deliveries in all instances. All patients and their attending physicians are alerted to the possible eventual need for adrenal as well as other types of hormonal replacement. In addition, all patients are given cards to carry explaining this possible need under conditions of stress, such as infection, surgery or injury. We ask them to join Medical Alert.[24]

It is reasonable to expect that, along with the improvement observed in the metabolic picture, there will also be an extension of comfortable and chronological life in these patients to normal or nearly normal for their age group and for a group of people with similar incidence of vascular disease or other independent disease processes. There is a high incidence of cardiovascular complications in patients with acromegaly. Many of the patients referred to us for treatment had been considered by both their physicians and us to be poor risks for other therapeutic procedures such as surgery, cryosurgery or radioactive implants (3 patients were referred for heavy-particle therapy after surgical procedures had been attempted and abandoned because of complications arising during surgery). The increased incidence of deaths due to cardiovascular and cerebrovascular causes, which had been noted in other studies,[13, 14] was also apparent in our series. Only 13 of the 191 patients treated during the past 15 years have died, and 5 of the deaths were due to cardiovascular disease, with all 5 patients having had cardiomegaly and hypertension prior to heavy-particle therapy. It is interesting to note also that in the patients treated by us, the median duration of their acromegaly was 8 years (range 1–40 years) at the time we treated them. The median durations were the same for males and females, although the males were younger on the average at the time of treatment – 39.0 years (range 17–60) compared to 46.2 years (range 20–68). If lowering the growth hormone level to normal is effective in extending duration of comfortable life, then these patients should be treated much earlier in the course of their acromegaly.

In addition to the 5 patients who died of cardiovascular complications, there are 8 patients who died of varying causes including suicide, acute myeloblastic leukemia, an accidental overdose of barbiturates 5 years after treatment, complications of a bleeding duodenal ulcer, septicemia with *Histoplasma capsulatum*, and acute vascular collapse during surgery for an unrelated condition. One died 11 years after completion of therapy from a meningioma in an area of the brain estimated to have received 300 rads. It seems unlikely that a cause-effect relationship between therapy and tumor was present. The last of the 13 deceased patients died from complications following a second transfrontal craniotomy.

The incidence of complications after heavy-particle therapy has been very low in our series, in part the result of our selection criteria. We feel strongly that in cases where extrasellar extension of the pituitary adenoma is present, serious consideration of surgical treatment is required. Suprasellar extensions were found in several patients who did not have visual field cuts, but only after carefully conducted tomographic pneumoencephalography. Therefore, this procedure is routinely carried out prior to accepting a patient for heavy-particle treatment in order to rule out the presence of suprasellar extension. In many cases arteriograms are also done, and in some cases cavernous venograms are valuable.

Seven patients who had very large suprasellar tumor extensions were not treated by us, but were referred for surgical hypophysectomies. Four patients were treated with heavy particles after having undergone surgical removal of their suprasellar extensions. We believed one other patient with a small suprasellar extension should have had this surgically excised prior to heavy-particle therapy, but he wanted to avoid surgery. Even though we did not consider him an ideal candidate, we treated him initially with heavy-particle pituitary irradiation (7500 rads/11 days) in October 1964. Initially, he improved with a fall in growth hormone level from 20 to 16 mμg/ml. However, he subsequently relapsed, and 2 years after heavy-particle therapy his growth hormone level was again 28 mμg/ml. Dr. Bronson Ray subsequently performed a surgical hypophysectomy, and this patient is currently doing well (growth hormone level down to 6 mμg/ml).

A total of 22 of the 191 patients we have treated had previously undergone a surgical procedure. In addition to the 4 already mentioned (who had suprasellar extensions surgically excised prior to heavy-particle therapy), there were 2 who had partial hypophysectomy followed by heavy-particle therapy within 5 months (and one of these had also undergone cryohypophysectomy 4.5 years prior to the second surgical procedure). Sixteen other patients had prior surgical hypophysectomies: 2 had cryohypophysectomy, 6 had transfrontal hypophysectomies, 5 had transsphenoidal hypophysectomies, and 3 had undergone 2 prior surgical procedures (one had cryohypophysectomy followed in 4.5 years by transfrontal hypophysectomy and the other had 2 transsphenoidal hypophysectomies within 3 months). However, all 16 patients had persistent or recurrent elevation in growth hormone levels and activity of the acromegalic signs and symptoms, and they were therefore treated with heavy particles on the average of 18 months after the surgical procedure (range 6 months to 3 years). Ten of these 16 patients were treated during the past year and follow-up information is not available yet; the remaining 6 were treated from 1 to 3 years ago, and they have all shown symptomatic improvements and their growth hormone levels have fallen.

Three patients in our series have undergone subsequent transsphenoidal hypophysectomies. One patient had an initial response to heavy particles, but later had a recurrence of high growth hormone levels. The second patient developed diplopia and her growth hormone level was still elevated at 6 months posttherapy when the hypophysectomy was performed. We would have preferred to observe the patient for a longer period of time, since our experience has indicated that periods of greater than 6 months are often required before optimal effects of heavy-particle therapy are observed. Sixteen months after transsphenoidal hypophysectomy the growth hormone level was down to 7 mμg/ml and she had improved significantly. The diplopia had disappeared immediately after surgery. The third has recently undergone surgical hypophysectomy and no details are available yet.

Another factor in our selection criteria is that since 1961 we have not accepted any patients for heavy-particle therapy who have received prior pituitary irradiation, since an increased incidence of mild ocular complications was noted among a few such patients whom we had accepted prior to that time. Six of the patients referred between 1958 and 1960 had already received from 1 to 3 courses of X-ray therapy (total doses ranging from 2000 to 5270 rads), but because they still had active and progressive acromegaly they were accepted, although reluctantly, for heavy-particle therapy. Mild non-progressive ocular complications subsequently developed in 3 of these 6 patients: in 2, transient diplopias occurred 14 months following heavy-particle therapy (both patients are doing well today, 13 years since treatment); in the third, a quadrant cut occurred one year after heavy-particle therapy, which did not progress (this patient died 9 years after treatment from a cerebral vascular accident at the age of 68). These mild ocular complications are presumed to have resulted from therapy, and their occurrence further reinforced our belief that heavy-particle therapy should be limited to those patients who have not received previous radiation therapy. As previously mentioned, we have followed this policy since 1961.

Mild ocular complications developed in 2 other patients in the group treated prior to 1961. The pituitary was very large in each of these cases, and therefore a large aperture was used in treatment. Bilateral small upper-field cuts developed in one patient 10 months after therapy, and these have remained stable for the past 10 years. The other patient complained of transient diplopia at 3 weeks and of difficulty in focusing his eyes when driving at 8 weeks posttherapy; symptoms compatible with uncinate seizures developed at 15 months posttherapy, but these were not constant and the patient has been seizure-free for 8 years. Both these patients are currently doing well, it being over 11 years since treatment.

Using our current selection criteria, which means not accepting patients who had received prior radiation therapy or who have extrasellar tumor extensions (and requiring pneumoencephalography and tomography to rule out the presence of the latter), we have limited the dosage delivered to the brain tissue surrounding the pituitary gland and to the cranial nerves to less than 3500 rads/6F/11 days. Of the 170 patients treated since 1961, 162 were treated with the plateau portion of the alpha-particle beam using a biplanar rotational technique; we have experienced no neurological complications in this large group.

Five patients with very large pituitary tumors were treated with the Bragg peak (which we have occasionally employed since 1968), because it is not possible by the present rotation technique to give a sufficient dose to a very large pituitary unless the Bragg peak is employed. Twelve portals were used in treating 2 of these patients, and they have each had an excellent response with no evidence of side effects. The other 3 were treated with 6 portals; in 2 patients transient diplopias developed, and in the third a transient unilateral scotoma developed. The scotoma may have been unrelated to the treatment, since it cleared rapidly and the patient has no sign of ocular difficulty 18 months following treatment. One patient who had transient diplopia developed uncinate seizures which were controlled by anticonvulsant therapy. Three additional patients were recently treated with a combination of plateau and Bragg peak heavy particles, but we have no follow-up information yet.

Our total experience using heavy particles to treat this large number of patients (191) over a 15-year period is encouraging, and it indicates that good control of acromegaly can be achieved by this safe method with a very low incidence of side effects.

Cushing's disease and Nelson's syndrome

In 1932, Cushing described a clinical syndrome he called the pluriglandular syndrome (which we now call Cushing's disease), a disorder he believed to be caused by a basophilic adenoma of the anterior lobe of the pituitary.[26] Actually, as an intern in surgery at the Peter Bent Brigham Hospital, I (J.L.) did the work-up on the first patient Dr. Cushing diagnosed as having basophilic adenoma.[27] When similar clinical findings were observed in patients with benign or malignant adrenal tumors or with adrenocortical hyperplasia, many investigators were led to believe that the condition was usually due to primary adrenal hyperfunction. When adrenocorticosteroids became available for replacement therapy, surgical adrenalectomy was successfully performed in many patients with Cushing's disease.

However, more recent findings are again causing clinicians to attack the pituitary gland first. When ectopic ACTH-producing tumors, adrenal adenomas, or cortisone-producing adrenal carcinomas can be ruled out as the cause of the syndrome, the pituitary gland or the hypothalamic-pituitary axis is the primary site of overactivity leading to adrenal hyperplasia and Cushing's syndrome. The evidence for this has been provided by the use of sensitive bioassay and radioimmunoassay methods for measuring plasma ACTH levels and thus revealing that small amounts of ACTH are released by these patients in spite of their high circulating levels of hydrocortisone.[28, 29] Also, roentgenologically detectable pituitary tumors were found in 15–25 % of the cases, with the additional observation that many of these tumors were not detectable until after bilateral surgical adrenalectomy. Furthermore, the incidence of Nelson's syndrome,[30] which sometimes develops following total adrenalectomy and is characterized by deep pigmentation of the skin similar to that seen in Addison's disease, was noted to be lower in those patients who had received pituitary irradiation prior to their adrenal surgery.[31] Since 1959, we have treated 27 patients to control adrenal hypersecretion through the administration of heavy particles to the pituitary gland. An additional 8 patients had previously been treated elsewhere for Cushing's syndrome by bilateral adrenalectomy, and were referred to us for heavy-particle treatment to the pituitary gland when Nelson's syndrome had developed.

Most of the 27 patients treated with heavy particles for primary adrenal hyperplasia received maximum pituitary doses from 9000 to 15,000 rads in 6 fractions over 11 days (one patient received only 6000 rads/11 days). Previous unsuccessful adrenal surgery had been carried out in 4 patients. One had undergone bilateral adrenalectomy, but subsequently developed Cushing's syndrome presumably from accessory adrenal tissue. Three had undergone subtotal adrenalectomies. With the exception of some of the patients with prior adrenal surgery, all patients could be characterized as having elevated urinary 17-hydroxycorticosteroids. In most patients the plasma cortisol was modestly to markedly elevated; in all patients the diurnal rhythm was abnormal, and the steroid responses to ACTH and to the oral or intravenous administration of metyrapone were exaggerated. Those patients who had adrenal remnants or accessory adrenal tissue were maximally ACTH stimulated and, as expected, their responses to suppression and stimulation tests were more like those observed in patients with adrenal adenomas. Dexamethasone suppression was determined in most patients; all showed suppression of greater than 50% at the high dose (8 mg/day), but few showed suppression at the low dose (2 mg/day). The ACTH levels (available only in the recent patients) were not markedly elevated, which is the expected finding in patients with bilateral adrenal hyperplasia.

Nineteen patients were treated more than one year ago (1959 to 1971), and follow-up studies reveal a significant fall in the 17-hydroxycorticosteroids (17-OHCS) following treatment. The exaggerated steroid response to metyrapone, which had been seen in all patients who had not undergone prior adrenal surgery, was also dramatically obliterated by heavy-particle therapy. Partial or complete remissions occurred in 18 of these 19 patients, but our analysis of the cases indicated a higher percentage of lasting results in patients treated with higher doses. Among the 7 patients who were treated in the lower-dose range (6000–10,000 rads/11 days), remissions were observed in 6. The other patient, who had previously undergone unilateral adrenalectomy, did not return for follow-up evaluation, but studies elsewhere demonstrated failure to respond. Without consultation with us, he subsequently had total adrenalectomy there, 9 months after our treatment. If a longer waiting period had been allowed, this might not have been necessary. Two patients had only transient remissions and later relapsed and underwent total adrenalectomies at 7 months and 38 months respectively. One patient in this group (D.M.), who had been in clinical remission for 6.5 years, died of infection.

All 12 patients who were treated in the higher dose range (11,000–15,000 rads/11 days) have had partial or complete remissions, and only 2 subsequently relapsed. One of these later had a total adrenalectomy. The pathology report revealed bilateral adrenal hyperplasia rather than nodular change in the adrenals. The other patient died 11 months after treatment, presumably from a cardiovascular or cerebrovascular accident (no autopsy performed).

The response rate in these 19 patients for whom we have one or more years of follow-up information appears to be significantly better than that obtained in patients treated with conventional radiation (a recent paper reported 20 % of the patients cured with such radiation therapy).[32] In addition, this form of treatment is a direct approach to the pathological secretion of ACTH, and therefore has the additional advantage of preventing the subsequent development of pituitary tumors in the rare patient who may have to have adrenalectomy later. None of the patients with Cushing's disease whom we have treated initially with heavy particles to the pituitary has subsequently developed pigmentation or evidence of pituitary tumor following therapy. A possible disadvantage lies in the fact that other trophic hormones are at risk, and the problem of infertility must be considered. Only one patient has thus far developed hypoadrenalism. This patient had undergone total adrenalectomy in 1964, but because of recurrent Cushing's disease (accessory adrenal still present) he was referred for heavy-particle therapy in 1966. He responded well to treatment, but later required cortisone replacement therapy. A few patients have developed hypogonadism or hypothyroidism. None of the patients has developed any signs of other radiation side effects, although one developed an incomplete third nerve palsy 7 years after treatment, which cleared coincidentally following a cavernous sinus venogram.

As mentioned earlier, 8 patients had undergone total adrenalectomy elsewhere and were subsequently referred to us for heavy-particle therapy when Nelson's syndrome developed. Six of these patients had enlarged sellas, the enlargement occurring after bilateral adrenalectomy. Three of the patients with enlarged sellas had surgical excisions of suprasellar extensions prior to heavy-particle therapy. The heavy-particle doses for this group ranged from 5000 to 10,000 rads delivered in 11 days. All patients had elevated plasma ACTH levels prior to treatment; a fall in serum ACTH level was observed in the 2 cases for whom we have both pre- and post-treatment radioimmunoassay ACTH determinations. A stabilization or decrease in pigmentation was observed in all 6 patients treated more than one year ago.

One patient with Nelson's syndrome had an invasive pituitary tumor and died 4 years after treatment following difficult surgery to relieve a large suprasellar extension. This patient had shown dramatic loss of pigmentation and fall of serum ACTH levels following therapy. However, the immunoreactive ACTH level again increased to over 2500 pg/ml just prior to her transfrontal cranial surgery. Postmortem examination revealed a malignant pituitary adenoma which had extended superiorly to involve the optic chiasm, left optic nerve and tract, and inferior portion of the internal capsule. The intrasellar portion of the pituitary adenoma showed radiation fibrosis, but there were areas of well-preserved tumor tissue invading bone laterally. The tumor had the appearance of the chromophobe tumors which are often associated with patients with Cushing's disease treated with bilateral adrenalectomy (except for pleomorphism of some of the cells), and no distant metastases were found.

The above-described case points out the tendency to invasiveness and malignancy of these tumors and emphasizes the need for aggressive management of these patients.[32-36] It also supports our previous statement that in patients with Cushing's disease (when ectopic ACTH-producing tumors and adrenal adenomas or adrenal carcinomas can be ruled out), the initial therapy should be directed to the pituitary and *not* to the adrenals. Currently the experts feel that Cushing's disease is usually due to hyperactivity of the hypothalamic-pituitary-adrenal axis, and at present the pituitary should be the target for its treatment. When a sufficient radiation dose is delivered to the pituitary, a much higher percentage of patients with Cushing's disease will respond to pituitary therapy.

In summary, because of the demonstrated efficacy, the capability of administering higher doses with heavy particles, and the role of pituitary irradiation in the prevention of later development of postadrenalectomy hyperpigmentation, heavy particles are an effective treatment for Cushing's disease and can now be considered an established method of treatment.

Chromophobe adenoma

During the past 12 years we have used alpha particles to treat 23 patients with non-functioning or chromophobe adenomas of the pituitary gland. This series is necessarily limited because our selection criteria exclude patients with suprasellar extension or with massive enlargement of the sella turcica. The method of treatment is the same as described for acromegalic patients, with the range of maximum pituitary doses being 4000–8000 rads delivered in 6 fractions over 11 days (except for one patient who received 4600 rads in 3 fractions over 5 days).

Seven patients were panhypopituitary at the time of treatment; 5 of these had undergone previous transfrontal decompressive surgery, and one had a 25-year history of hypopituitarism. Although the remaining 16 patients were not clinically hypopituitary, most of them did have diminished growth hormone responses to provocative testing. Eight of this group subsequently developed hypothyroidism, and 4 of these 8 developed secondary adrenal insufficiency. One patient subsequently had further intrasphenoidal extension of his tumor requiring transnasal surgical decompression 3 years after heavy-particle therapy. Three patients in the group have died, 2 from unrelated cardiovascular complications and one from complications following a transnasal hypophysectomy, performed at another institution in an attempt to relieve intractable headaches. A longer experience with a larger number of patients will be necessary to assess the comparative value of this form of therapy in patients with chromophobe adenomas.

Summary and comments

Heavy-particle therapy provides a form of treatment with no mortality and extremely low morbidity. Its use in treating pituitary disorders has resulted in dramatic improvement in the signs and symptoms of patients with acromegaly and with Cushing's disease (adrenal hyperplasia). In general, patients with Cushing's disease require larger amounts of radiation than those with acromegaly (12,000–16,000 rads/6F/11 days compared to 4500–6500 rads/6F/11 days). Heavy-particle treatment in Nelson's syndrome appears effective but less favorable. This finding emphasizes the need for prevention of this disorder. Heavy-particle treatment of patients with chromophobe adenoma appears to compare favorably with conventional methods of treatment, but our selection criteria limit the series and interfere with a satisfactory evaluation of results. However, with the higher doses that can be delivered using heavy particles, one would expect to obtain better results and a longer average survival. A larger series followed for a longer period of time will be necessary to determine this.

Although we have used the Bragg peak for many years in the treatment of other neoplasms and pituitary lesions, we have used it for pituitary tumors in only a few patients with acromegaly whose sellas turcicas were extremely enlarged. The majority of patients received treatment administered with a biorotational technique using the plateau portion of the heavy-particle beam. In view of the negligible complications observed in the large series of patients treated with the plateau,we feel that it is the optimal method in the case of small or moderately enlarged sellas. Until we apply the method for accurately locating the Bragg peak within the skull,[37] we think that Bragg peak therapy must be employed cautiously, especially so in cases where there is marked asymmetry or difficulty in discerning the lateral margin of the tumor. The means of locating the Bragg peak within the body involves the phenomenon of 'autoactivation', the Bragg peak being located by determining the depth-activation distribution of positron emitters such as carbon-11 and nitrogen-13.[37] When accurate localization is possible, the Bragg peak using multiaxial rotation of multiple fields will provide the optimum treatment for lesions requiring larger doses of radiation and for those with vulnerable normal tissue in the vicinity. However, for the treatment of patients with acromegaly, the required dose is relatively low so that the rotation technique using the plateau is usually quite adequate. The Bragg peak of the heavy-particle beam would be advantageous in treating cases of Cushing's disease, delivering higher doses above 15,000 rads/11 days.

Finally, with the newly available very heavy, high energy, heavy particles (carbon, nitrogen, neon, etc.) which produce very dense ionization in tissue,[11] a new field of irradiating many incurable neoplasms elsewhere in the body may develop. Unlike gamma rays, the heavy-particle induced dense ionization affects cells regardless of their hypoxic state.

Groups using cyclotrons at Harvard University,[16, 17] the University of Uppsala,[40, 41] and the Joint Institute for Nuclear Research in Dubna and the Institute for Theoretical and Experimental Physics in Moscow[42, 43] are already using heavy particles in medicine.

References

(1) LAWRENCE, J. H., NELSON, W. O. and WILSON, H. (1937): Roentgen irradiation of the hypophysis. *Radiology, 29*, 446.
(2) HAMWI, G. J., SKILLMAN, T. G. and TUFTS Jr, K. C. (1960): Acromegaly. *Amer. J. Med., 29*, 690.
(3) CHRISTY, N. P. (1969): When to hospitalize in acromegaly. *Hosp. Pract., 4*, 54.
(4) ROTH, J., GORDEN, P. and BRACE, K. (1970): Efficacy of conventional pituitary irradiation in acromegaly. *New Engl. J. Med., 282*, 1385.
(5) TOBIAS, C. A., ANGER, H. O. and LAWRENCE, J. H. (1952): Radiological use of high-energy deuterons and alpha particles. *Amer. J. Roentgenol., 67*, 1.
(6) TOBIAS, C. A., VAN DYKE, D. C., SIMPSON, M. E., ANGER, H. O., HUFF, R. L. and KONEFF, A. A. (1959): Irradiation of the pituitary of the rat with high-energy deuterons. *Amer. J. Roentgenol., 72*, 1.
(7) LAWRENCE, J. H. (1957): Proton irradiation of the pituitary. *Cancer (Philad.), 10*, 795.
(8) TOBIAS, C. A., LAWRENCE, J. H., BORN, J. L., McCOMBS, R. K., ROBERTS, J. E., ANGER, H. O., LOW BEER, B. V. A. and HUGGINS, C. (1958): Pituitary irradiation with high-energy proton beams; preliminary report. *Cancer Res., 18*, 121.
(9) LAWRENCE, J. H., TOBIAS, C. A., LINFOOT, J. A., BORN, J. L., LYMAN, J. T., CHONG, C. Y., MANOUGIAN, E. and WEI, W. C. (1970): Successful treatment of acromegaly: metabolic and clinical studies in 145 patients. *J. clin. Endocr., 31*, 180.
(10) LINFOOT, J. A., LAWRENCE, J. H., TOBIAS, C. A., BORN, J. L., CHONG, C. Y., LYMAN, J. T.

and MANOUGIAN, E. (1970): Progress report on the treatment of Cushing's disease. *Trans. Amer. clin. climat. Ass., 81*, 196.

(11) TOBIAS, C. A., LYMAN, J. T. and LAWRENCE, J. H. (1971): Some considerations of physical and biological factors in radiotherapy with high-LET radiations including heavy particles, pi mesons, and fast neutrons. In: *Progress in Atomic Medicine: Recent Advances in Nuclear Medicine, Vol. 3*, pp. 167–218. Editor: J. H. Lawrence. Grune and Stratton, Inc., New York, N.Y.

(12) LINFOOT, J. A., CHONG, C. Y., GARCIA, J. F., CLEVELAND, A. S., CONNELL, G. M., MANOUGIAN, E., OKERLUND, M. D., BORN, J. L. and LAWRENCE, J. H. (1971): Heavy-particle therapy for acromegaly, Cushing's disease, Nelson's syndrome, and non-functioning pituitary adenomas. In: *Progress in Atomic Medicine: Recent Advances in Nuclear Medicine, Vol. 3*, pp. 219–238. Editor: J. H. Lawrence. Grune and Stratton, Inc., New York, N.Y.

(13) EVANS, H. M., BRIGGS, J. H. and DIXON, J. S. (1966): The physiology and chemistry of growth hormone. In: *The Pituitary Gland, Vol. 1*, pp. 439–491. Editors: G. W. Harris and B. T. Donnovan. University of California Press, Berkeley, Calif.

(14) WRIGHT, A. D., HILL, D. M., LOWY, C. and FRASER, R. (1970): Mortality in acromegaly. *Quart. J. Med., 39*, 1.

(15) HAMBERGER, C. A., HAMMER, G., NORLEN, G. and SJOGREN, B. (1960): Surgical treatment of acromegaly. *Acta oto-laryng. (Stockh.), Suppl. 158*, 168.

(16) RAY, B. S., HORWITH, M. and MAUTALEN, C. (1968): Surgical hypophysectomy as a treatment for acromegaly. In: *Clinical Endocrinology, Vol. II*, pp. 93–102. Editors: C. B. Astwood and C. E. Cassidy. Grune and Stratton, Inc., New York, N.Y.

(17) MOLINATTI, G. M., CAMANNI, F., MASSARA, F., OLIVETTI, M., PIZZINI, A. and GUILIANI, G. (1962): Implantation of yttrium-90 in sella turcica in sixteen cases of acromegaly. *J. clin. Endocr., 22*, 599.

(18) KAUFMAN, B., PEARSON, O. H., SHEALY, C. N., CHERNAK, E. B., SAMAAN, N. and STORAASLI, J. P. (1966): Transnasal transsphenoidal yttrium-90 pituitary implantation in the therapy of acromegaly. *Radiology, 86*, 915.

(19) JADRESIC, A. and POBLETE, M. (1967): Stereotaxic pituitary implantation of yttrium-90 and iridium-192 for acromegaly. *J. clin. Endocr., 27*, 1503.

(20) FRASER, T. R. and WRIGHT, A. D. (1968): Treatment of acromegaly and Cushing's disease by yttrium-90 implant for partial ablation of the pituitary. In: *Clinical Endocrinology, Vol. II*. Editors: E. B. Astwood and E. B. Cassidy. Grune and Stratton, Inc., New York, N.Y.

(21) RAND, R. W. (1966): Cryosurgery of pituitary in acromegaly: Reduced growth hormone levels following hypophysectomy in 13 cases. *Ann. Surg., 164*, 587.

(22) ZERVAS, N. T. (1969): Stereotaxic radiofrequency surgery of the abnormal pituitary gland. *New Engl. J. Med., 280*, 429.

(23) HARDY, J. and WIGSER, S. M. (1965): Transsphenoidal surgery of pituitary fossa tumors with televised radiofluoroscopic control. *J. Neurosurg., 23*, 612.

(24) Medical Alert, Medical Alert Foundation, P.O. Box 1009, Turlock, Calif. 95380, U.S.A.

(25) GARCIA, J. F., LINFOOT, J. A., MANOUGIAN, E., BORN, J. L. and LAWRENCE, J. H. (1967): Plasma growth hormone studies in normal individuals and acromegalic patients. *J. clin. Endocr., 27*, 1395.

(26) CUSHING, H. (1932): The basophil adenomas of the pituitary body and their clinical manifestations (pituitary basophilism). *Bull. Johns Hopk. Hosp., 50*, 137.

(27) LAWRENCE, J. H. and ZIMMERMAN, H. M. (1935): Pituitary basophilism: report of a case. *Arch. intern. Med., 55*, 745.

(28) NEY, R. L., SHIMIZU, N., NICHOLSON, W. E., ISLAND, D. P. and LIDDLE, G. W. (1963): Correlation of plasma ACTH concentration with adrenocortical response in normal human subjects, surgical patients, and patients with Cushing's disease. *J. clin. Invest., 42*, 1669.

(29) BERSON, S. A. and YALOW, R. S. (1968): Radioimmunoassay of ACTH in plasma. *J. clin. Invest., 47*, 2725.

(30) NELSON, D. H., MEAKIN, J. W. and THORN, G. W. (1960): ACTH-producing pituitary tumors following adrenalectomy for Cushing's syndrome. *Ann. intern. Med., 52*, 560.

(31) LIDDLE, G. T. (1967): Cushing's syndrome. In: *The Adrenal Cortex*, pp. 523–551. Editor: A. B. Eisenstein. Little, Brown and Co., Boston, Mass.

(32) ORTH, D. N. and LIDDLE, G. W. (1971): Results of treatment in 108 patients with Cushing's

disease. *New Engl. J. Med.*, *285*, 243.

(33) PLOTZ, C. M., KNOWLTON, A. I. and RAGAN, C. (1952): Natural history of Cushing's disease. *Amer. J. Med.*, *13*, 597.

(34) ROVIT, R. L. and DUANE, T. D. (1969): Cushing's syndrome and pituitary tumors: Patho-physiology and ocular manifestations of ACTH-secreting pituitary adenomas. *Amer. J. Med.*, *46/3*, 416.

(35) FRASER, R., DOYLE, F. J., JOPLIN, G. F., BURKE, C. W. and ARNOT, R. (1971): The treatment of Cushing's disease by pituitary implant of Y-90 or Au-198. In press.

(36) WELBOURN, R. B., MONTGOMERY, D. A. D. and KENNEDY, T. L. (1971): The natural history of treated Cushing's disease. *Brit. J. Surg.*, *58*, 1.

(37) TOBIAS, C. A., CHATTERJEE, A. and SMITH, A. R. (1971): Radioactive fragmentation of N^{7+} ion beam observed in a beryllium target. *Phys. Letters*, *37A*, 119.

(38) KJELLBERG, R. N., SHINTANI, A., FRANTZ, A. G. and KLIMAN, B. (1968): Proton beam therapy in acromegaly. *New Engl. J. Med.*, *278*, 689.

(39) KJELLBERG, R. N., NGUYEN, N. C. and KLIMAN, B. (1972): Le Bragg Peak protonique en neuro-chirurgie stéréotaxique. *Neuro-chirurgie*, *18*, 235.

(40) FALKMER, S., FORS, B., LARSSON, B., LINDELL, A., NAESLUND, J. and STENSON, S. (1962): Pilot study on proton irradiation of human carcinoma. *Acta radiol. (Stockh.)*, *58*, 33.

(41) LARSSON, B., LEKSELL, L. and REXED, B. (1963): The use of high energy protons for cerebral surgery in man. *Acta chir. scand.*, *125*, 1.

(42) DZHELEPOV, B. P. and BOL'DIN, L. L. (1969): The use of the existing charged heavy-particle accelerators and the possibilities of creating new domestic ones for radiation therapy. Paper presented at: Symposium on Problems in the Development of Radiation Therapy Techniques in Oncology, Moscow 1969.

(43) ABAZOV, V. I., ASTRAKHAN, B. V., BLOKHIN, N. N., BLOKHIN, S. I., BUGARCHOV, B. B., DZHELEPOV, B. P., GOLDIN, L. L., KISELEVA, V. N., KOMAROV, V. I., KLEINBOCK, Y. L., KHOROSHKIV, V. S., LOMANOV, M. F., MINAKOVA, E. I., MOLOKANOV, A. G., ONOSOVSKY, K. K., PAVLONSKY, L. M., RUDERMAN, A. I., RESHETNIKOV, G. P., SALAMOV, R. F., SHMAKOVA, N. L., SAVCHENKO, O. V., STEKOLNIKOV, V. P., SHIMCHUK, G. G., VAJNBERG, M. S., VAJNSON, A. A. and YARMONENKO, S. P. (1971): Use of proton beams in the USSR for medical and biological purposes. In: *Communications of the Joint Institute for Nuclear Research (JINR)*, *Dubna 1971*, No. E-5854.

Discussion

DR. BAKER: Dr. Backlund will open the discussion with a brief summary of the indications for and results of treatment with stereotaxic radiosurgery, a new technique employing ^{60}Co.

DR. BACKLUND: Cerebral radiosurgery makes possible the achievement of well-localized, sharply demarcated lesions in the depth of the brain by means of a stereotaxic technique with single radiation doses and without opening the skull.[1] Radiosurgery was first applied to cases in the field of functional neurosurgery using proton beams.[2] Subsequently, a simpler technique using gamma radiation from multiple Cobalt-60 sources has been worked out and is now in routine use at the department of neurosurgery, Karolinska Sjukhyset. A thorough description of the technique has been published.[3] The procedure is performed by cross-firing of the target region by well-collimated beams from 179 Cobalt-60 sources distributed within a spherical sector. The beams are radially directed toward the centre of this sector in which the predetermined target point is positioned by means of conventional stereotaxic technique. The dose distribution around the target is disc-shaped and has a steep gradient. Lesions obtained in the gray matter of the brain have been shown to satisfy the demands of precision. When these well defined brain lesions were studied, the possibility became apparent of treating inaccessible brain tumours such as pinealoma and craniopharyngioma, as well as some of the adenomas.[4] Some cases of this type have now been treated, but the number is still limited because the dose distribution hitherto available was too small for larger tumours. However, a summated dose distribution can be obtained if two or more target points are used. On the other hand, it has been possible to treat selectively those areas of tissue which reasonably could be assumed responsible for the patient's clinical condition.

The first cases were treated according to a stereotaxic treatment program for craniopharyngiomas which has been routine for these tumours since 1966.[5] This includes intracystic administration of colloidal Yttrium-90 to cause gradual shrinkage of the cystic portions, and radiosurgery to the residual solid portion after the cyst obliteration.

The first case treated with gamma irradiation was a young man with an apparently inoperable craniopharyngioma. In 1967, a single dose of 2000 rads at the target point was delivered to the solid and calcified tumour portion. Unfortunately, he died 4 months later from a tonsillar herniation, due to obstruction in a ventriculoatrial shunt, inserted 5 months previously. The autopsy showed extensive destruction of the tumour, with a sharply demarcated crescent of surviving craniopharyngioma tissue at the periphery. Because of some distortion of the preparation at the autopsy, the spatial correlations between the physical dose distribution and the serial sections were somewhat difficult to determine. The reconstruction of the dose to the surviving areas of tumour tissue was thus somewhat approximate, but was estimated to be of the magnitude of some hundred rads only. The surrounding brain substance was reported to be completely normal. It now seemed obvious that solid portions of craniopharyngiomas were suitable objects for stereotaxic radiosurgery and were probably more sensitive to irradiation than had been assumed. Because of this, a further series of four cases have been treated with the same technique.[6]

One of these cases, a 23-year-old woman (ML), followed a very interesting course. Of her main initial symptoms, the visual disturbances disappeared and the diabetes insipidus was ameliorated after the complete shrinkage of a suprasellar cyst, treated with Yttrium-90, whereas the secondary amenorrhea remained unimproved. As the solid and calcified portion of the tumour was almost filling up the whole sella, the position of the pituitary gland could not be determined when this tumour portion was to be treated with radiosurgery, and the anterior lobe may well have received a considerable radiation dose when a target dose of 5000 rads was delivered. This possibility is supported by the decrease in cortisol and PBI values after the irradiation. Later on, these values became normal, and the pituitary apparently recovered, as the patient began to menstruate spontaneously, became pregnant and gave birth to a normal child. The observation time after the radiosurgery is now 4 years, and X-rays show that the growth of the tumour was apparently arrested by the treatment.

In two patients the observation period is too short to allow any conclusions concerning the clinical effect. The treatment, however, appeared to cause arrest of tumour growth within the irradiated area, in one case manifested as a shrinkage.

The results indicate that it is possible, without surgical risks, to treat selected portions of craniopharyngiomas and apparently, to obtain obliteration of the areas irradiated.

These encouraging experiences led to the selective irradiation of some pituitary tumours. The first of these was an acromegalic woman (MM), aged 58, with severe therapy-resistant arterial hypertension and cardiac failure which contraindicated surgery. She had a history of over 10 years and she had been treated previously with conventional X-rays without effect. The sella was only moderately enlarged, but its form was such that a microadenoma situated in its most anterior part was suspected. Pneumoencephalography showed no suprasellar extension. It was decided to irradiate the anterior third of the sella, and, because of the previous radiotherapy only 2000 rads were delivered to the target (Fig. 1a). During the first days after treatment, the patient's blood pressure fell. Within two weeks it was normal, and the patient even developed orthostatic hypotension. This was thought to be the result

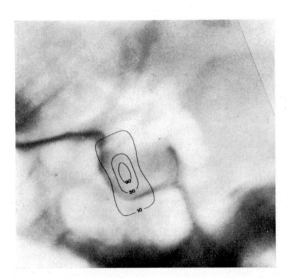

Fig. 1a   Case MM: The local bulging of the sellar floor anteriorly indicated the probability of a microadenoma in this region. The irradiated area is indicated by the 10, 50 and 90 % isodose curves.

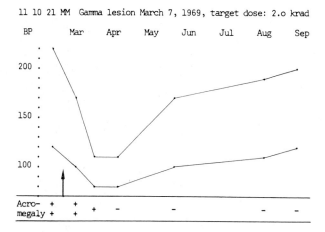

11 10 21 MM Gamma lesion March 7, 1969, target dose: 2.o krad

Fig. 1b Case MM: Graph showing the dramatic decrease of blood pressure (BP) after the radiosurgery (arrow) and the rate of disappearance of the acromegaly.

of secondary adrenal insufficiency due to a radiation-induced hypopituitarism, but the plasma
cortisol proved to be normal. Simultaneously, the symptoms of acromegaly began to disappear, and the growth hormone values became normal. During the following months the
hypertension gradually reappeared, but the symptoms of acromegaly have remained absent
(Fig. 1b). The patient has now been followed for 4 years without a recurrence of symptoms.

The last case presented was that of a 32-year-old woman (IMJ) with hyperactive acromegaly treated in 1968 with removal of a big mixed adenoma via the transsphenoidal route.
The symptoms reappeared and radiological examinations showed an irregular tumour mass

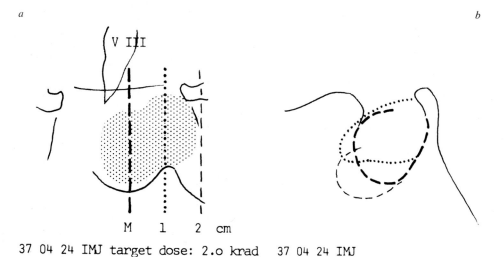

a   *b*

37 04 24 IMJ target dose: 2.o krad   37 04 24 IMJ

Fig. 2 Case IMJ: Sketches of X-ray findings. (a) antero-posterior and (b) lateral view, the latter
showing the asymmetry of the tumor, as indicated by the tomographic appearance of the
sella in three different sections, indicated in (a). The dotted area represents the area irradiated
with >10 % of the target dose, which in this case was 2000 rads.

extending parasellarly to the left. In addition to the acromegaly, the patient had a left-sided ophthalmoplegia which had developed gradually over 6 months. In March 1969 irradiation, using 4 targets, was performed (Fig. 2). The radiation dose in each of these was 2000 rads. After the treatment a gradual improvement of both the acromegaly and the ophthalmoplegia was observed. Within 3 months the oculomotor function was normal and has remained unchanged since then.

Conclusions

The clinical material available at present is still too small to allow the indications for radio-surgery in pituitary tumours to be formulated definitely. However, it is sufficient to establish that one has at one's disposal a completely safe and simple method, which allows closed selective radiosurgical treatment of microadenomas as well as of the portions of larger tumours, which may be held responsible for isolated symptoms e.g. cranial nerve involvement. The suitability for this type of surgery depends mainly upon whether a technique for accurate preoperative localization of microadenomas can be developed. In principle, radio-surgery has to be considered as an alternative to other types of therapy such as selective surgery. The pilot cases presented in this paper illustrate the principles and effects of radio-surgery as applied to pituitary tumours. The preliminary results indicate that even comparatively small radiation doses, delivered stereotaxically to selected portions of tumour, can obliterate the areas irradiated and eliminate isolated symptoms.

References

(1) LEKSELL, L. (1951): The stereotaxic method and radiosurgery of the brain. *Acta chir. scand.*, *102*, 316.
(2) LARSSON, B., LEKSELL, L. and REXED, B. (1963): The use of high energy protons for cerebral radiosurgery in man. *Acta chir. scand.*, *125*, 1.
(3) LEKSELL, L. (1971): *Stereotaxis and Radiosurgery*. Charles C. Thomas, Springfield, Ill.
(4) BACKLUND, E. O. (1969): Stereotaxic treatment of craniopharyngiomas. In: *Nobel Symposium 10: Disorders of the Skull Base Region*, p. 165. Editors: C. A. Hamberger and J. Wersäll. Almqvist and Wiksell, Stockholm.
(5) BACKLUND, E. O., JOHANSSON, L. and SARBY, B. (1972): Studies on craniopharyngiomas. II. Treatment by stereotaxis and radiosurgery. *Acta chir. scand.*, *138*, 749.
(6) BACKLUND, E. O. (1972): Stereotaktisk behandling av kraniofaryngiom med intracystiskt Yttrium-90 och extern Cobalt-60 bestrålning. Thesis (in Swedish), Stockholm.

Note The gamma radiation unit used in this study is manufactured by AB Motala Verkstad, Motala, Sweden.

Continuation of discussion

DR. ODELL: For me, one of the striking things to come from this symposium is the strong suggestion by Dr. Sheline's data that postoperative radiation has reduced the subsequent morbidity of the patient and progression of the disease.

DR. ANNE LAWRENCE: What is the effect of conventional radiotherapy on psychometric testing? We have seen occasional cases of what looks like temporal lobe epilepsy or of narcolepsy.

DR. KRAMER: That is an extremely interesting question, but unfortunately the answer is that there are practically no data available, and for relatively obvious reasons. It is extremely difficult to measure damage. I am convinced that some alteration to a portion of the brain does occur. It would be quite unrealistic to expect that it doesn't because we cause alteration that is measurable in almost every part of the body with doses in excess of 5000 rads. But in the brain it has seemed to be impossible to measure subclinical damage or damage to higher intellectual function.

We have rarely seen clinical damage from radiation therapy. I have made a fairly exhaustive study of the total available literature over the last 35 years, and I have come up with only 57 bona fide cases. Most of these patients have had fantastic doses of radiation, 20,000 rads or more.

I am not sure quite how you would evaluate this sort of irradiation damage in an animal system. Some work has been done on the taste effect, but there again, whether this is a local effect or whether this is a central nervous system effect I think is almost impossible to judge.

Now, there are a number of groups who are just beginning to determine what happens to normal brain not involved in the disease process that is being irradiated. For instance, we do incidentally irradiate a portion of the temporal lobe when we treat a nasopharyngeal cancer or a cancer of the maxillary antrum.

I think that intellectual impairment in children who have been irradiated is anecdotal. Those of us who are particularly interested in the irradiation of brain tumors in children have many, many instances of patients treated with very high doses. I have a group of over 20 craniopharyngiomas now that have been irradiated to a minimum dose of 5500 rads, and 6 of those consecutive cases are now alive 20 years later, and holding responsible positions in life. One is a Ph.D. in biology. Clearly their intellectual capacity would not appear to be affected.

DR. SHELINE: I agree with what Dr. Kramer has said. I think there are no reasonable data available. My experience in treating children with brain tumors other than the pituitary has been similar to his. We have not recognized any decrease in cerebral function attributable to irradiation.

DR. DI CHIRO: In the last two years I have been collecting information, partially from the literature and partially from patients' records, regarding post-radiation damage to the central nervous system, mostly in the spinal cord, but also in the chiasmatic region. I have been impressed by the protean nature of the post-radiation damage. Some of the post-radiation lesions are in fact cystic cavities under tension, and appear to have an expansive character. I would not rule out that certain types of visual field defects, including the bitemporal, can be caused by some unusual post-radiation tissue damage.

DR. HORWITH: The story we have heard for radiation therapy of acromegaly sounds rather encouraging. But I would like to point out that in our series of approximately 60 patients at New York Hospital treated with total hypophysectomy, about 50 % have had previous irradiation. These post-irradiation patients have continued evidence of activity and have continued elevation of growth hormone. The interval between irradiation and surgical therapy was an average of about four years.

It does point out that we can't really rely on radiotherapy in all patients with acromegaly and that these patients do have to be watched very carefully post radiation therapy.

DR. SHELINE: As I pointed out for our material, we have a 25 % failure rate, and, of course, if you collected the failures from enough treatment centers, you would easily assemble the number of irradiation failures described by Dr. Horwith.

DR. BENTSON: I have a technical question relative to volume of tissue irradiated. Suppose you have a patient with a relatively large supra-sellar extension of a tumor. He is operated upon and much, but not all, of the tumor is removed.

What region do you irradiate postoperatively? The volume where the tumor was, or where it is after the operation? If the latter is true, is this based on the surgeon's observations, or do you think the patient should have a limited pneumoencephalogram?

DR. KRAMER: Ideally, I would like to have a pneumoencephalogram done after surgery, but I am not sure that one is entitled to do it from the patient's point of view unless there are other indications. In the absence of a pneumoencephalogram, we irradiate the entire area occupied by the tumor initially.

DR. SHELINE: I do essentially the same thing, and I do not see a clinical need for a postoperative pneumoencephalogram.

I treat the original tumor volume for two reasons: first, in many cases I am not certain of the postsurgical confines of the lesion. Second, we are talking about radiation doses that are normally well tolerated, and there is very little hazard in being generous with the volume to be treated. It is better to treat a larger area than to miss a portion of the lesion and risk a recurrence.

DR. ORTH: I would like to summarize our experience with pituitary irradiation for Cushing's disease, or Cushing's syndrome caused by excessive secretion of pituitary ACTH. The primary treatment for Cushing's disease at Vanderbilt over the last 20 years has been conventional pituitary irradiation. We have treated 55 patients with Cushing's disease with conventional irradiation, usually 4200–4500 rads given over a period of a month via apposed bitemporal ports. Our results were published two years ago (Orth, D.N. and G.W. Liddle, *New Engl. J. Med.*, 1971, *285*, 243–247). About 20 % of these patients have had complete cure of their disease; daily steroid secretion fell to normal and all of the clinical abnormalities resulting from hypercortisolemia disappeared. They usually do not have a re-establishment of a normal diurnal rhythm in plasma cortisol, nor are they generally suppressible with low doses (0.5 mg every 6 hours) of dexamethasone. They frequently have had some evidence of mild loss of pituitary ACTH 'reserve', in that they do not respond perfectly normally to metyrapone. They do respond perfectly well, however, to various forms of stress and do not require glucocorticoid replacement therapy.

Another 25 to 30 % of these patients are sufficiently improved that we have been reluctant to subject them to more drastic forms of therapy. We have documented this improvement in terms of plasma cortisol levels of less than 13 $\mu g/100$ ml and correspondingly near normal urinary steroid values. Sometimes we have treated these patients with small doses of adrenal inhibitors, such as aminoglutethimide or metyrapone, in order to lower their cortisol values into the normal range.

The remaining patients have not been significantly improved and have been subjected to additional forms of therapy, usually bilateral total adrenalectomy.

Until two years ago, we had never had a complication from pituitary irradiation. All children who had been irradiated resumed normal growth once their cortisol values returned to normal, and all adults who subsequently tried to have children were able to do so. There were no neurological defects or deficiencies in other pituitary hormones. More recently, however, we have encountered complications in 4 patients who had been irradiated. One patient died with intractable high fever several months after irradiation. At postmortem examination, she had no evidence of infection and had what, in the opinion of the pathologists, was radiation vasculitis of the hypothalamus. Three others have become blind several months following irradiation. One of these, an acromegalic, was subjected to craniotomy and found to have no tumor encroaching upon the optic nerves. The nerves were swollen and had a yellowish discoloration which the surgeon felt was consistent with radiation-induced optic neuritis.

Thus, while we have had excellent results with conventional irradiation, we would now have to conclude that irradiation is not as innocuous as we had previously believed. There are at least two possible explanations for our recent experience. It is possible, of course, that statistical probabilities have simply caught up with us at last; we had had 51 patients treated over a period of 18 years without difficulty. It is also possible that some difference in technique is involved, and it would appear in retrospect that our radiotherapists have been somewhat more aggressive in the past few years than they had been previously.

DR. KRAMER: How high a dose did they go to with the cobalt and at what rate?

DR. ORTH: The total dose was approximately 5000 rads given at a dose of 250 rads per day over a total time period of 30 to 32 days, as I understand it.

DR. KRAMER: I think there are two things about this. First of all, if you go up to a thousand rads a week or a little less, you can give considerably higher doses, as I have mentioned before. We now have a series of 22 children who have had 5500 rads in 6 weeks for craniopharyngiomas and there has not been a single case of necrosis, and this series extends over 20 years now. If you increase the dose or decrease the number of fractions, then I think you are liable to get into trouble, and this has been very well documented. There are 2 or 3 such cases in the recent literature. So I don't think that is anything very specific.

Secondly, there does seem to be a small group of patients who seem specifically able to develop an acute demyelination even at a relatively low dose. We see this in the spinal cord, too, where patients develop a Lhermitte's sign often after what one would consider to be completely safe doses. It is quite likely that this may happen in the brain as well. So there is the extraordinary case, but it is certainly uncommon.

DR. SHELINE: If the radiation doses you are talking about are 5500 or 6000 rads given at a rate of 300 per day, this would be the equivalent of 6500 or 7000 rads given at a rate of 180 to 200 rads per day. Decreasing the number of treatment fractions, increasing the size of the individual fraction and increasing the dose all serve to increase the biological effect.

DR. ODELL: How many patients with Cushing's disease treated had a remission of Cushing's disease as defined by return of normal suppressibility? As an endocrinologist I don't know how to define Cushing's disease otherwise.

DR. KLIMAN: In our series normal suppressibility returned in 8 out of 10 patients during remission. The definition of dexamethasone suppressibility is difficult to interpret because the test response level is defined as 4 mg or less per 24 hours for 17-hydroxysteroids or 5 μg or less per 100 ml for plasma cortisol, and many of the patients who had a 'normal' test were already at that level before they were given dexamethasone.

Even these cases with normal basal steroid levels have shown further suppressibility. If their plasma cortisol was 10 to 15 μg/100 ml, it would fall below 5 on an overnight dexamethasone suppression test, or during a 48-hour 'low dose' test. These were patients who had abnormal tests before proton beam treatment, since we do not accept the diagnosis of pituitary dependent Cushing's syndrome unless there is evidence of resistance to 'low dose' test and definite suppressibility during the 'high dose' 8 mg dexamethasone per day. We have measured success by the remission of the clinical signs of the Cushing's disease, and these patients usually have had return to normal basal steroid function and normal suppressibility with dexamethasone.

I would like to add that some of the other discussants here, using other methods of pituitary radiation, have not found similar recovery of the dexamethasone test. On one side of the coin Dr. Krieger states that this test does not become normal despite a clinical remission in patients receiving X-irradiation in conjunction with a unilateral adrenalectomy. Contrariwise, Dr. Fraser, using implants of Yttrium-90 indicates that his patients also experience a loss of normal ACTH reserve as judged by metyrapone and insulin tolerance testing. It would appear that the different methods of therapy which produce clinical remission in Cushing's patients do not result in similar function tests. Whether there is hypothalamic damage with wide portal X-ray, whether there is more pituitary damage with localized implants or beads, for instance – these are hypotheses that might be tested by comparing the different function tests in the different groups.

DR. LINFOOT: Using plasma cortisols of less than 5 μg/100 ml in the morning as an indication of remission, our data with regard to proton beam therapy of Cushing's disease are essentially similar to that of Dr. Kliman's. The earliest thing we noticed was a decrease in the previously exaggerated response to metyrapone, a month or six weeks or two months after treatment, even before there has been much change in the basal blood level or in urinary levels of steroid.

Generally, the improvement in the dexamethasone suppression has been associated with a return of the metyrapone to either a normal or a subnormal level.

DR. FRANTZ: I would like to ask both Dr. Kjellberg and Dr. Linfoot if they are willing to accept patients with acromegaly who have had prior radiotherapy and in whom such therapy has failed.

DR. KJELLBERG: We want to make it clear that the complication rate is perhaps two times higher in patients with previous irradiation than in untreated patients. Fewer of our more recent patients have had conventional radiation than was the case with our early experience. Furthermore, the residuals are, in fact, quite mild – oculomotor effects are temporary, and the rare small field defects have not resulted in visual handicap.

Nevertheless, when we plan a proton hypophysectomy in a patient with prior radiation, we reduce the dose by 1000 to 2000 rads. We have consulted with a number of radiotherapists on this point, but it is difficult to add up doses of radiation at different times. In addition, the interval between exposures is important. We do not treat patients with protons until at least 24 months following an X-ray exposure or if they have received over 6000 rads previously. Conventional X-ray delivers radiation to the temporal lobes and surrounding structures very close to the limit of tolerance.

Nevertheless, the patients with continued activity of acromegaly do require specific and effective therapy and we continue to treat them either by proton beam, with the understanding that they have a slightly higher complication rate, or by surgical hypophysectomy.

DR. LINFOOT: We have not treated a patient who has had previous radiation therapy since 1961. As Dr. Kjellberg has mentioned, the complication rate is higher in that group.

DR. LEVIN: I would like to ask Dr. Kjellberg what percentage of his patients had fasting HGH levels of 10 ng/ml or below. Further, he mentioned all or many patients had reverted to normal glucose tolerance. Does this mean 'all' or no more than would be expected for a population of 230 non-acromegalic people, as far as glucose intolerance is concerned?

DR. KJELLBERG: Values for growth hormone between 5 and 10 ng/ml are variously used as 'normal'. About 70 or 80 % of our patients in the clinical category 'remission' were in the range of 10 ng/ml or less. It was very clear as we observed these patients, that some would demonstrate all the clinical indications of remission, but HGH remained above 10. However, such cases usually dropped to one-third or less of their pre-operative levels.

It should be pointed out that the post-treatment values as shown on the slide are those currently available to us, independent of the interval of follow-up. Many of the values shown are less than 24 months post-operative and will continue to fall. About half of the cases responding do so within the first year. Most of the remainder have exhibited clinical regression of acromegaly and HGH at 10 ng/ml or below by the second year, and a few cases have taken longer to fall below 10 ng/ml.

Dr. Kliman, could you discuss glucose intolerance in our acromegalic patients?

DR. KLIMAN: What is not immediately evident from the studies is that there is a limit to remission. Patients who have over 150 or 200 ng/ml of growth hormone do not usually achieve normal glucose tolerance. For example, one patient who required 180 units of insulin daily was later well controlled with oral diabetic therapy, whereas she was out of control previous to proton beam therapy.

There are some patients who are unlikely to experience improvement because of a family history of diabetes. There are only two cases in our series with a positive family history, and they showed no improvement in glucose tolerance or severity of the diabetes.

DR. DAUGHADAY: In individuals with early acromegaly, who have perfectly normal reproductive function, how many will lose that spermatogenesis or normal ovarian cycling with the therapy techniques you are using currently?

DR. LINFOOT: I think that is a very pertinent question. Most of our patients do not have to go on replacement therapy before two years and many of them much later than that. Nine pregnancies occurred within the first two years, and one or two patients have remained fertile for 4–5 years.

DR. KJELLBERG: Of 231 patients, we have detected 29 patients with any degree of suppression of their pituitary function at the time this review was made, which was completed at the end of November, 1972. Seven of these are partial, some patients require thyroid only, some require cortisone only. I do not recall exact numbers for how many patients have a documented reproductive alteration by itself, but it is less than 29 in 231 patients to date; perhaps Dr. Kliman does recall. Some of those may develop alterations in the future.

DR. KLIMAN: That comes very close in the overall series to the in-Boston patients, those who did return from local areas. The last time we surveyed it, the incidence of hypopituitarism in the acromegalic patients was 14 %.

I don't think that we have enough epidemiologic information to know how many of those would appear without therapy, but, assuming all those result from treatment rather than from the presence of the tumor, 14 % comes very close to the approximately 11 % reported from around the country, in all of the patients.

In some cases, the physicians may not have run tests and not reported it. But, we also have some over-reporting in the sense that some physicians will place a patient on pituitary replacement therapy without running all of the pituitary function tests that they should.

I think that reproductive function is the most common missing observation even from the best endocrinologists. We recommend regular measurements of the gonadotropin in both sexes, plasma testosterone for the male, and adequate menstrual histories in women.

DR. FRASER: I want to make a comment about the incidence of infertility arising from the treatment of acromegaly. Prior to treatment about 33 % of our patients are impotent or amenorrheic and LH-deficient. As I pointed out before, LH deficiency is an early sign of loss of pituitary function. Despite the fact that we have altered our treatment dose, the incidence of subsequent hypopituitarism of one sort or another has not correlated at all with the dosage, but correlated with the clinical status on arrival.

DR. PEARSON: One of the advantages of radiation therapy, I thought, was the fact that you could get rid of the hypersecretion and leave the rest of the pituitary functions intact. Is the incidence of hypopituitarism higher in patients receiving proton beam therapy than in those receiving conventional irradiation?

DR. LINFOOT: About a third of our patients are on some sort of replacement therapy.

DR. KJELLBERG: In the technique we use we seek to preserve one millimeter shells at the periphery of the glands with the object of trying to preserve normal pituitary function. My view has been that a 10 or 15 % incidence of patients with documented hypopituitarism requiring replacement is relatively low, considering the relatively high frequency of reversals of hyperfunction that are achieved with the Bragg peak method.

DR. KLIMAN: Could I just add very briefly that, unlike radioactive iodine therapy of the thyroid gland where the incidence of gland failure is cumulative over a long period of time, upwards of 10, 15, or 20 years, the appearance of the hypopituitarism following Bragg peak proton therapy occurs in the first 6 to 18 months after treatment. We have seen only rare patients where it has appeared after 24 months, and those have been patients with Cushing's syndrome without enlarged sellas, so they have a very concentrated intrasellar dose.

DR. KRAMER: Dr. Kjellberg, apparently you are using proton beam therapy both for destructive purposes in advanced carcinoma and other conditions, and for non-destructive purposes in pituitary tumors. Is this a difference in technique, or is it a difference in dose that allows you to choose between one and the other? I would also like to make a comment before you answer the question. It seems to me that today we have listened to and spoken to three rather disparate groups, each extolling the virtues of their particular form of management of pituitary tumors. In order to make a valid comparison of the results of the different forms of therapy, a comparative study should be organized with criteria for selection of patients and description of results.

DR. KJELLBERG: Concerning your comment, I couldn't agree with you more. I think it is entirely appropriate that this be part of the deliberations of a group like this. I think that the comparisons are indeed difficult because of differences in terminology, methods, frequency, and extent of follow-up.

With respect to total versus partial destruction, we have performed deliberate total hypophysectomy in patients with breast cancer and diabetic retinopathy. In those patients, we utilize larger doses (12,000 to 15,000 rads) and select beam sizes to induce radionecrosis in the entire anterior lobe.

In such patients, the interval from therapy to onset of hypopituitarism has a delay of 3 to 6 months. With breast cancer and diabetic retinopathy, such delay is a bit of a disadvantage.

Therefore, my current view is that I would rather use a transsphenoidal hypophysectomy for breast cancer and diabetic retinopathy because it is safe and reliable. The whole gland is visualized in the operative procedure and hypopituitarism is induced immediately. We have done in the past about 200 total ablations of the normal pituitary with protons, and it certainly does work. But the interval of delay erodes the frequency of good results because some of them have progression of their disease in the interval. Some of the cancer patients die, depending in part on the criteria of selection. The diabetics may lose more vision, depending on the winds of fortune that go along with bleeding in diabetic retinopathy.

With respect to dose, there are a few problems which I think we could discuss profitably in detail, but I will just outline these. It is not only a matter of absolute dose. Dose rate is important also. The doses that we used that are delivered in 30 to 40 min would be comparable to about two times that dose of X-ray, because of our high dose rate. That is, if we speak of 6000 rads delivered in 40 min, this is biologically about as effective as 12,000 rads of X-ray delivered in 4 to 6 weeks. This is not a precise figure because strict comparative analyses haven't been made.

We also alter the absolute value of the dose, depending on the size of the gland. Small glands get a higher absolute dose than large glands do, because we are confident from our experience and a variety of published studies that the volume of tissue irradiated, particularly in relatively small volumes, distinctly influences the amount of radiation biological effect. But I think that is a separate topic and not necessarily appropriate to much discussion here.

DR. BATZDORF: I, too, would like to see a formulation developed which would allow us to see which type of patient would be best helped by which type of therapy. This is one of the potentials that we see in the computerized method of assessing the patient's history, findings, laboratory, and X-ray data. I wondered whether you might think it appropriate to inquire to what degree there might be interest in the group to start a cooperative investigation into these questions, in a prospective fashion, taking in a large number of patients so we would be able to get some hard answers to some of these questions.

DR. CANARY: The first time that I recommended radiotherapy for a patient with Nelson's syndrome without a large sella, misgivings arose about the medical-legal implications of giving therapy to a 'normal' structure.

Following treatment in that patient, there was excellent reduction in skin pigmentation and loss of the neuromuscular syndrome which some patients show within a few weeks' time. Is the rate of favorable response usually that rapid? What would be the earliest and the usual onset of improvement in those patients who definitely do improve after irradiation? Are there problems or might one expect problems with a request for radiotherapy of the pituitary gland in patients without neurologic deficits and with a normal sella despite clear cut evidence of the presence of a Nelson's syndrome?

DR. KJELLBERG: We have considered one patient with Nelson's syndrome to be in remission in the sense that all of the pigmentation that had been evident in comparable photographs disappeared following proton beam treatment. It was much reduced in 1 month, almost gone in about 4 months, and undetectible in 7 months. This patient had her evolving hyperpigmentation a short interval, less than 6 months. The other cases with Nelson's syndrome were of many years' duration and were of very deep pigmentation. In a virtually black-skinned Nelson syndrome patient, we have never seen disappearance of all the pigment. They have always had residual pigment, but they have lightened.

DR. KLIMAN: Perhaps we can clarify that by saying that we have not accepted patients for treatment on the basis of the pigmentation. They have been accepted on the basis of chronic, severe headaches, and erosion of the sella, and in some cases serial X-ray films showing progressive expansion of the sella.

This group also included a patient who did have a suprasellar extension, but who was considered not a good candidate for surgery because of the preceding total adrenalectomy. If the patient had superimposed on this hypopituitarism and in particular diabetes insipidus, the patient's health and survival would be greatly at risk in a situation with both Addison's disease and hypopituitarism. While that patient has only slight decrease in pigmentation, her chronic headaches have ceased, and there has been no progression in terms of the size of the sella.

These patients are very difficult to do pneumoencephalograms on because of their adrenalectomy. For those of you who have wished to evaluate your patients to see if they do have a suprasellar mass, I advise that they be prepared with profuse intravenous saline and steroids for several hours before they go to the pneumoencephalogram room to avoid hypotension, which has been the most frequent problem in taking patients through this procedure with just the usual preparation with steroids alone.

DR. LINFOOT: I might speak to Dr. Canary's question. We have treated 2 patients with normal size sella, hyperpigmentation, and very high serum ACTH levels not suppressible with high levels of dexamethasone. They both had social problems as a result of their pigmentation. We treated them, and they lost much but not all of their pigmentation, but their ACTH values are still slightly elevated.

DR. KLIMAN: Have any of your patients with Nelson's syndrome come to hypophysectomy after proton beam treatment?

DR. LINFOOT: One required a hypophysectomy and fortunately tolerated the procedure well. She had a large suprasellar extension at the time of surgery.

DR. KLIMAN: None of our Nelson's syndrome patients have come to surgery or show any indication of requiring it. I think this is one instance where the surgeon is thankful not to operate.

VI. Miscellaneous ablative procedures for pituitary adenomas

Stereotaxic cryohypophysectomy: Ten year experience with pituitary tumors

ROBERT W. RAND, GUNNAR HEUSER and DONALD A. ADAMS

Departments of Surgery and Medicine, Division of Neurosurgery, UCLA School of Medicine, Los Angeles, Calif., U.S.A.

Destruction of the adenohypophysis and pituitary tumors in the sella turcica can be accomplished effectively by stereotaxic cryohypophysectomy. This has been used successfully since 1963 as palliative treatment of metastatic mammary cancer and of progressive proliferative diabetic retinopathy.[4–6] Selected non-secretory as well as secretory pituitary tumors causing clinical syndromes of acromegaly, hyperpigmentation and Cushing's disease have been arrested by cryohypophysectomy (Fig. 1).

a

b

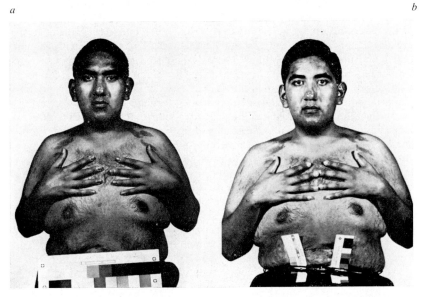

Fig. 1 Photographs (*a*) (before) and (*b*) (after). Mexican American with Nelson's syndrome following adrenalectomy for Cushing's disease. Pituitary adenoma biopsied and destroyed by stereotaxic cryohypophysectomy. Hyperpigmentation markedly improved. Note especially the fingernail beds.

In 1963, Cooper[1] was the first surgeon to destroy the pituitary gland in man by stereo-taxically directing a cryoprobe into the sella turcica using a transfrontal approach. This approach causes some damage to the frontal lobe from the tract of the cryoprobe, but more importantly carries the hazard of mechanical pressure against the optic nerves, chiasm and cerebral vessels at the time of probe insertion. Total hypophysectomy is not accomplished because movement and placement of the cryoprobe within the sella is limited. This is not the case using the stereotaxic transnasal transsphenoidal approach developed by Rand.[4]

The successful outcome of a stereotaxic cryohypophysectomy depends upon selection of patients, the use of an accurate stereotaxic instrument, a reliable cryosurgical unit which will achieve cryoprobe tip temperatures to —190 °C and finally patient cooperation. This latter is achieved by using agents that eliminate pain and anxiety while retaining the ability to test the optic and extraoptic nerve function during the actual freezing.

Patients whose diseases can be treated by cryohypophysectomy fall into 3 categories: those with metastatic mammary and prostate cancer, or with progressive proliferative dia-betic retinopathy or with selected pituitary tumors and related disorders.

Selection of patients

Neurosurgical criteria for the selection of patients include the following: (1) paranasal and sphenoid sinuses free of infection, (2) configuration of the sella turcica to allow accurate placement and movement of the cryoprobe, and (3) a desire by the patient to have cryo-hypophysectomy after thorough explanation of the procedure, its potential hazards and the postoperative medical management.

The neuroradiological anatomy of a particular *pituitary tumor* determines whether it is suitable for destruction by cryohypophysectomy. Suprasellar extension should be minimal as demonstrated by pneumoencephalography. The limit of suprasellar extension is about 10 mm above a line connecting the planum sphenoidale and the dorsum sellae.

Carotid angiograms are performed to determine the exact position of the internal carotid arteries within the cavernous sinuses in relation to the sella turcica, and to rule out aneurysms simulating pituitary tumors. A rare aneurysm of the basilar artery may occasionally simulate a pituitary tumor and therefore vertebral angiograms should probably be included in the work-up whenever feasible.

Irregularly lobulated non-secretory pituitary tumors as demonstrated by planigrams, cavernous sinus venograms and carotid angiograms are best treated by transfrontosphenoidal craniotomy or transnasal transsphenoidal approach and excision of the neoplasm with micro-neurosurgical techniques. The especially designed cryoprobe is a useful adjunct in destruc-tion of an unresectable pituitary tumor, under direct vision with the surgical microscope.

Patients with pituitary tumors are reluctant to undergo craniotomy as long as their vision is not impaired. Most acromegalic patients can be treated with reversal of the syndrome by stereotaxic cryohypophysectomy. Resolution of symptoms and signs begins within 2–5 days after cryohypophysectomy. The abnormally elevated growth hormone blood levels as measured by radioimmunoassay rapidly decrease to near normal or normal levels in the immediate postoperative period. Chromophobe adenomas limited to the sella turcica also lend themselves to destruction by cryohypophysectomy.

Instrumentation

The Rand-Urban stereotaxic instrument used to guide the twist drills, biopsy instruments and cryoprobes provides accuracy to ±0.5 mm and permits precise and positive adjustment. Each step in the operative procedure is verified by means of X-ray films and closed television fluoroscopy. The Rand-Urban stereotaxic instrument moves in the X, Y and Z axes with a double arc system having a common center. An accessory tangent movement on the large arc allows the cryoprobe to follow a path parallel to the normal arc radius. Vertical movement is provided in the arc quadrant independent of the head-holder system which has rotary action.

The radius of the original arc was 13.5 cm and it was found that in some patients it came over the mouth making it difficult for the anesthesiologist to suction the fluids and secretions. Consequently the new arc system by Rand and Urban has 16 cm arc radius to overcome this problem.

The patient's head is adjusted so that the desired surgical target is placed in the midline of the stereotaxic instrument (Fig. 2). Once the pituitary gland or pituitary adenoma has been located at the center point of the arc system, the cryoprobe can be advanced from any direction to this focal point because the two rotational arc systems are concentric.

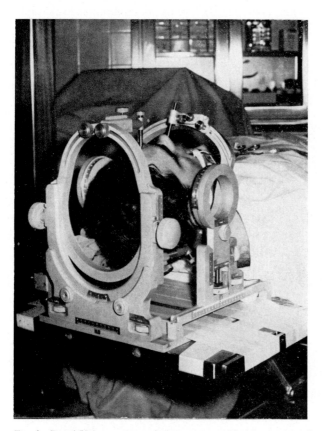

Fig. 2 Rand-Urban stereotaxic instrument with 16 cm arc radius to allow adequate room for the anesthesiologists. The instrument has movements in the X, Y and Z axes with a double arc system having a common center. Pituitary fossa is aligned to center of the double arc system by closed television fluoroscopy and teleroentgenography.

Collimated X-ray films verify target position. The radiopaque reticules replace the collimated target on both sides for the film exposure. The image size is the same for a series of film exposures thereby permitting the overlay principle to be utilized. In this manner progressive steps can be compared during the operation. Closed television fluoroscopy is employed in the lateral plane to allow for rapid adjustment of the drill cryoprobe and biopsy needle positions.

The cryosurgical unit

The Cooper Cryosurgical Unit CE-2 is employed for all stereotaxic cryohypophysectomy procedures and can produce steady cryoprobe tip temperatures of —180 °C to —190 °C for prolonged periods. Ultracold temperatures are required to destroy normal pituitary tissue and pituitary adenomas by disrupting cell membranes, altering the pH and electrolyte concentration of the cell, and stasis of blood supply.

Total anterior lobe necrosis can be accomplished if the temperature is lowered to —180 °C, for 10–15 min using the large 4.2 mm probe in a central position or the 2.7 or 3.2 mm cryoprobes in 2 lateral positions for 10 min each (Fig. 3). The risk of cerebrospinal rhinorrhea can be virtually eliminated by sealing the twist drill hole with silicone dowels.

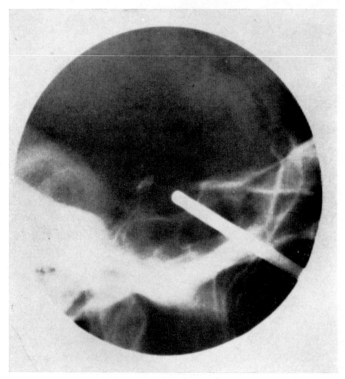

Fig. 3   Lateral X-ray of normal sella turcica with a small cryoprobe in position for final cryogenic lesion on one side. The Cooper cryosurgical unit CE-2 is employed to obtain and maintain cryoprobe temperatures down to — 186° C.

Anesthesia

The potential damage by freezing the adjacent cranial nerves III, IV, V and VI in the cavernous sinus laterally, and the optic chiasm and nerves superiorly, represents one of the serious potential risks of stereotaxic cryohypophysectomy. The patient must be cooperative during freezing so that the visual acuity, visual fields and extraocular muscle function can be tested as the production of the cryogenic lesion progresses.

The nasal cavities, pharynx, larynx and trachea are anesthetized with adequate topical anesthesia. To avoid aspiration of nasal blood and gastric contents, an endotracheal tube with inflatable cuff is passed. The patient is given tranquilizer drugs intravenously to allay anxiety and narcotics to stop pain. Additional amounts of these drugs are given during the operation as required. Nitrous oxide-oxygen or fluorothane is used to produce light sleep between the cryogenic lesions. A local anesthetic is injected into the scalp for pin fixation of the head in the stereotaxic instrument.

This anesthetic regimen allows the surgeon to test eye movements and to have the patient recognize, with hand signals, numbers held in front of each eye. Thus any dysfunction of the extraocular motor nerves and the optic nerves can be ascertained during the production of the cryogenic lesion. Incipient palsies of 1 or more of these cranial nerves have been observed in about 10 % of patients undergoing cryohypophysectomy. The early partial palsy is a reversible phenomenon only due to cooling of the cranial nerve below $+15\,°C$. Complete remission will occur if the cryosurgical unit is shut off immediately. Permanent nerve palsy has not occurred in any of our patients undergoing cryohypophysectomy.

Surgical technique

Prior to surgery the patient is prepared by using nasal cleansing with 0.25 % phenylephrine (Neo-Synephrine) hydrochloride nose drops and bacitracin solution, 500 units/ml. The anesthesia program and need of cooperation are discussed in detail with the patient.

The patient's head is aligned in the head-holding unit of the Rand-Urban sterotaxic instrument under local anesthesia so that the sagittal plane of the head is perpendicular to the base of the instrument and the transverse plane of the skull is in the axis of the arc system.

Teleroentgenographic films in the lateral view are taken and the arc system is adjusted in order that the focal point of the arc will lie in the desired area of the sella turcica. The relationship of the sagittal plane to the midline of the instrument is determined by appropriate films. The posterior border of the nasal septum serves as the primary midline osseous landmark. Compensation for slight misalignment of the head is made by adjusting the head holder or the cryoprobe holders on the large arc system to the appropriate side of the desired number of millimeters.

In the case of the normal pituitary gland, twist drill holes are made in the floor of the sella between 3–4 mm to the right and left of the midline. This allows passage of the small (2.7 mm) cryoprobe. Prior to making the twist drill holes, the nasal cavity is again prepared with phenylephrine, bacitracin and 4 % cocaine on cotton pledgets. The sphenoid sinus is irrigated with bacitracin solution.

Carotid angiograms and/or cavernous sinus venograms (Fig. 4a and b) demonstrate the exact relationship to the sella turcica in anteroposterior X-rays and are generally done as a preoperative procedure. The central beam should pass directly between the eyes in a true frontal projection for these angiograms.

The cryoprobe in its guide and holding system is inserted into the desired region of the pituitary gland or the pituitary tumor under closed television fluoroscopy. In the case of a normal pituitary gland the small vacuum type cryoprobe and CE-2 liquid nitrogen system have been routinely employed producing 2 overlapping cryogenic lesions 3–4 mm on either side of the midline and confining these lesions to the anterior two-thirds of the sella turcica. The cryoprobe tip temperature is gradually lowered to between —180 °C and —190 °C and held for 10–15 min to produce each of these multiple cryogenic lesions.

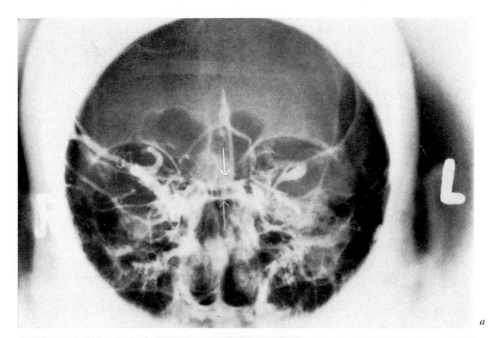

a

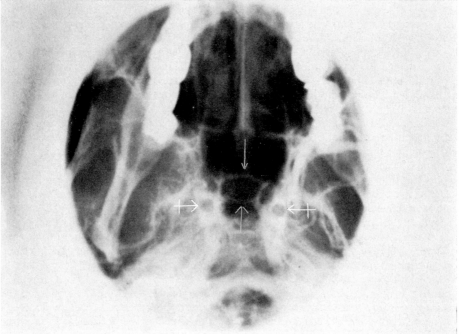

b

Fig. 4 (*a*) Anterior posterior view of cavernous sinus venogram using simultaneous retrograde injection of the jugular veins at the base of the skull which demonstrates a normal pituitary gland and carotid arteries.

(*b*) Basal view of same. Cavernous sinus venogram outlining normal pituitary tumor and relation to carotid arteries.

Secretory microadenomas of pituitary causing acromegaly, Cushing's disease can often be outlined by this technique.

The normal pituitary gland can be equally well destroyed by using the larger cryoprobe (4.2 mm) centrally placed in the anterior lobe of the hypophysis and making 2 overlapping cryogenic lesions each at —180 °C for 10 min. Twist drill holes should be sealed to prevent cerebrospinal rhinorrhea. This may be accomplished with fine silicone sponge dowels.

In the case of intrasellar pituitary adenomas, the small (2.7 mm), intermediate (3.2 mm) or large (4.2 mm) cryoprobes have been used. The selection of the particular cryoprobe diameter is dependent primarily on the size of the pituitary tumor. In a patient with acromegaly and a normal sized sella turcica, the small cryoprobe is usually employed. The intermediate sized probe is used with some enlargement of the sella turcica, and the largest cryoprobe for large sized tumors.

The cryoprobe tip is advanced 3–4 mm after each lesion until the anterior three-quarters of enlarged sella have been covered in the lateral view with overlapping cryogenic lesions. It is important to have the temperature at the tip of the cryoprobe return to +20 °C in order to avoid moving any ice mass. The distance the cryoprobe is placed from the midline is dependent upon the direction of growth of the tumor as determined by neuroradiological studies. Generally, pituitary adenomas confined to the sella turcica have been found to grow asymmetrically and, therefore, the center of the cryoprobe may be 4–5 mm from the midline on one side and 6–8 or more mm on the other side, depending upon these measurements of the tumor in the anterior planes.

Pituitary tumor biopsy

Irradiation therapy to an enlarged sella turcica, presumably containing a pituitary adenoma, has been the treatment of choice for years provided the function of the optic chiasm or the optic nerves is not compromised severely by compression. The fallacy of this reasoning is emphasized by publications which describe cerebral aneurysms of the internal carotid and basilar arteries producing sella turcica enlargement consistent with chromophobe adenoma and causing clinical hypopituitarism. Therefore, it continues to be our opinion that each patient with a suspected pituitary tumor and especially a chromophobe adenoma should have a complete neuroendocrinologic and neuroradiologic evaluation including carotid and vertebral angiograms, pneumoencephalograms and cavernous sinus venograms.

If irradiation therapy of non-secretory chromophobe adenomas appears to be what the patient and referring physician desire, at least a transsphenoidal stereotaxic tumor biopsy should be performed in order to establish the tumor cell type, and whether or not it is a cystic tumor.[6] If the adenoma is largely cystic, or if it turns out to be some neoplasm such as a craniopharyngioma or meningioma, radiation therapy will have little if any benefit. The biopsy of the intrasellar tumor would spare the patient any short- or long-term ill effects of pituitary fossa radiation which may be devastating to a few patients.

The stereotaxic biopsy is accomplished by using gentle syringe suction applied to a long, small diameter biopsy needle which has been placed into the center of the intrasellar tumor, using the Rand-Urban stereotaxic guide. The procedure is done in these circumstances under a general anesthesia provided cryohypophysectomy is not to follow. Such a biopsy procedure takes about an hour to perform. The nasal cavity preparation is similar to that for cryohypophysectomy. A routine biopsy has been taken in all cases with pituitary tumor just prior to the actual cryohypophysectomy. In 95 % of cases quite adequate tissue has been obtained by the needle biopsy technique and no ill effect of biopsy has as yet been observed during the 17 yr the authors have used the technique.

A tissue button is prepared and serial sections are stained with hematoxylin and eosin. Special stains are used in studying pituitary cytology and histochemistry.

If adequate tissue is not obtained, a special Urban roto-dissector can be substituted for the biopsy needle. This instrument has a small side hole near the blunt end of the outer shaft. An inner cannula with a cutting blade is rotated by a small electric engine. Tissue is drawn into the hole of the suction tip as suction is applied and it is cut off by the rotating blade. The tissue is trapped in a small bottle containing either a fixative solution or physiological saline.

Diagnostic studies

A pituitary tumor is suspected whenever one or more pituitary functions have become deficient. Neurological symptoms, especially visual field defects, do not usually become evident until later on in the development of the disease.

A full neuroendocrine work-up usually requires hospitalization and, if complete, is quite expensive. Therefore, our diagnostic approach is stepwise and only advances to the full work-up once the diagnosis of a pituitary tumor appears definite. If skull X-rays are abnormal (example given – double floor of the sella) a pneumoencephalogram and angiogram are mandatory. If FSH and LH levels are found to be low, a tumor is suspected even if skull X-rays are normal. At this time we proceed with additional studies including a metyrapone test and arginine stimulation of growth hormone. In males, we will obtain a testosterone measurement in addition to FSH and LH. The usefulness of prolactin measurements in not fully known at this time, but we always check for the presence of galactorrhea. A formal water deprivation test is done only when the patient shows clinical evidence of diabetes insipidus. When this develops, upward extension of the pituitary tumor is usually found.

Additional tests are now available for the more complete study of neuroendocrine function. These, however, are usually very costly to the patient and only rarely absolutely necessary. A determination of TSH can be very useful when done at the beginning of the investigation since elevated TSH levels point towards a primary thyroid deficiency whereas low TSH levels point towards the pituitary. Clomid stimulation of gonadotropin secretion has now been standardized in both male and female and is a good way of accessing the responsiveness of the hypothalamic pituitary system. The presence of releasing factors in the blood will in the future help to determine whether a disease process is primarily hypothalamic or pituitary.

Postoperative management

Endocrine replacement therapy

From the day of operation, the patient is treated with steroids. During the first 2 or 3 postoperative days, the patient is given dexamethasone which is later on switched to Solucortef which in turn is replaced by maintenance doses of cortisone within a week. We do not usually put a patient on thyroid immediately. Instead, blood tests of thyroid function are performed and the patient started on thyroid once tests of thyroid function show a definite decline.

Blood levels for testosterone are obtained 1–3 months after surgery, especially if the patient complains of decreased libido and potency. Treatment consists of Depotestosterone. We usually give 200 mg intramuscularly every week for 2 months to be sure that therapy is optimal. Thereafter, once the patient has shown definite response, injections are spaced out at intervals from 2–3–4 weeks depending upon the patient's preference.

In the female, we always initiate therapy with estrogens and progestins when menopausal symptoms develop following surgery. In the young female, this therapy is always initiated regardless of symptoms, provided that the patient remains amenorrheic and has no other contraindications.

Limited pneumoencephalography for posttreatment evaluation

Neurologists, neurosurgeons and ophthalmologists have generally depended upon the visual field examination to determine whether or not a particular pituitary tumor is recurring. We have come to the conclusion, after studying our series of pituitary tumors here at UCLA Hospital for the past 15 yr, that recurrent or progressive visual field or visual acuity deficits in patients harboring known pituitary tumors are a *late* sign of recurrence. Time and time again in patients who have been examined every 6 months with what appears to be a stable visual apparatus they suddenly begin to lose vision in 1 or both eyes. When the appropriate neuroradiological studies are carried out the physician is amazed at the size of the recurrence which had been unsuspected until the visual changes.

Consequently, we have developed a technique of selective partial pneumoencephalography which can be done as an outpatient procedure (Fig. 5a and b). The purpose of the study is simply to place a small amount of filtered oxygen or carbon dioxide in the chiasmatic cistern and anterior third ventricle under controlled TV fluoroscopy and then expose appropriate X-rays. The absorption of the gas will be quicker if carbon dioxide is used.

The patient is brought to the Surgical Outpatient Recovery Room Suite NPO. Appropriate interval history and a brief physical examination are carried out. Medication is ordered and given prior to the study. The patient is placed in the pneumoencephalograph chair and after the preoperative medication plus local anesthesia a lumbar puncture is performed with a small spinal needle gauge (23–25). Approximately 7–10 ml of filtered oxygen or carbon dioxide is then directed to the desired areas around the sella turcica and in the anterior third ventricle. AP and lateral planigrams can be taken in addition to regular AP and lateral films with the patient's head in a slightly extended position. The needle is removed and the

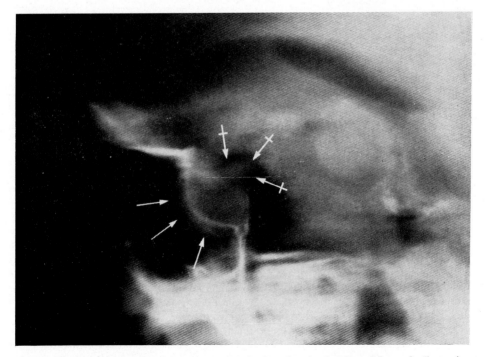

Fig. 5a   Sagittal laminograms of pneumoencephalogram showing bulging of floor of sella turcica into sphenoid sinus (arrow) and limited suprasellar extension (arrows).

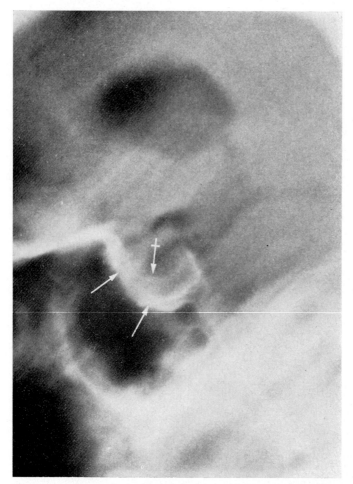

Fig. 5b   Limited pneumoencephalogram following successful stereotaxic cryohypophysectomy in acromegaly. Patient had complete remission of symptoms with growth hormone levels less than 5 ng. Floor of sella turcica has recalcified with no evidence of tumor recurrence.

patient is sent to the Surgery Recovery Room to be discharged later in the afternoon. No effort is made to fill the ventricular system totally because this has been previously done on the preoperative pneumoencephalograms. The examples of the selective type of pneumoencephalography are seen in Figure 5a and b.

It is our opinion that if selective pneumoencephalography is carried out every 12–18 months, any evidence of tumor recurrence will be found immediately and appropriate additional therapy can then be done. By using this technique as an outpatient procedure the patient has minimal expense and yet the maximum information as to the status of the pituitary tumor. It is very much easier to appropriately treat a recurrence of a pituitary tumor when it is early than when it becomes massive.

As one might expect, the patients are genuinely concerned about having another pneumoencephalogram because of the severe headaches with the first pneumoencephalogram. It has been our experience that minimal headaches occur following partial limited pneumoencephalographic studies. By using a small spinal needle, such as a 25 gauge, the risk of post-spinal headache is reduced. Generally, the patients have been cooperative with this program because of their concern that a tumor recurrence might occur. The reassurance that one can give the patient by demonstrating to them that there is no evidence of recurrence is an important psychological factor in the treatment of patients with pituitary adenomas.

Results

Destruction of normal pituitary tissue

Extreme freezing temperatures are necessary to accomplish total adenohypophysectomy. In the first 6 patients with metastic mammary cancer using the small (2.7 mm) vacuum cryo-probe, tip temperature was gradually lowered to —180 °C making a total of 5 cryogenic lesions (2 on the left side of the midline for 20 min each; 2 on the right side for 20 min each; and 1 central lesion for 9 min). This technique resulted in complete clinical and endocrino-logical hypophysectomy in these patients. Subsequently, the procedure has been standardized as discussed in the previous section, and results have been equally satisfactory.

It was observed at autopsy that in some of these patients who died of their cancer, the posterior lobe of the pituitary gland was only partially damaged or even totally spared from the effects of freezing. This phenomenon has been attributed to the rich vascular anastomoses between the superior and the inferior hypophyseal arteries in the region of the pars inter-media. This thermal barrier tends to protect the neurohypohysis against cryogenic necrosis, as the portal circulation does in the case of the pituitary stalk.

Treatment of non-functioning (chromophobe) adenomas

In the course of the development of this operation the opportunity arose to try its usefulness in chromophobe adenomas which have more than 15 mm extension above the diaphragm sellae as shown by pneumoencephalography.

In 1 patient, a young man of 32 yr, with a long-standing chromophobe adenoma previously treated by 2 craniotomies and cobalt therapy, the tumor extended at least 1.5–2.0 cm above the diaphragma sellae. He had only 1 small area of vision remaining in the left eye and a temporal field cut in the right eye. Overlapping cryogenic lesions were produced bilaterally. Vision was lost on the left side 12 hours later. At the time of craniotomy several weeks after cryohypophysectomy, viable tumor could not be identified within the enlarged sella turcica. However, it was still in the suprasellar position causing pressure on the right optic nerve and optic chiasm. The final pathological diagnosis in this case after comparing the specimens from the various operations was possibly malignant chromophobe adenoma. Therefore, it is not recommended to attempt stereotaxic cryohypophysectomy in pituitary tumors under the above circumstances because, although the tumor can be destroyed within the sella, its suprasellar extension is not appreciably influenced either by single or multiple cryogenic lesions.

On the other hand, a young woman previously treated by craniotomy and cobalt therapy had complete remission of recurrent bitemporal hemianopsia after stereotaxic freezing of her tumor. In addition, menstruation returned to normal and the hypophyseal adrenal axis has remained intact for over 3 yr. Her tumor (chromophobe adenoma) had extended only 10 mm above the diaphragma sellae. This patient experienced partial recurrence of her bitemporal hemianopsia and has since undergone another cryosurgical procedure. Vision has again returned to normal.

Treatment of acromegaly

Patients with acromegaly have in the past been faced with a decision to have conventional radiation therapy or craniotomy. Ray and Horwith[3] and others have demonstrated the rapid effectiveness of total surgical hypophysectomy. However, in our experience, both the patient with acromegaly and his personal physician would rather have radiation therapy, even if it is of limited benefit. These same patients will, on the other hand, generally submit to some type of transsphenoidal stereotaxic operation. If one uses radioactive yttrium[90], gold or irridium to destroy the pituitary tumor, potential late irradiation effects remain and the incidence of extraocular and optic nerve damage and cerebrospinal rhinorrhea with meningitis is significant.

Patients can be offered the surgical technique of stereotaxic cryohypophysectomy and although the potential risk of permanent optic nerve or extraocular nerve damage and the risk of cerebrospinal rhinorrhea with meningitis remain, the chance of such a complication is minimal, provided certain surgical principles are followed. The potential risk of producing latent ill effects comparable to those attributed to irradiation is eliminated.

Thirty-two patients with acromegaly have undergone stereotaxic cryohypophysectomy. Two of these 32 patients had subsequent transnasal transsphenoidal microsurgical operations and a transfrontal craniotomy without improvement. Three additional patients had serious complications following the surgery which led to their death; these included meningitis and cerebral hemorrhage (Fig. 6). The meningitis occurred because 1 of the silicone dowels

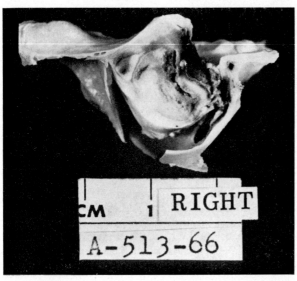

Fig. 6 Sagittal section of enlarged sella turcica harboring an eosinophilic adenoma causing acromegaly. The tumor was totally destroyed by cryohypophysectomy. The pituitary gland which was normal was left intact except for a small area of hemorrhage. Patient succumbed to gastrointestional hemorrhage secondary to meningitis.

slipped and cerebrospinal rhinorrhea developed. Today we would do an immediate transnasal, transsphenoidal microsurgical repair. Of the remaining 27 patients, 19 have shown growth hormone assays that are consistently less than 4 ng (Table I). In 7 patients the growth hormone levels vary between 5–10 ng. In 1 patient the growth hormone is between 10–15 ng.

Preoperative growth hormone evaluation in 17 patients who had been classified in the success group ranged from 19 to over 120 ng/ml. In 10 of these patients the postoperative growth hormone levels are less than 5, basically in the range of 1 or 2. In 5 patients the figures range between 5–7 and in 1 patient it was 12 ng/ml. All of the 27 patients who have been classified as 'success' appear to be in a clinical remission. Partial pneumoencephalo-

Table I   *Acromegaly data*

Type of surgery	No. done	Success	Failure	Complications	
Cryohypophysectomy	32	27	2	1	Meningitis case
				2	Cerebral hemorrhages
Craniotomy	5		5	1	Proton radiation at Berkeley
				4	Radiation therapy
Cryohypophysectomy plus craniotomy	1		1		Proton radiation at Berkeley (2 visits, too early to obtain results)
Cryohypophysectomy plus transsphenoidal hypophysectomy	1		1		Proton radiation at Berkeley (2 visits, too early to obtain results)

Time period: 18 November 1963 to 3 May 1971. Patients: 24 males, 21 females, total 45.

grams have been performed in 7 of these people and the sella is 'empty' and the floor has recalcified in most of these patients.

Between 1970 and 1972 we did not treat acromegaly with the stereotaxic cryohypophysectomy procedure because we felt that we should evaluate the results obtained for patients treated between 1964 and 1970. It is our current belief that stereotaxic cryohypophysectomy is the procedure of choice in the treatment of acromegaly in tumors that are confined to the sella turcica and are not excessively large and lobulated. In the latter cases the cryosurgical technique may be used, but would probably have to be supplemented with radiation to destroy or inhibit residual tumor tissue from producing growth hormone. It is well known that the less the amount of tumor tissue remaining the more satisfactory will be the radiation results.

If the pituitary tumor causing acromegaly does have suprasellar extension, then a trans-frontal-transsphenoidal operation will usually allow adequate exposure to radically excise or destroy the tumor. Frigitronics has designed a special cryoprobe system which is quite flexible and allows for discrete cryodestruction of any residual pituitary tissue that cannot be excised or resected in the usual manner. This technique we feel is superior to using any caustic solution such as Zenkers.

The patients who have undergone successful stereotaxic cryohypophysectomy for acromegaly have noted decrease of the puffiness of the soft tissue of the extremities and face after 24 hours and usually within 72 hours of the operation. During our follow-up period of up to 8 yr, the majority of these patients have experienced striking clinical benefit from cryohypophysectomy with concomitant lowering of growth hormone levels to normal or subnormal levels.

Summary

The indications for cryohypophysectomy, its technique and complications are discussed in detail. The results of this procedure in patients with pituitary tumors are presented.

In patients with acromegaly, cryohypophysectomy appears to be the procedure of choice as long as there is no marked upward extension of the tumor. Finally, cryohypophysectomy is also successful in patients with chromophobe adenoma.

Complete hypophysectomy can be achieved with the cryoprobe, with minimal risk to the patient and quick postoperative recovery. Even large tumors can be almost totally destroyed with this procedure. After 10 yr of using stereotaxic hypophysectomy, and of comparing it with other therapeutic modalities, we have found it a very satisfactory procedure for the destruction of the pituitary gland and its tumors. In properly selected cases, destruction, after the cryoprocedure, is as complete as after any other procedure, including craniotomy.

References

(1) COOPER, I. S. (1963): Cryogenic surgery. A new method of destruction or extirpation of benign or malignant tissues. *New Engl. J. Med., 268,* 743.
(2) CUSHING, H. P. (1912): Pituitary body and its disorders. In: *Clinical States produced by Disorders of the Hypophysis Cerebri.* Lippincott, Philadelphia, Pa.
(3) RAY, B. S. and HORWITH, M. (1964): Surgical treatment of acromegaly. *Clin. Neurosurg., 10,* 31.
(4) RAND, R. W. (1968): Cryogenic technique in stereotaxic neurosurgery. *Int. Surg. (Chic.), 15,* 319.
(5) RAND, R. W. (1968): Stereotaxic cryohypophysectomy. In: *Cryosurgery,* pp. 207–245. Editors: R. W. Rand, A. P. Rinfret and H. von Leden. Charles C. Thomas, Springfield, Ill.
(6) RAND, R. W., HEUSER, G., DASHE, A., ADAMS, D. and ROTH, N. (1969): Stereotaxic transsphenoidal biopsy and cryosurgery of pituitary tumors. *Amer. J. Roentgenol., 105,* 273.

Discussion

DR. ROSS: Drs. Levin and Zervas have agreed to present short summaries of their experience with cryohypophysectomy and thermal ablation of the pituitary.

DR. LEVIN: Drs. John Adams and Robert Seymour, in the Department of Neurosurgery at the University of California in San Francisco, have used transsphenoidal cryohypophysectomy to treat over 100 patients with acromegaly. This procedure is effective in a majority of patients, and the complications are minimal. Three instances of cerebrospinal fluid rhinorrhea all occurred among the first 25 patients.

Transient diabetes insipidus may occur in the first 48 hours. Extra-ocular muscle weakness and visual field defects occur in approximately 15 % of the patients and have always remitted by the end of the third week.

The incidence of adrenal insufficiency is approximately 20 %. We also have an incidence of decreased thyroid function in about 30 % of our patients after this procedure. This may appear long after treatment. Of 100 patients treated, one or two had hormonal recurrence with an elevation of the growth hormone to above 10 ng/ml after prior lowering to less than 10 ng/ml. Twenty-six patients have been followed for over 5 years.

In analyzing the data from the first 50 patients we found the mean fasting growth hormone (GH) was 52 ng/ml pre-operatively and 13 ng/ml post-operatively.

Thirty-eight patients (76 %) of this group post-operatively had growth hormone less than 10 ng/ml. When we grouped the patients according to preoperative growth hormone levels, we found fully 90 % of the patients with pre-operative levels of 40 ng/ml or less have post-operative GH reduction to 10 ng/ml or less; in contrast, only 50 % of the patients who had pre-operative levels above 40 ng/ml have post-operative values less than 10 ng/ml. These data suggested that a more extensive procedure has to be done in patients with high initial GH levels.

A very great advantage of cryosurgery is rapidity of response. Growth hormone, glucose, and insulin were significantly lowered 6 weeks after treatment in the group of patients who had an optimal metabolic response. There is not a great deal of difference as we follow them longer. At one year or more, the values remain unchanged from those seen at 6 weeks and were still within the normal range.

DR. ODELL: Drs. Brown and others (J. Brown, R. E. Ottoman, R. W. Rand, N. Matthews and S. D. Frasier: 'Treatment of acromegaly: Comparison of external radiation and cryohypophysectomy. *Endocr. Soc. 52nd Meeting*, 1970, *150*, 111) published an abstract concerning cryohypophysectomy. They indicated that growth hormone concentrations in acromegalic patients fell promptly following cryosurgery, but then gradually increased again over 3 to 5 years until they were no different from pre-operative values. As far as I can tell, this report has never been published as a full length paper. However, in as much as you performed the surgery on the patients they studied and it is such an important matter, would you update us?

DR. RAND: I discontinued the operation because of the data that you referred to by Drs. Brown and Gold in order to assess the long-term results in the initial group. On the basis of the growth hormone levels and clinical improvement I have reported here, we are now reinstituting our program of cryohypophysectomy.

DR. ZERVAS: Thermal ablation of pituitary adenomas using the stereotaxic transsphenoidal approach has the inherent capability of limiting tissue destruction to the tumor while sparing the surrounding visual pathways. (1) The optic chiasm and the oculomotor nerves are insulated from the pituitary adenoma by the intervening fluid pathways, namely the chiasmatic cistern above the tumor and the carotid arteries and the cavernous sinuses lateral to the tumor. In over 250 operations carried out to ablate the normal hypophysis for the treatment of breast carcinoma or diabetic retinopathy, these insulating channels were effective in preventing permanent visual damage due to heat except in one case. Ionizing radiation, on the other hand, has no special affinity for tumor tissue and decays according to geometric considerations. Surrounding structures are vulnerable to any errors of dosage or positioning of the source and are not protected by any of the anatomical characteristics of the sella turcica. Cryo methods prevent the dissipation of cold by freezing the vascular and cerebrospinal fluid circulation, thus permitting cooling of adjacent visual neural pathways. Visual loss or diplopia may occur with minimal lowering of temperature as the cold lesion spreads and thus obligates the surgeon to terminate the lesion before a deep freezing lesion can be made in the tumor itself. Efforts to control the extent of radiation or cold lesions in order to minimize visual injury may as a consequence preserve portions of the tumor.

We have performed stereotaxic thermal ablation in 18 patients with acromegaly. For the most part the tumors were of large size, corresponding to Grade III or IV adenoma as characterized by Hardy.[2]

The criteria for operation included: (1) laboratory demonstration of elevated human growth hormone on glucose tolerance testing; (2) active clinical disease with headache, acral enlargement, hyperhydrosis, glucose intolerance, hypertension or cardiomyopathy. Patients with minimal clinical symptoms wishing to avoid infertility were not chosen for operation.

All operations were performed under endotracheal anesthesia with patients awake so that visual function could be monitored. The radiofrequency heating electrode was introduced into the tumor using the transnasal transsphenoidal stereotaxic method.[1] With adenomas greater than 2 cm in diameter, bilateral punctures were made. The electrode consisted of a 1.8 mm insulated cannula with a central malleable stylet with a preformed curve that could be projected through a side hole at the tip of the cannula at right angles to its axis. This electrode could project up to 12 mm laterally from the axis of the electrode thus permitting the production of fully overlapping lesions in tumors up to 24 mm in diameter. The radial stylet was made of soft coiled wire with a blunt tip so as to prevent injury to nearby vascular structures. All lesions were made at 80° C for 30–60 seconds. Prior to the induction of these lesions electrical stimulation was carried out. If oculomotor motion was observed at less than 1.5 volts the electrode was readjusted. This electrode permitted the induction of a series of lesions around the circumference of the tumor in any coronal plane. In most cases it was necessary to use two to three coronal planes, one at the posterior margin of the tumor, one centrally and one anteriorly. Six to ten lesions in each plane were necessary. All lesions were monitored radiographically to be certain that the radial stylet did not penetrate above the diaphragma sellae. In 7 patients some suprasellar extension was present, and lesions made 2 to 3 mm above the diaphragma sellae were monitored carefully to prevent visual impairment.

Results

Immediate remission of headache, hyperhidrosis and diminution of acral enlargement were noted in all but 2 patients within one week following operation and without later recurrence. Headache continued in 1 patient who had a postoperative HGH of 6 ng/ml. Glucose intolerance was severe in 6 patients and subsided in all 6 after operation. Human growth hormone fell slowly over a period of 6–12 weeks. The average reduction of HGH was 88 % and levels greater than 10 ng/ml were noted in only 2 patients of the 17 patients who had total ablations (Fig. 1). Two patients with reductions of HGH to normal levels still continued to have severe painful osteoarthritis and were dissatisfied at the result. One other patient with normal HGH level following operation was disappointed at the wrinkling of the face that occurred postoperatively.

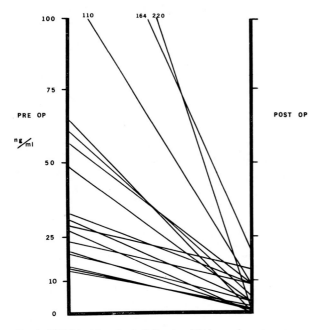

Fig. 1 HGH in 17 patients following RF hypophysectomy.

Three of the patients had received radiation therapy at some time prior to operation. Two patients with very large invasive adenomas were administered radiation therapy following operation.

No death occurred in the immediate postoperative period, but one patient died 6 months following operation of a myocardial infarction. Diabetes insipidus occurred transiently in 2 patients. Neither cerebrospinal fluid rhinorrhea, meningitis nor other infection occurred in any patient. One patient developed a partial oculomotor nerve palsy which subsided completely within 18 days. One patient developed an intrasellar hemorrhage causing visual loss and diplopia within 24 hours following operation. Prompt evacuation of the hemorrhage by stereotaxic aspiration brought about prompt and total cessation of all signs of visual impairment.

The follow-up period has been 6 months to 6 years, and recurrence has not been observed as yet in any but the very first patient. This woman with HGH levels well above 500 ng/ml was not treated using the radial electrode, but had simply a number of straight electrode punctures with lesions made in four quadrants of a giant adenoma. Cardiomyopathy in this woman subsided moderately and postoperative growth hormone levels fell below 50 ng/ml, but more recently have again begun to rise.

When thermal ablation is designed to destroy as much tumor tissue as possible it inevitably will result in panhypopituitarism. In most of our patients we attempted to spare the most superior posterior medial wedge of tissue within the sella so as to diminish damage to the pituitary stalk. This tactic was successful in that minor transient diabetes insipidus occurred in only one patient. On the other hand, panhypopituitarism did develop in all but one patient.

The foreknowledge that panhypopituitarism is an inherent complication of thermal hypophysectomy would preclude the use of this technique in patients who desire to remain fertile if possible. However, these results support the use of thermal ablation as a predictable and safe means of producing prompt relief in all patients with acromegaly. In particular, the effects of thermal ablation are not diminished with tumors of large size, since even patients with giant adenomas had a satisfactory result. Moreover, strong consideration has to be given to producing total ablation in tumors of only moderate size even at the risk of producing panhypopituitarism since any lesser effort may prevent later definitive treatment. Microadenomas may be an exception, but with proper identification of the exact position of the nodule, it should be a simple matter to destroy the nodule and spare the normal pituitary using a simple well placed lesion.

Acknowledgement

All the endocrine determinations were carried out in the laboratory with Dr. Johanna Pallota, who was also responsible for the clinical assesment of all patients.

References

(1) ZERVAS, N. T. (1969): Stereotaxic radiofrequency surgery of the normal and the abnormal pituitary gland. *New Engl. J. Med.*, *280*, 429.
(2) HARDY, J. (1973): This Volume, pp. 179–194.

VII. Medical treatment of pituitary tumors

Alternatives to ablative therapy for pituitary tumors

A. M. LAWRENCE and T. C. HAGEN

University of Chicago Pritzker School of Medicine, Chicago, Ill., U.S.A.

'Alternatives to ablative therapy for pituitary tumors' in this chapter is meant to be synonymous with medical or pharmacologic approaches to pituitary adenomatous disease. Clinical experience with such modalities is still meager. The entire area is in its developmental infancy as regards both cumulative experience and specific approaches. The rationale for even considering medical therapy is based on both the desire to develop better, more specific and less morbid 'cures' for pituitary tumor disease, as well as on a body of credible information which seems to offer rationale for exploring pharmacologic approaches to adenomatous hyperplasia in the pars distalis.

In this chapter a general discussion of the basis for this rationale is offered, possible drug approaches are explored and an attempt is made to review the small but important experience with medical therapies in patients with various forms of pituitary tumor disease.

It is generally acknowledged that pituitary tumors should be treated. These patients are at definite risk for damage to surrounding structures, hypopituitarism, or visible morbidity or mortality from excess ACTH, TSH, growth hormone or prolactin secretion. Therapeutic approach to pituitary overgrowths was at one time a relatively simple choice between transcranial hypophysectomy and megavoltage X-ray therapy to the pituitary. Variations on these modalities are now legion. No one approach is consistently perfect nor do any lack real or potential morbid complications.[1] The clinical dilemma of what, where, when and how to treat is further confounded by new data which pose questions as to what is precisely meant by the diagnosis of a pituitary tumor, whether these tumors are reversible in some cases and whether they are caused in some instances by extrapituitary factors potentially amenable to control.[2]

There are, for example, even uncertainties when attempting to identify patients at risk for developing morbidity directly attributable to tumorous overgrowth within the anterior pituitary. The diagnosis of a pituitary tumor is admittedly an arbitrary one. Although clinicians are emotionally attached to radiographic evidence of enlargement or contour deformity of the sella turcica this is an uncertain criterion at best. It should be chastening to reflect on the many patients with so-called 'empty sellas' who received radiotherapy to the pituitary fossa before pretreatment pneumoencephalography became a more routine procedure.[3] Although these particular patients can now be sorted from others being considered for therapy the question as to the pathogenesis of the large but empty sella remains. A significant percentage of patients with acromegaly show no obvious distortion of the sella turcica on either ordinary or tomographic X-ray projections but here clinical and laboratory data allow the comfortable conclusion that a pituitary tumor is present. It must be asked, however, whether this assumption is always correct. Although few patients with pituitary-

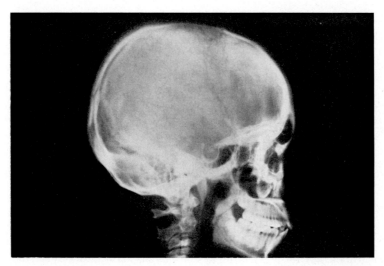

Fig. 1   Example of an enlarged sella turcica in an 18-year-old female with primary hypothyroidism and intact pituitary function. Followed for 7 years on replacement thyroid. No progression in sella size or deterioration in pituitary function.

dependent Cushing's disease have measurable enlargement of the sella turcica it is moot to argue that the pathogenesis of their disease differs in any essential respect from that of the patient with Cushing's disease and no enlargement of the pituitary fossa. Indeed, following adrenalectomy for Cushing's disease some of these same patients will ultimately show sufficient enlargement to allow them entry into the pituitary tumor or adenoma category.[4, 5] The child with juvenile acquired primary hypothyroidism and an enlarged pituitary certainly does not have a pituitary tumor in the accepted sense since reduction in raised TSH levels and normalization of sella size with advancing years and thyroid therapy are seen.[6] Adult patients with the same syndrome (Fig. 1) do not show regression in sella size even though TSH levels decline on thyroid therapy.[7] What of the 20 % or more of pituitary micro-adenomata seen in autopsy material? Are we missing treatable disorders? Do our patients with non-puerperal galactorrhea and no discernible pituitary enlargement all have prolactin secreting adenomata? How frequently does an enlarged sella represent the presence of reversible hyperplasia rather than the presence of a relatively autonomous and growing neoplasm? Clearly our designation and understanding of the clinical significance of all pituitary enlargements is limited.

Identifying patients with pituitary overgrowth and deciding to treat are relatively simple tasks for most clinicians, but choosing a given therapeutic modality is not in many instances. A safe, simple, effective approach designed to preserve maximum pituitary function is an optimum goal. Since no therapy available in 1973 is consistently effective nor lacking totally in potential morbidity, the search for better therapies continues. Until we have clarified our understanding of the pathogenesis of these growths, our approaches to therapy must of necessity be simplistic. Ablative attacks upon the pituitary, partial or complete, clearly serve a useful purpose if reduction in pituitary size or removal of excessive secretions is sought. Recently, however, the speculation that some pituitary tumors owe their inception to disturbances originating in the hypothalamus has led to a consideration of possible pharmacologic or medical approaches to treatment. [8–11]

There is now general accord that the master of anterior pituitary function lies within the hypothalamus, and that the median eminence and its elaborate and rich portal vascular plexus carry signals from above to either stimulate or inhibit pituitary peptide synthesis and release. Many release factors have been identified; certain ones, luteinizing hormone releasing hormone (LHRH) and thyrotrophin releasing hormone (TRH), have been characterized and synthesized. These peptides, releasing and inhibitory hormones or factors, appear to be formed enzymatically within hypothalamic neurons. Secretions from these neurons are probably carried axonally into the median eminence portion of the neurohypophysis where concentrations of transmitter agents are highest. There these terminals come into contact with portal vessels leading toward and into the anterior pituitary. These vessels are fenestrated in a fashion similar to that seen in all tissues of absorptive and secretory function. These granule laden terminals vary in morphology and in the nature of their chemical content as well. Histochemical staining indicates the presence of such neurotransmitters as dopamine, norepinephrine, serotonin, acetylcholine and others. The portal vessels of the median eminence seem to distribute themselves zonally within the anterior pituitary. Secretion of factors from the hypothalamus is also modulated by synaptic neurotransmission from other brain areas and by the negative feedback effect of target gland hormones. Significant alterations in pituitary hormone release are noted following various modes of administering cholinergic drugs, amines or their precursors, or during alpha- and beta-adrenergic stimulation or blockade. Several excellent discussions of these many investigative areas have now been published.[12-15] Provided sufficient and convincing data can be marshalled to implicate the hypothalamus in the development of some pituitary tumors, pharmacologic manipulation of the chemistry of this portion of the brain may lead to specific therapies for non-autonomous pituitary overgrowths or hyperplasias.

Hypothalamic factors

Even given the certain knowledge that the hypothalamus synthesizes materials which modulate stimulated and inhibited release of hormones from the anterior pituitary it can be asked what evidence is there for believing disordered signaling from above the pituitary might play a role in the development of some pituitary tumors? In established, pituitary-dependent Cushing's disease, impaired suppressibility of ACTH secretion by cortisone has argued for a corticotrophin releasing hormone (CRH) locus relatively insensitive to the negative feedback effects of circulating cortisol.[11, 16] A corollary to this belief is the appearance of clinically significant hyperpigmentation, increased ACTH and MSH secretion and enlargement of the pituitary fossa following adrenalectomy and replacement cortisone therapy in some Cushing's disease patients.[4, 5] Here it is reasoned that in the absence of elevated cortisol levels, sufficient to feed back negatively upon a disordered hypothalamus, chronic and excessive hypothalamic stimulation of pituitary ACTH and MSH secretion with resultant hyperpigmentation and pituitary enlargement eventually develop. Continued loss of diurnal cortisol secretory rhythm and abnormal responses to administered pyrogen in patients 'cured' by radiotherapy to the pituitary have also provided evidence for a basic disorder centered within the hypothalamus in this disease.[16]

In acromegaly, too, relative non-autonomy of growth hormone secretion has been taken as some evidence for continuing hypothalamic control of growth hormone secretion.[8,9] Frequent paradoxical growth hormone responses are suggestive of hypothalamic disease as well.[8,9] A raised threshold for a negative feedback effect of growth hormone can be demonstrated in some patients before as well as following clinically effective pituitary irradiation (Fig. 2) reminiscent of what occurs in some patients with Cushing's disease.[17,18] A factor possessing growth hormone releasing properties has been demonstrated in the serum of patients with active acromegaly.[19] The occurrence of so-called 'pituitary apoplexy' with the development of hypothalamic hypopituitarism in one of our acromegalic patients adds, we believe, to the belief that a hypothalamic disturbance may be the cause of acromegaly in certain cases.[20] In this particular patient an acute vascular accident spontaneously developed within the hypothalamopituitary axis. Abatement of active acromegaly followed soon thereafter as did hypopituitarism. Growth hormone was measurable (3–6 ng/ml) but did not rise with provocation. Prolactin levels were high, however. Unmeasurable TSH levels rose significantly during the intravenous administration of TRH. Evidence for a significant amount of responsive pituitary tissue suggested that autocure of this particular patient's acromegaly was secondary to interruption of hypothalamic influences following the vascular event. Similar cases are on record.[21, 22]

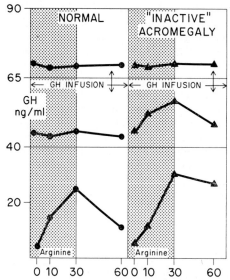

Fig. 2 Demonstration of an apparent raised threshold for autoregulation of growth hormone secretion in a patient with 'inactive' acromegaly. Abolition of an arginine provoked rise in growth hormone was noted in the normal subject when a growth hormone infusion raised circulating levels to 40–44 ng/ml. In the 'cured' acromegalic this effect was not achieved until levels were raised above 60 ng/ml. Prior to successful radiotherapy, mean basal growth hormone levels in this patient were 54.6±4.3 ng/ml.

In addition to these observations in Cushing's disease and in acromegaly, there is a growing appreciation of a possible role of target gland deficiency in the generation of exaggerated hypothalamic signals leading to pituitary enlargement. It is generally assumed that target gland secretions exert a negative feedback effect on the hypothalamopituitary axis. Studies in humans and in monkeys confirming this assumption are few, but do nevertheless lend credence to this classical dogma.[23–25] Given these considerations, it could be predicted that loss of a target gland secretion could lead to uninterrupted secretion of a hypothalamic factor with resultant hyperplasia of the appropriate cells within the pituitary gland. Many rodent species develop gross neoplastic growths within the anterior pituitary following surgical or radioiodine ablation of the thyroid, for example.[26] Although an equivalent phenomenon has been recognized in some children with primary hypothyroidism,[6] it is only recently that a similar syndrome has been appreciated in certain adults with primary hypothyroidism.[7] Many of these adults have had Hashimoto's thyroiditis. Not very long ago, but prior to today's more extensive endocrinologic evaluation of patients with pituitary disease, many individuals with primary hypothyroidism and pituitary enlargement were given a diagnosis of chromophobe adenoma and a course of pituitary irradiation. Clinical history of hypothyroidism is variable and in some, of relatively short duration.[7] Wider application of the TSH immunoassay has shown significant numbers of euthyroid patients with Hashimoto's thyroiditis with grossly elevated TSH levels.[27] This finding raises the possibility that chronic hypersecretion of TSH, presumably due to faltering thyroxine production, may account for subsequent enlargement of the pituitary. Most, presumably, are not autonomous adenomas since elevated TSH levels fall to normal when euthyroidism is achieved on replacement thyroxine therapy; other parameters of pituitary function have been normal in cases which have been studied.[7] Pituitary enlargement in patients with gonadal failure has also been reported.[28, 29] In the main these have also borne the clinical diagnosis of chromophobe adenoma. Although elevated bioassayed urinary gonadotrophin levels have been measured in such cases, most of the patients were reported in an era prior to the advent of sensitive and specific radioimmunoassays. It can be anticipated, however, that with more in-depth endocrinologic evaluation of patients with pituitary tumors, additional patients with enlargement of the sella and elevated gonadotrophin levels will be discovered and reported.

Other considerations arise when attempting to invoke target gland failure in the development of some pituitary tumors. Although it was originally concluded that overproduction of one hypothalamic release factor should result in hypertrophy and hyperplasia of 1 line of cells within the pituitary, this may not be so. Rodent tumors from thyroidectomized animals, grown in tissue culture, almost invariably manufacture TSH, but examples of gonadotrophin or growth hormone-like production have been reported.[30] Chromophobe adenomas in patients with primary gonadal failure[28, 29] may have been LH, FSH producing tumors, but acromegaly[31] and Cushing's disease[32] have been seen as well. We have been impressed by the number of acromegalic women who, by history, developed their first signs and symptoms of acromegaly soon after surgical castration or spontaneous menopause, following pregnancy or antiovulatory medications without resumption of menstrual cycles (Table I). Immunoassayed LH and FSH levels have been raised to levels consistent with

Table I *Development of acromegaly in 18 women: temporal relationship to estrogen deficiency*

No.	Circumstances
7	1–3 yr following oophorectomy-hysterectomy. No estrogen therapy.
4	2–6 months following parturition – persisting amenorrhea.
2	Perimenopausal period.
2	Taking antiovulatory steroids – persisting amenorrhea and signs of acromegaly after 'pills' discontinued.
3	Incomplete histories.

primary gonadal failure in most. Furthermore, experience with TRH administration in humans has indicated that these hypothalamic factors are not as strictly specific as originally believed. There are now reports, and we have also observed, that some normal subjects[33] and several patients with pituitary tumors[34] (Fig. 3) demonstrate a brisk rise in growth hormone when TRH is administered.

Pharmacologic approaches

Given these kinds of considerations, what possible kinds of pharmacologic approaches are potentially available for patients with pituitary adenomas? In this context there is reason to neglect medical approaches which would result in clinical abatement of the disease process by simply interfering with peripheral responsiveness to secreted hormones (estrogen therapy in acromegaly) or by accelerating catabolism of the offending hormone (Dilantin in Cushing's disease). Such treatment could theoretically lead to progression in size of the pituitary tumor

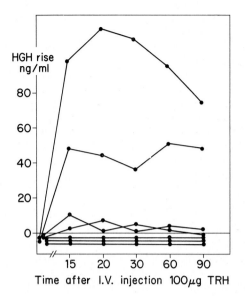

Fig. 3 Unusual and rapid growth hormone release following intravenous TRH (100 μg) in 7 male acromegalics.

if the negative feedback system did in fact require higher than normal levels of circulating hormones for suppression of hypothalamic stimulation. Years ago estrogen therapy in acromegaly may have been abandoned because of a report[35] which suggested progression of pituitary size despite regression of clinical stigmata of active acromegaly, now believed secondary to diminished peripheral responsiveness to growth hormone caused by high tissue levels of estrogen.[36]

At the level of the pituitary, drugs may be developed which will either selectively destroy specific pituitary cells or compete more favorably for membrane binding sites for specific hypothalamic releasing factors (ergot alkaloids in the case of prolactin secreting tumors, for example). Although attention is focused on *stimulation* of ACTH, growth hormone and gonadotrophin release by factors from the hypothalamus, there is reason to believe that dual inhibition and release may exist for each of these peptides. It is known, for example, that the major influence of the hypothalamus on prolactin secretion is an inhibitory one, but TRH does stimulate a rise[37] and this may explain the phenomenon of galactorrhea seen in some patients with primary hypothyroidism. A major breakthrough has recently been reported from Guillemin's group. These workers have isolated, characterized and synthesized a biologically active growth hormone inhibitory factor of hypothalamic origin.[38] Thus it may be possible to administer such agents to inhibit secretory activity and further growth of hypertrophic cells in select patients with pituitary adenomatous hyperplasia. Indeed, if the hypothalamus does play a significant role in the pathogenesis of some pituitary tumors, it is reasonable to wonder whether some disturbance in the balance between release and inhibition does not occasionally occur.

At the level of hypothalamic loci responsible for secretion of release and inhibitory hormones, pharmacologic or therapeutic approaches seem potentially at hand and deserve study. Since these hypothalamic factors are enzymatically formed within the hypothalamus,[39] better understanding of their synthesis and degradation may lead to the development of drugs which can interfere with synthesis or which would hasten metabolism. Furthermore, much evidence attests to the importance of adrenergic and cholinergic neurotransmission from other centers of the brain and within the hypothalamus as well. Membrane alpha or beta receptors may further determine the path of cellular responsiveness. Some evidence links hypothalamic synthesis of prostaglandins in this chain of events.[40] Thus studies are needed which will methodically investigate the results of pharmacologic manipulation of amine storage, synthesis and metabolism, of alpha and beta receptor stimulation and blockade, and of prostaglandin synthesis, inhibition of action or blockade of response by competitive inhibition of membrane receptors. The effect of cholinergic blockade requires study. In certain instances dual adrenergic-cholinergic, inhibition-stimulation may be involved. Pharmacologic means which may increase one phase of neurochemotransmission while blunting another may lead to unusual but therapeutically effective approaches to certain kinds of pituitary disorders including pituitary adenomata caused by hypothalamic disease of one sort or another.

Medical approaches to treatment

Medical approaches to treatment of pituitary tumors in man have only recently been reported and discussed. Growth of certain chromophobe adenomas can be checked if appropriate target gland hormones are provided in patients with primary end-organ failure.[6, 7] L-DOPA and monoamine oxidase inhibitors have been considered in the treatment of pituitary-dependent Cushing's disease.[1, 41] L-DOPA,[42,44] certain of the ergot alkaloids[45–48] and clomiphene[49] have enjoyed a modicum of therapeutic success in patients with galactorrheic syndromes. High dose progestin[50–52] or phenothiazine[52] administration has been associated with clinical and laboratory improvement in a few patients with active acromegaly. Results of treatment are often inconsistent and attempts to reproduce results recorded by one laboratory have failed altogether in the hands of others.[53,54]

'Chromophobe adenoma'

From previous discussions it seems abundantly clear that certain patients with primary target gland failure can develop an enlarged pituitary. In the absence of clinical evidence for Cushing's disease, acromegaly or galactorrhea, such patients are generally designated as having a chromophobe adenoma. Experience in children with primary hypothyroidism treated with maintenance thyroid therapy alone has not, to our knowledge, seen any progression in size of the tumor or disturbance in pituitary function. Recognition of this phenomenon in adults is of fairly recent origin but we have followed such patients for more than 8 yr without noting progression in size of the 'tumor' or alteration in pituitary function. Radiotherapy to the pituitary in these patients has been withheld and treatment has consisted of maintenance thyroid therapy. Recently, too, patients with an enlarged pituitary fossa and primary gonadal failure have been recognized. Previously such adult patients were considered instances of chromophobe adenomata and frequently underwent a full course of radiotherapy to the pituitary gland. Our patients with this syndrome are now being followed on maintenance sex steroid therapy alone, provided no suprasellar extension or visual field encroachment are evident.

Cushing's disease

3,4-Dihydroxyphenylalanine (L-DOPA) and certain monoamine oxidase inhibitors have been tried as therapy in Cushing's disease.[11, 41] Control of hypothalamic synthesis and secretion of corticotrophin releasing hormone (CRH) is believed by some workers to be inhibited by a central hypothalamic adrenergic system.[55, 56] It is uncertain whether this is the result of a direct limbic system neurotransmitter to hypothalamic cells synthesizing CRH or whether, in addition, increased synthesis of norepinephrine or its precursors within the hypothalamus may cause unusual responsiveness of corticotrophs to CRH. Several studies have demonstrated sympathomimetic inhibition of stress-induced ACTH release. In animals, L-DOPA administration has had a similar effect. Several of the pathophysiologic features of Cushing's disease in man are seen in rats treated with drugs which will deplete the concentration of stored catecholamines.[57] These include loss of diurnal cortisol or ACTH secretory rhythms and a raised threshold for glucocorticoid suppression of ACTH secretion. The administration of L-DOPA reverses such effects and, in certain animal studies, inhibits stress-induced ACTH release as well.[55, 57] Results of L-DOPA administration to humans with Cushing's disease have not proven successful in one series, even with doses as high as 5 g daily.[11] Others have reported that certain monoamine oxidase inhibitors may return glucocorticoid suppressibility of ACTH towards normal in some patients with Cushing's disease.[41] It seems that considerably more refinement in understanding dopaminergic or noradrenergic inhibition of CRH secretion and ACTH release is needed before it can be assumed that relative lack of adrenergic inhibitory tone is the basic defect in Cushing's disease.

Prolactin

There are those who strongly believe that all cases of non-puerperal galactorrhea harbor pituitary adenomata. Non-puerperal lactation is encountered in some patients on drugs such as reserpine, methyldopa, morphine or phenothiazines.[58] Galactorrhea may be seen in primary hypothyroidism. Many instances without sellar enlargement are designated as idiopathic. With discernible enlargement of the pituitary fossa various titles are applied.[59]

The hypothalamus is known to exert an inhibitory tonus upon pituitary prolactin release by secretion of prolactin inhibitory factor (PIF). That this phenomenon is probably adrenergically mediated is supported by studies in animals which find that pituitary prolactin synthesis and secretion rises with maneuvers which either directly deplete the hypothalamus of amines and their precursors or prevent their normal synthesis and transmission.[60, 61] Drug associated galactorrhea in man occurs with agents known to lower catecholamine concentration within the hypothalamus.[58] Drugs such as phenobarbital which may interfere with central adrenergic transmission or agents which may cause dendritic receptor blockade such as the phenothiazines have also been associated with galactorrhea. Since TRH can cause prolactin release in normal man,[37] the galactorrhea in some primary hypothyroid individuals is likely secondary to this phenomenon, but this effect may be amplified by a general lowering of sympathetic tonus associated with the hypothyroid state.

In addition to adrenergic neurotransmission, the state of activity of the hypothalamic loci which synthesize and secrete LHRH and FSH-RH also seem of importance in the overall hypothalamic regulation of pituitary prolactin secretion.[62] More often than not amenorrhea or anovulatory cycles are present in patients with non-puerperal galactorrhea. Drugs which cause galactorrhea regularly interfere with normal cycles.

Castration in animals leads to an accelerated rate of amine synthesis within the hypothalamus and decreased prolactin secretion.[63] Progesterone administration is associated with diminished hypothalamic amine synthesis and turnover[64] and decreased LH secretion.[65] Prolactin secretion is likely increased. Many cases of persisting amenorrhea and galactorrhea are seen in women who have taken antiovulatory compounds,[66] a kind of pseudo Chiari-Frommel syndrome. Thus the cause of galactorrhea in association with these compounds may be related to an initial disturbance in LH and FSH secretion.

Medical approaches to the treatment of non-puerperal galactorrhea have included discontinuing drugs implicated in its causation and the administration of thyroid to hypothyroid patients. Many weeks may be required before prolactin levels are lowered and lactation ceases.[58] In some, presumably drug associated cases, increased prolactin secretion persists despite discontinuance of the medication. In these instances, L-DOPA,[42-44] ergot derivatives[45-48] or clomiphene[66] have been used with variable success. In animals, the anti-estrogenic compound clomiphene causes a marked increase in hypothalamic amine turnover in intact and in castrate rats; a sharp rise in LH and a drop in prolactin release are observed.[67] Thus the success of clomiphene therapy in patients with amenorrhea and lactation may be related to its ability to stimulate aminergic neurons within the hypothalamus and thereby re-establish the critical balance necessary for increased cyclic LH and FSH secretion and greater inhibition of prolactin release.

L-DOPA, orally or intravenously, causes an abrupt drop in circulating prolactin levels[42-44] and some have reported clinical benefit in galactorrheic states.[42-43] One problem with L-DOPA, which presumably works by augmenting the adrenergic influence to PIF secretion, is its short duration of action. Nevertheless, its use and the availability now of serum immunoassayed prolactin levels to better quantitate the effect of therapy have opened avenues for the development of other agents capable of similar induction of a high adrenergic or dopaminergic tone within the hypothalamus. Ergot alkaloids, however, may prove of greater and more enduring benefit in idiopathic and non-acromegalic pituitary tumor patients with galactorrhea. Several groups have now extended observations from animals and in vitro pituitary studies to galactorrhea in man and have discovered that the ergot compounds ergonovine and ergocryptine may result in cessation of galactorrhea and resumption of normal menstrual cycles in those women in whom amenorrhea has developed.[45-48] A drop in high serum prolactin levels in a series of galactorrheic women receiving 2-Br-alpha-ergocryptine has recently been reported.[47] The exact mechanism of action of ergots in these galactorrheic states is not clearly understood although studies drawn from animals suggest both a hypothalamic dopaminergic stimulation to PIF release as well as a direct effect of ergots on pituitary prolactin secreting cells.[67] At the level of the pituitary, ergots may cause specific cytotoxic effects or may result in atrophy and disappearance of prolactin secreting cells because of interference with reception of hypothalamic influences.

Acromegaly

Our laboratory has concentrated particularly on medical approaches to treatment of acromegaly. Proton beam bombardment is occasionally unsuccessful and long-term effect on pituitary function is yet to be learned. More conventional radiotherapy to the pituitary may not be as innocuous as previously believed if more careful psychometric testing before and after therapy were to be analyzed on a broad scale. Transsphenoidal microdissection or intrahypophyseal instillation of ionizing radiation sources or cryoprobes may generate unexpected bleeding in the most experienced hands and result in less than optimum therapy or hastily executed surgery which may thoroughly injure normal pituitary reserve.

Hypothalamic stimulation of growth hormone release seems to be alpha-adrenergically mediated. Propranolol, a beta blocker, enhances growth hormone release to provocative stimuli[68] and the oral administration of 0.5 g of L-DOPA has become a useful stimulatory test which is presumed to indicate functional intactness of the hypothalamus and to show the pituitary's ability to respond to growth hormone releasing factor.[69] In animals, maneuvers which act to augment adrenergic neurotransmission result in increased secretion of growth hormone.[70] Further, stimulation of extrahypothalamic areas in rats such as the hippocampus, the basolateral amygdala and mesencephalic interpeduncular nucleus[71] can also cause growth hormone release. These and other observations have led to preliminary attempts to alter growth hormone secretion in acromegaly with agents known to depress adrenergic tone within the hypothalamus: progestins[50-54] and phenothiazines.[52-72] Alpha-adrenergic blockade of L-DOPA stimulated growth hormone release has been reported[73] but to our knowledge has not been tried therapeutically in acromegaly. Recently, L-DOPA was reported to cause a paradoxical lowering of growth hormone secretion in some patients with active disease[74] highlighting the likelihood that hypothalamic mediation of somatotroph hyperplasia may be extraordinarily variegated and ultimately require a tailored therapeutic approach in any given patient.

We proposed that progesterone therapy might benefit some patients with active acromegaly.[50] In the course of analyzing endocrine function in our patients it was apparent that many developed acromegaly following situations associated with a sharp decline in sex steroid concentrations, surgical or spontaneous menopause, discontinuance of birth control pills or conclusion of pregnancy (Table I). Since castration in animals is associated with a rapid increase in amine synthesis within the hypothalamus[63] we have become suspicious that in certain predisposed women this phenomenon might lead to unchecked and chronic secretion of high levels of hypothalamic growth hormone releasing hormone (GHRH). Ultimately such mechanisms might lead to acromegaly. The administration of progesterone to castrate rats results in a diminished rate of catecholamine synthesis within the hypothalamus[63] and is likely due to decreased tyrosine hydroxylase activity which follows such therapy.[63] This enzyme represents a rate limiting step in the synthesis of catecholamines. Since growth hormone secretion appears to be adrenergically mediated via the hypothalamus, it was reasoned that progestagens might suppress growth hormone secretory responsiveness. Indeed, others have shown that the oral progestin medroxyprogesterone acetate can lower growth hormone secretory responsiveness to an arginine infusion,[75] limits the growth hormone rise in response to insulin induced hypoglycemia,[76] attenuates the hormone rebound following oral glucose administration[77] and dampens sleep associated growth hormone secretion.

Administration of the orally active progestin, medroxyprogesterone acetate (MPA), to individuals with active acromegaly has met with singularly variable results.[50-54] In our initial series of 12, 75 % demonstrated significant lowering of elevated basal levels into or near the normal range over a 6-day period while receiving MPA, 10 mg 4 times daily. Several morning samples were obtained in each patient in this group and the wide fluctuations frequently commented upon in acromegaly were not seen. In addition to an apparent drop in basal growth hormone secretion, peak growth hormone rises in response to an arginine infusion were considerably attenuated in both normal volunteers and in 9 of 11 acromegalic subjects receiving MPA.[50]

Ten of our patients with active acromegaly have taken MPA 40 mg daily for 1–38 months. Clinical improvement consisting of regression in soft tissue hyperplasia, e.g. ability to wear rings and shoes which had become too small, disappearance of a tendency to perspire about the head and upper thorax, and alleviation of headache, occurred in 7. However, growth hormone levels drawn basally in the hospital and randomly in the outpatient clinic were consistently within the normal or near normal range in only 3 of this group. Pretreatment values in these patients ranged between 25–35 ng/ml and while on therapy dropped to between 5–12 ng/ml. Growth hormone suppressibility, by induced hyperglycemia, did not return and is reminiscent of similar findings in patients 'cured' by pituitary irradiation where abnormal patterns of growth hormone secretion persist despite apparent subsidence of the disease process (Fig. 4). In the other 4 patients who experienced clinical improvement while receiving MPA, a 40 to 70 % lowering of growth hormone levels from mean pretreatment levels was noted. Random values on therapy, however, plateaued above 30 ng/ml. In 1 patient of this group, values which had initially dropped from greater than 100 to 30 ng/ml rose again to pretreatment levels over the course of 4 months on therapy.

In 1 woman with active disease, MPA therapy was associated with a drop in measured growth hormone levels from 25 ng/ml to less than 8 ng/ml under basal conditions. Little if any clinical improvement was noted, however. Indeed worsening of her arthritis ultimately prompted her physician to advise a course of radiotherapy. A year later growth hormone levels were within the normal range and her arthritis stable. Three patients were judged to show no effect from MPA therapy; mean basal growth hormone levels were very slightly

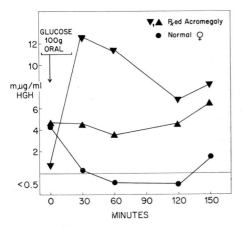

Fig. 4   Example of the preservation of abnormal growth hormone secretory responses even after successful radiotherapy in acromegaly.

lower in 2 over the course of an 18-month period, but radiotherapy to the pituitary had been received 3 and 5 yr earlier.

MPA therapy was interrupted in the 3 who showed marked growth hormone lowering and in 1 whose values dropped from greater than 100 to 30 ng/ml. A remarkable rebound was seen in all. In the last patient values rose to pretreatment levels, but in the other 3 levels greatly exceeded pretreatment measurements. One woman underwent a subtotal thyroidectomy for a non-functioning thyroid nodule and was off therapy for 1 week postoperatively when re-evaluation was undertaken. Basal values which had never exceeded 35 ng/ml and which had dropped to less than 10 ng/ml while on MPA rose to 78 ng/ml and remained in this range for the 7-day testing period. Also, more marked stimulation of GH release was seen during oral glucose tolerance testing and arginine infusion. Over the course of 3.5 months, while back on MPA therapy, random resting values dropped to less than 10 ng/ml.

Other experience with MPA therapy in acromegaly, reported in the English literature, has ranged from positive or partial effects in some[51, 52] to absence of any discernible effect.[53, 54] Malarkey and Daughaday studied mean growth hormone concentrations in 11 patients with active acromegaly and noted clinical benefit and significant lowering of growth hormone in 3.[51] Sherman and Kolodny noted both lowering of raised growth hormone levels and suppression with glucose in their one patient placed on MPA therapy.[52] Jackson and Ormston, however, found no significant alteration in clinical signs or in growth hormone levels in their 11 patients treated in similar fashion for several months.[53] Finally, Rake and his associates have followed 12 patients with active disease receiving MPA daily for 3 months.[54] Growth hormone levels were measured at 2 weeks and at 3 months when patients returned to a clinic setting. In 3 a significant reduction in circulating growth hormone levels was noted, from 200 to 39, from 45 to 18 and from 57 to 27 ng/ml. Apparently only the first of these noted clinical improvement. Despite lack of any significant improvement in growth hormone levels in 7 of this group, a rather marked drop in hydroxyproline excretion occurred in the group as a whole while on MPA. With these inconsistent and at times uncertain results of therapy with MPA, several authors have pleaded for a more carefully monitored approach to any therapeutic claim pointing out that very careful assessment over a long period of time before and during therapy is important in order to arrive at a justified conclusion. Our experience with rebound elevations in growth hormone levels in patients who stop MPA has also pointed to the importance of assessing timed effects of long- and short-acting drugs in this disease.

Recognition of the clinical association of galactorrhea and phenothiazine therapy prompted others to suggest that these agents might be therapeutically effective in active acromegaly. Drug associated galactorrhea is presumed to result from lessened hypothalamic adrenergic neurotransmission.[58] Since the release of growth hormone releasing factor is either noradrenergically or dopaminergically mediated it was reasoned that the phenothiazines might act to lower elevated titers in active acromegaly. Kolodny and Sherman reported a single patient[52] in whom both MPA and chlorpromazine appeared to effect normalization of basal growth hormone levels. Growth hormone suppression in response to oral glucose administration was also restored. Application of this single experience to larger series has not borne out any universal therapeutic benefit, however.[72] We have effected significant clinical benefit and laboratory lowering of growth hormone levels in 1 patient with chlorpromazine but this had to be discontinued because of unacceptable side effects. Substituting other phenothiazines caused similar effects and MPA therapy was reinstituted in this particular patient. Following a full course of radiotherapy, 6000 R to the pituitary, growth hormone levels remained above 100 ng/ml. Five years after radiotherapy no laboratory or clinical change had occurred. MPA therapy was associated with regression in tissue fullness, headaches disappeared and excess perspiration abated. Growth hormone levels which definitely dropped remained higher than normal and plateaued between 46–52 ng/ml despite apparent well-being.

Current pharmacologic or medical approaches to treating acromegaly and other pituitary adenomatous diseases are far from perfect. This form of treatment is in its developmental infancy, however (Table II). Radiotherapy, introduced at the turn of the century, despite

Table II

Tumor	Potential medical therapies in 1973	Refs.
Chromophobe	Target gland replacement	6, 7
Galactorrhea	Ergocryptine	45, 47
	Ergonovine	48
	Clomiphene	49, 66
	L-dopa	42, 43, 44
	PIF	
Cushing's disease	? L-dopa	11
	? Monoamine oxidase inhibitors	41
Acromegaly	Medroxyprogesterone	50–54
	Phenothiazines	52, 72
	L-dopa	74
	GHIF	38

innumerable refinements, is still an uncertain approach. Twenty per cent or more of acromegalic patients so treated have active disease years later. Indeed, it is not entirely certain why radiotherapy does work and it may be that its effect is felt more at the level of the median eminence than within the pituitary.[11]

Formidable advances in neuroendocrinology have been made during the past decade.[12–15] Even so it is apparent that acquisition of more data will be necessary in order to translate this new knowledge to therapeutic developments for diseases of the pituitary in man. To ignore these burgeoning areas of new research because of therapeutic inconsistencies and uncertainties would be to ignore the therapeutic challenge which faces those who care for these patients. Pharmacologic approaches to disorders of pituitary function and to treatment of adenomatous hyperplasia will of necessity depend a great deal on developments in basic neuroendocrinology. We feel confident in predicting that the future will recognize promising new medical approaches to the treatment of pituitary adenomata and probably a host of iatrogenically induced disorders of pituitary function as well.

References

(1) LAWRENCE, A. M., PINSKY, S. M. and GOLDFINE, I. D. (1971): Conventional radiation therapy in acromegaly: a review and reassessment. *Arch. intern. Med., 128*, 369.

(2) LAWRENCE, A. M. (1971): Medical management of acromegaly. In: *Les Adénomes Hypophysaires Sécrétants*, pp. 197–202. Masson et Cie, Paris.

(3) CAPLAN, R. H. and DOBBEN, G. D. (1969): Endocrine studies in patients with the 'Empty sella syndrome'. *Arch. intern. Med., 123*, 611.

(4) NELSON, D. H., MEAKIN, J. W. and THORN, G. W. (1960): ACTH producing pituitary tumors following adrenalectomy for Cushing's syndrome. *Ann. intern. Med., 52*, 560.

(5) ROVIT, R. L. and DUANE, T. D. (1969): Cushing's syndrome and pituitary tumors. Pathophysiology and ocular manifestations of ACTH secreting pituitary adenomas. *Amer. J. Med., 46*, 416.

(6) VAN WYCK, J. J. and GRUMBACH, M. M. (1960): Syndrome of precocious menstruation and galactorrhea in juvenile hypothyroidism: an example of hormonal overlap in pituitary feedback *J. Pediat., 57*, 416.

(7) LAWRENCE, A. M., WILBER, J. and HAGEN, T. C. (1973): The pituitary and primary hypothyroidism: enlargement and unusual growth hormone secretory responses. *Arch. intern. Med., 132*, 327.

(8) CRYER, P. E. and DAUGHADAY, W. H. (1969): Regulation of growth hormone secretion in acromegaly. *J. clin. Endocr., 29*, 386.

(9) LAWRENCE, A. M., GOLDFINE, I. D. and KIRSTEINS, L. (1970): Growth hormone dynamics in acromegaly. *J. clin. Endocr., 31*, 239.

(10) SHERMAN, L. and KOLODNY, H. D. (1971): The hypothalamus, brain-catecholamines, and drug therapy for gigantism and acromegaly. *Lancet, 1*, 682.

(11) KRIEGER, D. T. (1973): Lack of responsiveness to L-dopa in Cushing's disease. *J. clin. Endocr.*, in press.

(12) MEITES, J. (Ed.) (1970): *Hypophysiotropic Hormones of the Hypothalamus: Assay and Chemistry*. Williams and Wilkins Co., Baltimore, Md.

(13) MARTINI, L., MOTTA, M. and FRASCHINI, F. (Eds) (1970): *The Hypothalamus*. Academic Press, New York-London.

(14) MARTINI, L. and GANONG, W. (Eds) (1971): *Frontiers in Neuroendocrinology 1971*. Oxford University Press, New York-London-Toronto.

(15) KNIGGE, K. M., SCOTT, D. E. and WEINDL, A. (Eds) (1972): *Brain-Endocrine Interaction – Median Eminence Structure and Function*. S. Karger, Basle.

(16) KRIEGER, D. T. and GLICK, S. M. (1972): Growth hormone and cortisol responsiveness in Cushing's syndrome. Relation to a possible central nervous system etiology. *Amer. J. Med., 52*, 25.

(17) LAWRENCE, A. M., HAGEN, T. C. and KIRSTEINS, L. (1971): Regulation of growth hormone secretion in normals and in acromegaly. In: *Abstracts, II International Symposium on Growth Hormone, Milan 1971*. Excerpta Medica, Amsterdam.

(18) LIPMAN, R., TAYLOR, A., SCHENK, A. and MINTZ, D. H. (1972): Acromegaly: a disorder of growth hormone feedback. *Clin. Res., 20*, 432.

(19) HAGEN, T. C., LAWRENCE, A. M. and KIRSTEINS, L. (1971): In vitro release of monkey pituitary growth hormone by acromegalic plasma. *J. clin. Endocr., 33*, 448.

(20) LAWRENCE, A. M., GORDON, D. L., HAGEN, T. A. and SCHWARTZ, M. A. (1973): Hypothalamic hypopituitarism following 'pituitary apoplexy' in acromegaly. Unpublished data.

(21) TAYLOR, A. L., FINSTER, J. L., RASKIN, P., FIELD, J. B. and MINTZ, D. (1968): Pituitary apoplexy in acromegaly. *J. clin. Endocr., 28*, 1748.

(22) RIGOLOSI, R. S., SCHWARTZ, E. and GLICK, S. M. (1968): Occurrence of growth hormone deficiency in acromegaly as a result of pituitary apoplexy. *New Engl. J. Med., 279*, 362.

(23) SAKUMA, M. and KNOBIL, M. (1970): Inhibition of endogenous growth hormone secretion by exogenous growth hormone infusions in the rhesus monkey. *Endocrinology, 86,* 890.

(24) ABRAMS, R. L., GRUMBACH, M. M. and KAPLAN, S. L. (1971): The effect of administration of human growth hormone on the plasma growth hormone cortisol glucose, and free fatty acid response to insulin: evidence for growth hormone autoregulation in man. *J. clin. Invest., 50,* 940.

(25) HAGEN, T. C., LAWRENCE, A. M. and KIRSTEINS, L. (1972): Autoregulation of growth hormone secretion in normal man. *Metabolism, 21,* 603.

(26) FURTH, J., DENT, N. N., BURNETT, W. T. and GADSDEN, E. L. (1955): The mechanism of induction and the characteristics of pituitary tumors induced by thyroidectomy. *J. clin. Endocr., 15,* 81.

(27) MAYBERRY, W. E., GHARIB, H., BILSTAB, J. M. and SIZEMORE, G. W. (1971): Radioimmunoassay for human thyrotrophin. Clinical value in patients with normal and abnormal thyroid function. *Ann. intern. Med., 74,* 471.

(28) CAUGHEY, J. E. (1958): Hypogonadism and pituitary tumors. Report of case of dystrophia myotonica with hypogonadism in acromegaly. *N. Z. med. J., 57,* 482.

(29) KELLY, L. W., Jr (1963): Ovarian dwarfism with pituitary tumor. *J. clin. Endocr., 23,* 50.

(30) RUSSFIELD, A. B., FRIEDLER, G. and FRENKEL, J. K. (1963): Biological characteristics of two transplantable pituitary tumors of Syrian hamsters. *Cancer Res., 23,* 720.

(31) WILLERNSE, C. H. (1962): A patient suffering from Turner's syndrome and acromegaly. *Acta endocr. (Kbh.), 39,* 204.

(32) BASSØE, H. H., GADEHOLT, H., RONOLD, K. and STØA, K. F. (1965): Cushing's disease in a patient with gonadal dysgenesis and pituitary tumor. *Acta endocr. (Kbh.), 48,* 72.

(33) ROTHENBUCHNER, G., VANHAELST, L., BIRK, J., GOLDSTEIN, J., VOIGT, H. K., FEHM, H. L., LOOS, U., WINKLER, G., SCHLEYER, M., RAPTIS, S. and PFEIFFER, E. F. (1971): Blood levels of TSH, HGH, cortisol, and ACTH after synthetic thyrotropin releasing factor. *Horm. Metab. Res., 31,* 139.

(34) IRIE, M. and TSUSHIMA, T. (1972): Increase of serum growth hormone concentration following thyrotropin-releasing hormone injection in patients with acromegaly or gigantism. *J. clin. Endocr., 35,* 97.

(35) HURXTHAL, L. M., HARE, H. R., HORRAX, C. and POPPEU, J. L. (1949): The treatment of acromegaly. *J. clin. Endocr., 9,* 126.

(36) SCHWARTZ, E., ECHEMENDIA, E., SCHIFFER, M. and PANARIELLO, V. A. (1969): Mechanism of estrogenic action in acromegaly. *J. clin. Invest., 48,* 260.

(37) JACOBS, L. S., SNYDER, P. J., WILBER, J. T., UNGER, R. D. and DAUGHADAY, W. H. (1971): TRH stimulation of prolactin secretion in man. *J. clin. Endocr., 33,* 996.

(38) BRAZEAU, P., VALE, W., BURGUS, R., LING, N., BUTCHER, M., RIVIER, J. and GUILLEMIN, R. (1973): Hypothalamic polypeptide that inhibits the secretion of immunoreactive pituitary growth hormone. *Science, 179,* 77.

(39) MITNICK, M. and REICHLIN, S. (1972): Enzymatic synthesis of thyrotropin-releasing hormone (TRH) by hypothalamic 'TRH synthetase'. *Endocrinology, 91,* 1145.

(40) ITO, H., MOMOSE, G., KATAYAMA, T., TAKAGISHI, H., ITO, L., NAKAJIMA, H. and TAKEI, Y. (1971): Effect of prostaglandin on the secretion of human growth hormone. *J. clin. Endocr., 32,* 857.

(41) NICOLESCU-CATARGI, A., CRISTOVEANU, A., STAN, M. and BERCEANU, A. (1970): The re-establishment of the dexamethasone depressive effects in Cushing's disease by a monoamine oxidase inhibitor. In: *Abstracts, III International Congress on Hormonal Steroids, Hamburg 1970.* Excerpta Medica, Amsterdam.

(42) MALARKEY, W. B., JACOBS, L. S. and DAUGHADAY, W. H. (1971): Levodopa suppression of prolactin in nonpuerperal galactorrhea. *New Engl. J. Med., 285,* 1160.

(43) TURKINGTON, R. W. (1972): Inhibition of prolactin secretion and successful therapy of the Forbes-Albright syndrome with L-dopa. *J. clin. Endocr., 34,* 306.

(44) FRIESEN, H., GUYDA, H., HWANG, P., TYSON, J. and BARBEAU, A. (1972): Functional evaluation in prolactin secretion: A guide to therapy. *J. clin. Invest., 51,* 706.

(45) LUTTERBECK, P. M., PRYOR, J. S., VARGA, L. and WENNER, R. (1971): Treatment of non-puerperal galactorrhea with an ergot alkaloid. *Brit. med. J., 3,* 228.

(46) VARGA, L., LUTTERBECK, P. M., PRYOR, J. S., WENNER, R. and ERB, H. (1972): Suppression of puerperal lactation with an ergot alkaloid: A double-blind study. *Brit. med. J., 2,* 743.

(47) DEL POZO, E., BRUN DEL RE, R., VARGA, L. and FRIESEN, H. (1972): The inhibition of prolactin secretion in man by CB-154 (2-Br-α-ergocryptine). *J. clin. Endocr.*, *35*, 768.

(48) LAWRENCE, A. M. and HAGEN, T. C. (1972): Ergonovine therapy for nonpuerperal galactorrhea. *New Engl. J. Med.*, *287*, 150.

(49) GAMBRELL Jr, R. D., GREENBLATT, R. B. and MAHESH, V. B. (1971): Postpill and pill-related amenorrhea-galactorrhea. *Amer. J. Obstet. Gynec.*, *110*, 838.

(50) LAWRENCE, A. M. and KIRSTEINS, L. (1970): Progestins in the medical management of active acromegaly. *J. clin. Endocr.*, *30*, 646.

(51) MALARKEY, W. B. and DAUGHADAY, W. H. (1971): Differential response of human acromegaly to medroxyprogesterone acetate. *J. clin. Endocr.*, *33*, 424.

(52) KOLODNY, H. D., SHERMAN, L., SINGH, A., KIM, S. and BENJAMIN, F. (1971): Acromegaly treated with chlorpromazine. *New Engl. J. Med.*, *284*, 819.

(53) JACKSON, I. M. D. and ORMSTON, B. J. (1972): Lack of beneficial response of serum GH in acromegalic patients treated with medroxyprogesterone acetate (MPA). *J. clin.Endocr.*, *35*, 413.

(54) RAKE, J. S., HAFI, S. A., LESSOF, M. H. and SNODGRASS, G. J. A. I. (1972): A trial of medroxyprogesterone acetate in acromegaly. *Clin. Endocr.*, *1*, 181.

(55) GANONG, W. F. (1970): Control of adrenocorticotropin and melanocyte stimulating hormone secretion. In: *The Hypothalamus*, pp. 313–333. Editors: L. Martini, M. Motta and F. Fraschini. Academic Press, New York, N.Y.

(56) GANONG, W. F. (1972): Evidence for a central noradrenergic system that inhibits ACTH secretion in brain. In: *Endocrine Interaction*, pp. 254–266. Editors: K. M. Knigge, D. E. Scott and A. Weindl. S. Karger, Basle.

(57) VAN LOON, G. R., HILGER, L., KING, A. B., BORYCZKA, A. T. and GANONG, W. F. (1971): Inhibitory effect of L-dihydroxyphenylalanine on the adrenal venous 17-hydroxycorticosteroid response to surgical stress in dogs. *Endocrinology*, *88*, 1404.

(58) TURKINGTON, R. W. (1972): Prolactin secretion in patients treated with various drugs. *Arch. intern. Med.*, *130*, 349.

(59) YOUNG, R. L., BRADLEY, E. M., GOLDZIEHER, J. W., MYERS, P. W. and LE COCQ, F. R. (1967): Spectrum of nonpuerperal galactorrhea: report of two cases evolving through the various syndromes. *J. clin. Endocr.*, *27*, 461.

(60) BIRGE, C. A., JACOBS, L., HAMMER, C. and DAUGHADAY, W. H. (1970): Catecholamine inhibition of prolactin secretion by isolated rat adenohypophysis. *Endocrinology*, *86*, 120.

(61) NICOLL, C. S. (1971): Aspects of the neural control of prolactin secretion. In: *Frontiers in Neuroendocrinology*, pp. 291–330. Editors: L. Martini and W. Ganong. Oxford University Press, New York–London–Toronto.

(62) MEITES, J. (1970): Direct studies of the secretion of the hypothalamic hypophysiotropic hormones (HHH). In: *Hypophysiotropic Hormones of the Hypothalamus: Assay and Chemistry*, pp. 261–278. Editor: J. Meites. Williams and Wilkins, Baltimore, Md.

(63) ANTON-TAY, F., ANTON, S. M. and WURTMAN, R. J. (1970): Mechanism of changes in brain norepinephrine metabolism after ovariectomy. *Neuroendocrinology (Basel)*, *6*, 265.

(64) BEATTIE, C. W., RODGERS, C. H. and SOYKA, L. F. (1972): Influence of ovariectomy and ovarian steroids on hypothalamic tyrosine hydroxylase activity in the rat. *Endocrinology*, *91*, 276.

(65) FRANCHIMONT, P. and LEGROS, J. J. (1970): The control of gonadotropin secretion in the human. In: *The Hypothalamus*, pp. 351–364. Editors: L. Martini, M. Motta and F. Fraschini. Academic Press, New York, N.Y.

(66) FRIEDMAN, S. and GOLDFIEN, A. (1969): Amenorrhea and galactorrhea following oral contraceptive therapy. *J. Amer. med. Ass.*, *210*, 1888.

(67) HÖKFELT, T. and FUXE, K. (1972): On the morphology and the neuroendocrine role of the hypothalamic catecholamine neurons. In: *Brain-Endocrine Interaction, Median Eminence: Structure and Function*, pp. 181–223. Editors: K. M. Knigge, D. E. Scott and A. Weindl. S. Karger, Basle.

(68) BLACKARD, W. G. and HEIDINGSFELDER, S. A. (1968): Adrenergic receptor control mechanism for growth hormone secretion. *J. clin. Invest.*, *47*, 1407.

(69) BOYD, A. E., LEBOVITZ, H. E. and PFEIFFER, J. B. (1970): Stimulation of human growth hormone secretion by L-dopa. *New Engl. J. Med.*, *283*, 1425.

(70) MACLEOD, R. M., FONTHAM, E. H. and LEHMEYER, J. E. (1970): Prolactin and growth hormone

production as influenced by catecholamines and agents that affect brain catecholamines. *Neuroendocrinology (Basel)*, *6*, 283.

(71) MARTIN, J. B. (1972): Plasma growth hormone (GH) response to hypothalamic or extra-hypothalamic electrical stimulation. *Endocrinology*, *91*, 107.

(72) DIMOND, R. C., BRAMMER, S., HOWARD, W. J., ATKINSON, R. L. and EARLL, J. M. (1972): Chlorpromazine treatment of acromegaly. *Clin. Res.*, *20*, 424.

(73) KANSAL, P. C., BUSE, J., TALBERT, O. R. and BUSE, M. (1972): The effect of L-dopa on plasma growth hormone, insulin, and thyroxine. *J. clin. Endocr.*, *34*, 99.

(74) LIUZZI, A., CHIODINI, P. G., BOTALLA, L., CREAMASCOLI, G. and SILVESTRINI, F. (1972): Inhibitory effect of L-dopa on GH release in acromegalic patients. *J. clin. Endocr.*, *35*, 941.

(75) SIMON, S., SCHIFFER, M., GLICK, S. M. and SCHWARTZ, E. (1967): Effect of medroxyprogester-one acetate (MPA) upon stimulated release of growth hormone in men. *J. clin. Endocr.*, *27*, 1633.

(76) GERSHBERG, H., ZORRILLA, E., HERNANDEZ, A. and HULSE, M. (1969): Effects of medroxy-progesterone acetate on serum insulin and growth hormone levels in diabetics and potential diabetics. *Obstet. Gynec. (N.Y.)*, *33*, 383.

(77) BHATIA, S. K., MOORE, D. and KALKHOFF, R. K. (1972): Progesterone suppression of the plasma growth hormone response. *J. clin. Endocr.*, *35*, 364.

(78) LUCKE, C. and GLICK, S. M. (1971): Effect of medroxyprogesterone acetate on the sleep induced peak of growth hormone secretion. *J. clin. Endocr.*, *33*, 851.

Discussion

DR. ROSS: Dr. Gorden is going to present a summary of the experience he and Dr. Roth have gained with the use of high dose estrogen therapy for acromegaly.

DR. GORDEN: Some clinical features of acromegaly can be ameliorated by the administration of large doses of estrogen. The effect of estrogen appears to be exerted at the site of action of growth hormone (GH) or on the hormone molecule itself since no consistent alteration in the concentration of circulating growth hormone has been observed with estrogen administration.

While subjective improvement in symptoms such as headache, acral pain, or paresthesias has been seen in some patients, there are no systematic double blind studies to evaluate these effects. Objective changes have been clearly demonstrated, however; these include a decrease in urinary calcium excretion, reduction in bone accretion rates, decrease in serum phosphorous[1] and amelioration of glucose intolerance[2, 3] (Figs. 1 and 2).

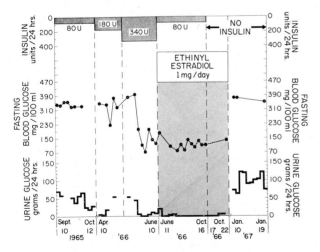

Fig. 1a   Effect of oral estrogen on insulin requirements, and on blood and urine glucose in a 53-year-old female patient with acromegaly.

The effect of estrogen on glucose tolerance represents the most dramatic clinical application of this agent to the treatment of acromegaly. Estrogen therapy may be useful in selected female patients awaiting reduction in GH from the primary therapy, e.g. irradiation, or when large doses of insulin are required and difficult to administer, or when the major modes of therapy have failed to reduce the GH concentration.

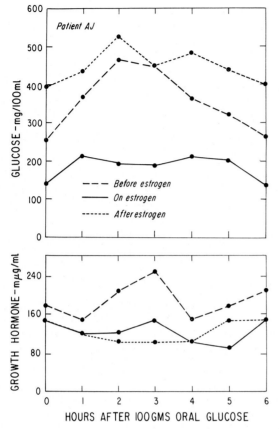

Fig. 1b Blood glucose and plasma growth hormone during 100 g oral glucose tolerance test in the patient shown in Fig. 1a.

Severe fasting hyperglycemia and glycosuria may be ameliorated with 1 mg of ethinyl estradiol per day. This amount of estrogen may completely obviate the need for very large doses of insulin (Figs. 1a, b). The improvement in glucose tolerance is associated with a reduction towards normal of the insulin concentrations but with no consistent change in the plasma GH (Fig. 2) (Fig. 1b). These changes in acromegalic subjects whose glucose intolerance is secondary to elevated plasma GH are in contrast to normal subjects who may increase their plasma GH and independently become glucose intolerant with the administration of estrogen.

Three female patients have been treated for several months to several years with 1 mg of ethinyl estradiol per day. We have uniformly noted improvement in glucose tolerance in those patients with glucose intolerance, decrease in serum phosphorus, improvement in acral pain and paresthesias, and possible decrease in sebaceous hyperactivity. Large doses of estrogen are required to produce the desired therapeutic effects and to prevent break-through bleeding. When large doses are used, it is difficult to cycle the patient and generally continuous therapy must be given; progesterone may be given simultaneously to prevent endometrial hyperplasia. Initially all of our patients have experienced nausea and breast enlargement which usually subsides as therapy continues. All estrogen treated patients have a decrease in the concentration of serum albumin which was correlated with a gain in body

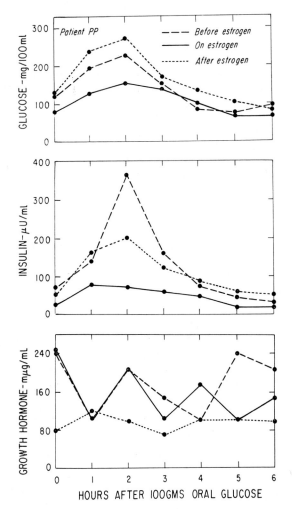

Fig. 2   Blood glucose, plasma insulin, and plasma growth hormone during 100 g oral glucose tolerance test in a 33-year-old acromegalic female.

weight, presumably due to an increase in extracellular fluid volume. There may be a slight
increase in blood pressure but none of the patients reported had other untoward effects such
as vascular thrombosis or neoplasia.

Although estrogen should not be considered a primary form of therapy in acromegaly,
it may be used in selected cases to treat specific manifestations of the disease.

References

(1) SCHWARTZ, E., ECHEMENDIA, E., SCHIFFER, M. and PANARIELLO, N. A. (1969): Mechanism of
     estrogenic action in acromegaly. *J. clin. Invest.*, *48*, 260.
(2) McCULLOGH, E. P., BECK, J. C. and SCHAFFENBURG, C. A. (1955): Control of diabetes and
     other features of acromegaly following treatment with estrogens. *Diabetes*, *4*, 13.
(3) MINTZ, D. H., FINSTER, J. L. and JOSIMOVICH, J. B. (1968): Effect of estrogen therapy on car-
     bohydrate metabolism in acromegaly. *J. clin. Endocr.*, *27*, 1321.

Continuation of discussion

DR. NOEL: Dr. Hardy mentioned that he had operated on 20 patients with galactorrhea and amenorrhea, most of whom had microadenomata. A rather surprising feature of those patients was the very large percentage in whom galactorrhea and amenorrhea seemed to be associated with the use of oral contraceptives, which raises the question of whether there might be an etiologic relationship between oral contraceptives and prolactin-producing microadenomata.

It has been our experience that most patients with galactorrhea who do not have sellar enlargement, visual impairment, or other evidence of a pituitary tumor have such mild symptoms that we have hesitated to recommend either surgery or radiotherapy. Indeed, we have rarely been able to get these patients to take suppressive agents such as L-DOPA for more than a few weeks: in most the degree of galactorrhea and the amenorrhea were simply not enough of a problem to make them willing to put up with taking pills several times a day.

Since there have been recent reports of ergot preparations restoring menses and stopping galactorrhea both in patients with pituitary tumors and in those with apparent 'functional' galactorrhea, I wonder if Drs. Hardy and Friesen treated any of their galactorrhea patients before performing surgery. Perhaps a fairly long-acting preparation like CB-154 (2-Br-alpha-ergocryptine) might restore menses and terminate galactorrhea making surgery unnecessary.

DR. FRIESEN: We have not investigated most patients before surgery, but we have examined prolactin values after surgery. In one patient with a prolactin concentration pre-operatively between 5000–7000 ng/ml, post-operatively, values were 2000 ng/ml.

After one week of CB-154 therapy prolactin values declined to 50 ng/ml. I think the ergot drug is better tolerated than L-DOPA and, more importantly, the duration of action of CB-154 is much longer than that of L-DOPA.

DR. LAWRENCE: One other factor in the prolactin story that I neglected to comment on is experience with clomiphene. In patients with amenorrhea and galactorrhea associated with birth control pills, there has been success with clomiphene.

Whether the effect of clomiphene is due to alteration of the adrenergic tonus in the hypothalamus thereby causing increased secretion of PIF I do not know, but it is effective. Galactorrhea ceases and periods return.

DR. DAUGHADAY: Our experience with the use of L-DOPA in the treatment of the hyperprolactinemia is very similar to Dr. Noel's. I think the major symptom in these patients was a wet bra occasionally and they do not like to be nauseated to have it corrected. The dynamics of the drug are such that escape of prolactin levels occur regularly, somewhere between 4 and 6 hours. To maintain a 24 hour suppression of prolactin requires frequent administration. Unfortunately, patients with tumors and high prolactin levels are frequently quite refractory to L-DOPA administration.

DR. KULIN: I should like to ask Dr. Lawrence whether there is direct evidence for the existence of a chromophobe adenoma in the adult patients with primary hypothyroidism and an enlarged sella?

DR. LAWRENCE: These are all patients in whom there is unequivocal enlargement of the sella and some deformity of the floor contour but no bulging above the diaphragma sella in pneumoencephalograms. Two had some air in the center of a large intrasellar mass.

These patients had perfectly normal pituitary function. All had high TSH levels which became normal after they became euthyroid. Growth hormone responsiveness was abnormal when patients were hypothyroid but became normal in the euthyroid state.

VIII. General discussion: case presentations of patients with problems in management

Case presentations

DR. ODELL: We have had the opportunity to hear summaries of the experiences of our various experts. We would now like to get opinions about specific management problems. The patients presented are hypothetical, but representative of those encountered by clinicians.

> The first patient is a 21-year-old woman who has secondary amenorrhea and galactorrhea. Careful questioning revealed that she took no medication, specifically no tranquilizers or oral contraceptives, and did not have headaches.
> Physical examination was entirely normal, except for the galactorrhea. There were no suggestions of acromegaly and no visual field defects. Fat globules were found on microscopic examination of the breast fluid.

There are two diagnostic areas of concern: (1) the endocrine assessment and (2) the X-ray evaluation. Dr. Daughaday, what further procedures would you like for the endocrine evaluation of this patient? She is asymtomatic except for minimal galactorrhea.

DR. DAUGHADAY: Actually, we have learned that this is a rather common situation, and as we get experience, we find more and more examples of this. The combination of amenorrhea and galactorrhea indicates a high probability that the patient will be found to have hyperprolactinemia. The endocrine diagnosis depends primarily on establishing which hormones are in excess, and whether it is a functional or a pathologic elevation. We should start with measurements of basal prolactin levels. If basal prolactin levels are elevated, we would follow-up with procedures designed to stimulate prolactin secretion such as chlorpromazine or TRH administration. These would be followed by pharmacologic agents such as L-dopa that suppress prolactin secretion.

We would consider the etiology to be functional in those individuals who have modest elevations of prolactin and who respond appropriately to pharmacologic testing.

The etiology is more likely to be a pituitary tumor in patients whose prolactin levels are chronically elevated to greater than 50 ng/ml and who are relatively refractory to pharmacologic maneuvers.

DR. ODELL: Supposing there was an abnormality in growth hormone control systems, as tested by insulin or arginine, or both, and the rest of the pituitary function studies were normal, what would you do with that information?

DR. DAUGHADAY: Growth hormone responses to testing are usually normal in patients such as this. However, the presence of a hormonal deficit does not alter your fundamental approach to therapy in hypersecreting pituitary adenomas.

DR. ODELL: Dr. Daughaday has suggested a thorough endocrine evaluation be performed with emphasis on prolactin concentrations and control systems. What else would you like if anything in the endocrine diagnostic evaluation of this patient?

DR. A. LAWRENCE: A patient with secondary amenorrhea, galactorrhea and no evidence of primary hypothyroidism deserves an evaluation of pituitary function. I suppose we differ about what should be included. Measurements of LH and FSH are fairly routine and would establish some understanding of why the patient had secondary amenorrhea. In addition to the endocrine evaluation there is no question that a tomographic X-ray of the sella would be appropriate in such a patient.

DR. ODELL: Commonly serum LH and FSH concentrations are perfectly normal in these patients. They just do not show the fluctuations with midcycle LH-FSH surge and so forth as they would in the normal menstruating woman. Thus, frequently the absolute concentrations, even obtained several days in a row, do not add to further endocrine assessment, except to indicate that primary ovarian failure is not the cause of amenorrhea.

The second area that you would investigate would be the assessment of sella volume or sella outline by tomographs or whatever X-ray procedures seemed appropriate. In addition to the AP and lateral skull films and tomograms of the sella, would further neuroradiographic studies be indicated?

DR. A. LAWRENCE: There is one entity we have not covered when considering galactorrheic syndromes. That is the association of galactorrhea with primary hypothyroidism.

DR. RANDALL: In some patients, even though the plain films of the skull have been normal, we have gone ahead and done pneumoencephalograms and have picked up instances of suprasellar extensions of the tumor not yet big enough to cause a visual field defect. So I think that the question of pneumoencephalography with tomography ought to be considered.

DR. ZERVAS: Dr. Randall, are you influenced by the fact that your patients generally come from a distance and you really have to arrive at a diagnosis on the initial visit? If they were close by would you still recommend pneumoencephalography for patients with normal sella films?

DR. RANDALL: We are indeed influenced by the fact that our patients do not always live next door to us and we have to come to some decision within a short period of time. We have followed people from nearby, and have not done the pneumoencephalograms initially.

DR. ODELL: Dr. Randall, if the sella were enlarged would you routinely do an arteriogram since you cannot rule out an aneurysm by the pneumoencephalogram?

DR. RANDALL: In general, if the sella is enlarged we will do an arteriogram, because usually we are going to institute some type of treatment.

DR. ODELL: To proceed with the evaluation of this patient, further studies indicated that visual fields were entirely normal. This patient had a normal sella except for an asymmetrical floor. No suprasellar extension was observed on the pneumoencephalogram, and an arteriogram was normal. The growth hormone responses were normal to provocative tests. Prolactin concentrations were 250 ng/ml (normal <30 ng/ml).

Now Dr. Hardy, how would you treat this patient?

DR. HARDY: First, I would look at the films of the sella, to localize the asymmetry of the floor to one side if possible.

DR. ODELL: The asymmetry was on one side.

DR. HARDY: It is alway lateralized because prolactin tumors are always in the lateral wing of the gland. It is obvious that there is no suprasellar extension. I would suggest a microsurgical exploration of the sella transsphenoidally and selective removal of the lesion, because I think the major problem in this patient is not galactorrhea, but infertility. She will want to have children, and we can decompress her normal pituitary gland so that she can resume normal menstruation shortly and probably be able to conceive.

DR. ODELL: Dr. Sheline, how would you treat this patient?

DR. SHELINE: I have had very little experience with treating lesions so identified. I suspect that we have treated similar lesions but have included them with the general category of chromophobes. May I ask a question?

We have been talking a great deal about slightly asymmetrical sella floors. Would anyone care to comment on how frequently the floor of the sella in the normal individual is a little asymmetrical?

DR. KAUFMAN: The sella floor is not infrequently asymmetrical. I cannot give you the exact figures, but a very rough estimate would be 10 to 15 %. The harder one looks, the more asymmetrical floors one will find. They should be distinguished from local erosive changes when there is a local, small mass present. This distinction can be accomplished on some radiographs, depending on the X-ray projections and the quality of the films.

DR. BAKER: My impression is that asymmetries in the floor of the sella occur in 25 to 30 % of normal people.

DR. ODELL: Dr. Hardy, based on the data available and these statements that many normal people have sellar asymmetries, do you think people with asymmetrical sellas have micro-adenomata that are producing no symptomatology?

DR. HARDY: I think so, yes, but the patient under discussion had symptomatology.

DR. LEVIN: Dr. Hardy, if you did not have that prolactin level available, would you still have suggested microdissection?

DR. HARDY: Sure. The major problem is not galactorrhea but amenorrhea, and you have to decompress the normal gland. She has some lesion there that prevents gonadotropin secretion.

DR. ODELL: Dr. Hardy, would you still operate on that patient if the sella were perfectly normal and no asymmetry was found?

DR. HARDY: If I read it as normal myself, although she might certainly have a lesion, I would wait another six months.

DR. ODELL: Dr. Fraser, with the information we have given how would you treat this patient?

DR. FRASER: In the first place, we would agree that the evidence suggests a small prolactin producing tumor. Regarding the question of asymmetry of the sella floor, it is true that some asymmetry is seen in normals. However, an obviously abnormal asymmetry is recognizable here. As the asymmetry was abnormal, we would first define the diaphragma by PEG. We would put 2 yttrium implants giving 20,000 rads to the periphery of the gland, a dose which hardly ever interferes with normal function. Such patients have subsequently lost their galactorrhea and have been able to have children. That would be our normal approach, but from what we have heard here, I think we might contemplate putting the yttrium only on the abnormal side to assure even better the preservation of normal function.

DR. KJELLBERG: Do you think it is reasonable to distinguish a so-called normal asymmetry from pathologic asymmetry? Is this a reasonable distinction to make?

DR. BAKER: This is very difficult. I think that if you have an asymmetry with a high hormonal level, it is very easy to say, with one eye on the chemical studies and one eye on the X-ray, that this is an abnormal asymmetry. But if you are looking at X-rays without the endocrinologic data, then it becomes very difficult to say whether asymmetry is abnormal or not.

I would ask you about the arteriograms being normal. Was there a magnification arteriogram? There are many arteriograms in the past that we have thought normal, but going back over them now with our experience with magnification, we see that we were overlooking many things such as small arteries that opacify tumors in the pituitary. We now see hypertrophy of the perisellar arteries and things of that sort which we did not see 5 years ago.

DR. HARDY: I would like to comment on the use of angiograms. If the sella is not enlarged and there is just a slight asymmetry typical of a microadenoma, not just a sloping floor but a little convexity, I would not do the magnification angiograms because it is not necessary in such cases since it is obvious that this is not an expanding lesion.

DR. RAND: The cavernous sinus venograms will show asymmetry in a case such as we are discussing better than angiograms. At least our experience has led us to that conclusion. I would recommend a cavernous sinus venogram.

DR. HARDY: Because the lesion is less than 10 mm in diameter, the venography will be normal.

DR. DI CHIRO: I think that we have to clarify some of the disagreements and discrepancies which have occurred in this discussion. Dr. Hardy commented on the localized indentations in the sellar floor, as for instance 'a niche' excavated by a microadenoma. I do not believe, on the other hand, that Dr. Hardy was referring to the slightly slanted sellar floor seen in the frontal projections and often reported by radiologists as evidence of asymmetrical sella.

I would agree with Dr. Rand, that at this stage, at least, the most sensitive type of procedure to establish a lateral extension of a pituitary tumor is the cavernous sinus angiography. Lately, however, I have been impressed by Dr. Baker's work regarding the frequency of small vessel changes and angiographic blushes in pituitary adenomas.

DR. RANDALL: We have treated some of these patients successfully with external irradiation. One patient subsequently became pregnant. Does anyone else have experience with conventional irradiation?

DR. ODELL: From time to time we have seen such a response. In past years, many of us, given this patient with a normal arteriogram, normal pneumoencephalogram and slight asymmetry of the sella floor, would have followed her carefully without treatment.

DR. KJELLBERG: I would treat the patient with protons on the basis that the prolactin elevation indicates a tumor.

DR. ANNE LAWRENCE: I would suggest clomiphene or even an ergot preparation as a first therapy. If the patient's clinical syndrome reversed itself, I would feel that intrusive maneuvers to the pituitary were unwarranted.

DR. NOEL: I would also like to make a second suggestion. Although the discussion of therapeutic approaches to this patient has emphasized the probability that she has a pituitary tumor, there are other major etiologies which have not been ruled out and which would require an altogether different course. First, she could have a high prolactin because of a hypothalamic or functional disorder; secondly, she could have some form of interruption of the stalk connections between the hypothalamus and the anterior pituitary. The suggestions made by Dr. Friesen and his collaborators in their article in the *Journal of Clinical Investigation* (1972, *51*, 706–709), should be given greater emphasis in choosing patients most likely to benefit from surgery. For most patients galactorrhea with or without amenorrhea is a mild disorder and, in the absence of a clear-cut pituitary adenoma, a full endocrinologic evaluation and perhaps a period of observation are warranted before surgery or radiotherapy are considered.

DR. ODELL: The second patient has the same history as the first patient but different results were found with the diagnostic procedures. The skull films revealed symmetrical enlargement of the sella with a volume that was 2,000 cu. mm. The pneumoencephalogram showed no extrasellar extension. Visual fields and acuity were within normal limits and serum prolactin was not available to the doctors taking care of this patient. Growth hormone response to arginine and insulin were abnormal. Metyrapone, TRH and clomiphene stimulations were within normal limits. Would this change anybody's treatment?

DR. ANNE LAWRENCE: I think that with unequivocal evidence of abnormal sella enlargement one has to consider arteriograms as well as pneumoencephalograms before proceeding with definitive therapy to the pituitary gland.

My personal prejudice is for conventional radiotherapy. There are many patients with this syndrome who show no further growth of the tumor, cessation of lactation and resumption of normal menstrual periods.

With a gland this large, further growth of tumor needs to be halted by some definitive form of treatment.

DR. PEARSON: Up until very recently, I think we would approach the patient conservatively. We would like to have seen the Kaufman maneuver (*This volume* p, 100) to make sure this wasn't an empty sella. If the diaphragma sella or the airsoft tissue interface on pneumoencephalography is convex upwards, then the findings are certainly in favor of a tumor.

At present, I think we would favor microsurgical excision of the prolactin producing tumor.

DR. KJELLBERG: With definite enlargement of the sella beyond reasonable limits, we would treat with our lower-dose adenoma treatment, because it is without risk and it is simple and easy, and it works.

DR. ODELL: Would anyone recommend not treating this patient now, and follow her carefully? Since all of you are shaking your heads, it appears that everyone would treat this patient after completing the neuroradiologic studies.

Now, this patient was treated with four-port supravoltage X-ray with an estimated tumor dose of 5,000 rads. She was followed for 5 years with X-rays taken every 6 months. Slow, steadily progressive increase in sella size was observed until it was clearly increased to 3,300 cu. mm. She had now bitemporal hemianopsia. Now, how would you treat the patient, Dr. Fager?

DR. FAGER: Traditionally, this patient would be a candidate for a transfrontal excision of the tumor. The chances are that we would follow that excision, depending on what we found at surgery and how much we were able to accomplish, with a second course of supervoltage irradiation, perhaps another 2,000 roentgens. This is the treatment we would have instituted. But I think as neurosurgeons gain more skill with the transsphenoidal operation, that would be preferable as the prime treatment.

DR. KJELLBERG: In the presence of the visual field loss, we would use transsphenoidal hypophysectomy.

DR. ODELL: Two votes for transsphenoidal. Dr. Baker?

DR. BAKER: I must again rise to defend diagnostic radiology. At least, we should do a pneumoencephalogram on this patient before these procedures are undertaken, I think, and the possibility of doing an angiogram should be considered.

DR. ODELL: Were you taking it for granted that both of those procedures would be done before surgery? I think most were.

DR. FAGER: We understood that.

DR. ZERVAS: We have encountered a number of cystic tumors that still have not caused any visual field defect. I would think that at the very least a transsphenoidal biopsy would have been in order prior to radiation.

DR. RAND: I would like to underscore Dr. Zervas' comments about stereotaxic biopsies prior to giving radiation. We have advocated this for a number of years because you may be irradiating a cystic lesion or other disease not responsive to radiation.

If the suprasellar extension was not enormous, I would also agree, a transnasal, transsphenoidal approach, using microsurgical techniques, would be appropriate.

If it was very large, I would use a transcranial operation combined with the transsphenoidal approach through the planum sphenoidale.

DR. KJELLBERG: I favor open microsurgical methods over stereotaxic methods by the transsphenoidal route.

DR. ODELL: Dr. Guiot, would you like to comment on how you would treat the patient at this stage?

DR. GUIOT: By the transsphenoidal approach. The fact that she has been amenorrheic for more than 5 years makes it unlikely that she will become pregnant.

DR. DAUGHADAY: I should comment that endocrinologists aren't entirely impotent in restoring fertility by replacement gonadotropin therapy.

DR. SHELINE: Why in the face of obvious radiation therapy failure was the patient watched for 5 years without further treatment?

DR. ODELL: This is a hypothetical case. Let us say that there was variation in the volume of the sella as interpreted by the radiologist over these years, and it was not absolutely certain that her tumor was increasing until this period had gone by. It was clear she had not resumed normal menses, however, and her galactorrhea had continued.

DR. HARDY: I have a little doubt about the differential diagnosis in this patient. Despite intensive radiotherapy, the sella progressively increased in size. It is most important to make an exploration, to rule out another kind of lesion. In the 20 cases I report here, there were incidental findings in 2 patients: one had a small craniopharyngioma and another one had a Rathke pouch cyst. This might explain why the tumor didn't shrink with radiotherapy.

DR. ODELL: Those were not delineated by other diagnostic procedures.

DR. HARDY: No, they are too small.

DR. ODELL: Now, we have further information about this patient. Hypophysectomy was performed by the transfrontal approach and the patient developed further visual field loss after surgery. The prolactin level remained markedly elevated.

We call in our experts for their treatment recommendations now. Let me just ask, who would take her as a patient at this stage and what would you do?

DR. FAGER: This is one of the tragic things that is not generally appreciated. When you operate on patients from above, you occasionally – and I underline the word 'occasionally' – do produce damage to the optic system. Obviously, the tumor was not completely removed and the patient suffered loss of vision.

DR. ODELL: Dr. Hardy, would you accept this patient and how would you treat her?

DR. HARDY: If this is a patient who has had radiotherapy, I am afraid the result will not be satisfactory. Nevertheless, I think we should explore the sella. We will find scar tissue, fibrotic reaction, all sorts of mixed tissue that will be very hard to differentiate from normal tissue.

Unfortunately, we will probably be obliged to make a radical excision of all the intrasellar content. It is too late for this patient to be improved from the endocrinological point of view.

DR. ODELL: Dr. Rand, would you accept this patient at this stage and what would you do?

DR. RAND: For the past 10 years, we have used the surgical microscope through the transfrontal surgical approach to explore the pituitary and suprasellar area. Under these conditions, you can see the blood supply of the optic nerves and the hypothalamus. In our experience further visual deterioration has not occurred.

If you use the microscope with a transfrontal approach and combine this with the transsphenoidal approach to get under the optic chiasm, you are combining the best surgical exposures. You can see the top of the tumor, the bottom and the sides of the tumor and avoid trauma to the visual system.

At this point, I might consider a transsphenoidal operation if I thought I could help the patient's visual loss.

DR. KJELLBERG: I think it should be mentioned that since the patient had a transfrontal craniotomy, the likelihood that there is residual suprasellar tumor is not very good. It seems to me that the choice of therapy depends on the definition of reasonable goals to be achieved by any procedure. I think a pneumoencephalogram would do a substantial amount to clarify the anatomic arrangement around the sella. If the pneumoencephalogram excluded suprasellar extension, this would indicate that there is not much you can do about the fields. The visual fields are gone, and further transfrontal surgery is probably contraindicated. The great amount of radiation the patient has had pretty well excludes further radiation therapy. The high prolactin levels indicate residual adenoma and the tumor has a high prospect for growth in view of its past history. The prospect of removing the tumor by transsphenoidal route remains the only reasonable objective of therapy.

DR. LEBOVITZ: This is a very illustrative case. This patient was a girl and had amenorrhea which drew attention to the problem. Now if the patient had been a young man 21 years of age, how would we diagnose this syndrome at an early stage to obtain the kind of results which Dr. Hardy described? Does this mean that every male who has a mild decrease in libido should have a prolactin level? And if so, will that be elevated and provide us the kind of data which we need to diagnose prolactin-secreting tumors in males? In the past we have usually measured gonadotropins and said that if they were normal, the decrease in libido must be psychogenic.

DR. DAUGHADAY: You are asking a question which is an important one from the endocrine point of view. I suspect that we are going to be called upon to do this.

An elevated prolactin doesn't necessarily mean a functioning pituitary tumor. Prolactin measurement is the 'sed rate' of the endocrinologists. There are a host of functional and organic disturbances of the hypothalamus and pituitary which elevate serum prolactin. However, serum prolactin elevation would be a very important finding in a patient with a suspicious sella turcica.

DR. NOEL: We have seen males with pituitary tumors with prolactins as high as 10,000 ng/ml without any manifestations of excess prolactin secretion, such as galactorrhea or gynecomastia.

DR. ODELL: The third patient can be dealt with very briefly. A 15-year-old girl who presented to her physician with growth retardation and classic history and physical findings of Cushing's syndrome. Laboratory data revealed the standard ACTH-dependent Cushing's disease. Urinary 17-hydroxysteroids suppressed with high dose dexamethasone, and the skull films were entirely normal.

Several forms of treatment are currently available including bilateral adrenalectomy, drugs, pituitary irradiation, and hypophysectomy. How would you treat her, Dr. Randall?

DR. RANDALL: Under our current system of treatment, we would do a total bilateral adrenalectomy on this patient. We are currently examining this approach in an attempt to decide whether it is the appropriate one. In view of what we have heard here, this may well not be the appropriate approach in the future.

DR. ODELL: Dr. Sheline, how would you treat this patient?

DR. SHELINE: I would irradiate the pituitary in much the same manner that has been reported from Vanderbilt in their earlier series, reserving adrenalectomy for irradiation failure.

DR. ODELL: Dr. Horwith, how would you treat this patient?

DR. HORWITH: The severity of the Cushing's syndrome, including the degree of cardiovascular and skeletal involvement and psychosis is terribly important. If we felt we had to move rapidly, we would certainly do bilateral adrenalectomy.

DR. ODELL: The psychiatric manifestations in this patient were nil. Her main manifestation was that her growth rate had slowed. The physical findings were subtle but definite. There was no rush in treatment. How would you treat that patient?

DR. KJELLBERG: I think this is an excellent case for protons. With the Bragg peak technique the remission rate is about 2.5 or 3 times higher than with conventional radiation and our improvement rate is in the same proportion. I would like not to render such a patient hypopituitary, which is a substantial risk even with microsurgical approaches at this stage of her illness.

DR. ODELL: Dr. Hardy?

DR. HARDY: There is no surgical risk in exploring the sella turcica transsphenoidally. This patient could certainly harbor a tiny intrapituitary basophilic adenoma located in the central mucoid wedge of the gland that might be selectively removed with preservation of the normal pituitary gland.

DR. KJELLBERG: I would like to comment. There is a fair amount of information on studies of the pituitary in Cushing's disease that for some reason has been largely ignored. Plotz and others in the early 1950's studied a large number of autopsy specimens from patients with Cushing's disease. As I recall, 80 % of the patients showed abnormalities of the pituitary of the nature of basophilism. Many showed discreet adenomas, but many others showed diffuse invasion of the anterior lobe by basophils, and would not, I fear, benefit from selective removal.

DR. A. LAWRENCE: The patient is 15 and we do not like to render the patient Addisonian for life. We are all concerned with the small incidence of hypopituitarism that occurs from almost any attack on the pituitary gland. Our habit is to individualize them and we do not have a single approach. In the main, in the very ill patient, we would treat with medical therapy until the patient was well enough to undergo bilateral adrenalectomy. We reserve radiotherapy to the pituitary until there is evidence of Nelson's syndrome having developed, but we keep changing our approach as new information appears.

DR. ORTH: I also think you have to individualize the treatment of these patients. We recently treated a patient similar to this with severe growth retardation. We believed the growth situation was important enough to warrant a bilateral adrenalectomy, followed by conventional pituitary irradiation. In a retrospective analysis of over two dozen cases receiving similar treatment, we have not seen the development of Nelson's syndrome. Prevention of Nelson's syndrome is desirable since the established syndrome is difficult to treat. This particular girl, like the four others in our series, has resumed or started normal menses, and has grown since these procedures were performed. As everyone else here, we have been impressed with the microsurgical techniques and now would consider that alternative form of therapy.

DR. KJELLBERG: The frequency of the development of Nelson's syndrome after bilateral adrenalectomy appears to be proportional to the duration of observation. Preoperatively the sellas are abnormal in about 5 % of patients; postoperatively in about 10 %.

If you follow the patients long enough that percentage does indeed rise. We understand that the long-term figure for sellar enlargement in a large series may be 30 %. That is a substantial risk in a patient with the prospect of a long-term survival. Therefore, it seems reasonable to prevent the development of Nelson's syndrome and avoid secondary treatment.

DR. ROTH: Since patients with hyperadrenocorticism have such a high risk of complications, I think it should be standard procedure for us to try to restore their steroid levels to normal for a reasonable time period before subjecting them to any surgical procedures. Aminoglutethimide, with or without metyrapone, would be the best choice. I think that the rationale is quite analogous to the standard procedure of administering thyroid blocking drugs to restore the euthyroid condition before any surgery is undertaken on patients with hyperthyroidism. In some patients one might consider drugs such as metyrapone, aminoglutethimide, or op'DDD as an alternative to surgery.

DR. BATZDORF: Dr. Hardy, have you ever had a negative exploration in instances in which you suspected a microadenoma to be present?

DR. HARDY: Our cases have all been verified histologically and several have also had electron microscopic studies.

DR. BATZDORF: The electron microscopic studies would not be available to you at the time of surgery. If you were operating on a patient and did not find an anatomically recognizable lesion peroperatively what would you do?

DR. HARDY: If I did not find it, I would close!

DR. CANARY: We continue to be plagued infrequently by patients with clear-cut features of Cushing's syndrome who respond to high dose and low dose decadron suppression and to metyrapone as if the disease were hyperplasia, but who have an adrenal adenoma. I am, therefore, unwilling to recommend immediate irradiation of the pituitary without definition of the presence or absence of an adenoma in the adrenal. Would you comment on the usefulness of ACTH measurements?

DR. ODELL: ACTH levels are difficult to use at the moment because they fluctuate so much. ACTH is secreted in a pulsatile fashion and serum levels vary widely from moment to moment. When a minimum of 4 or 5 ACTH determinations are made and correlated with serum cortisol levels, they may be useful.

Let me also emphasize that there are a number of tumors that produce either corticotropin or a corticotropin releasing factor and can be mistakenly identified as Cushing's disease.

DR. LINFOOT: We are now doing iodocholesterol scans to rule out an adrenal adenoma in patients with Cushing's syndrome. I would hope better adrenal scanning agents will soon be available.

DR. ODELL: The final patient is a 19-year-old female who presented to her physician with classic Turner's syndrome. Serum LH and FSH were both elevated and skull films revealed a symmetrically enlarged sella turcica with a volume of 2500 cu. mm.

DR. DAUGHADAY: This might be hyperplasia secondary to end organ deficiency. I would place the patient on replacement levels of estrogen for a period of three weeks to a month and see whether the markedly elevated gonadotropin levels fall. If you get a rapid decrease and the rest of the endocrine work-up is normal, I would be willing to follow the patient over a period of time to see whether there was any progressive change in pituitary size.

DR. ODELL: The patient was placed on estrogen plus progestogen, and the gonadotropins fell to low normal concentrations and remained there.

DR. DAUGHADAY: I would be quite satisfied with that and careful clinical follow-up.

DR. ODELL: And the diagnosis you would make would be pituitary hyperplasia secondary to end organ deficiency. Any other diagnostic procedures?

DR. RANDALL: Would you do a pneumoencephalogram before going on with this program?

DR. DAUGHADAY: Only if there were some abnormality other than enlargement of the sella turcica on X-ray.

DR. A. LAWRENCE: My only concern in this patient is that pituitary enlargement seen in Turner's syndrome has generally occurred in adults. Although it is intriguing to invoke end organ failure as a causative agent, I am not certain that that is the case. Because she is 19, I would do exactly what Dr. Daughaday proposed and follow her closely because she is a little young for the hyperplastic gland to have occurred.

DR. ODELL: For exactly the reasons outlined by Dr. Lawrence, she was treated with estrogen and progesterone. Later, a pneumoencephalogram revealed that she had empty sella.

DR. PEARSON: Could I just ask if anybody has ever heard of a pituitary tumor producing excess FSH or LH?

DR. ODELL: I have not seen or heard of any. Has anybody else?

DR. HORWITH: We have one under study now. Unfortunately, the tumor has not been biopsied. The patient was assumed to have a chromophobe adenoma and was treated with irradiation. The data came back after irradiation had been started. Plasma FSH and LH were both elevated. Our clinical impression was that this patient was hypogonadal. Plasma testosterone was low.

DR. LEVIN: There is a case reported of a patient with an enlarged sella who had high level total urinary gonadotropins (Gordon and Moses, *Ann. int. Med.*, 1965, *63*, 313). However, the patient did not have endocrine responses to exogenous ACTH, TSH, or HCG, so end organ failure must be considered.

DR. KLIMAN: A case of possible gonadotropin-secreting tumor or sella enlargement secondary to prolonged physiological gonadotropin stimulation in a hypogonadal man was reported by Bower (*Ann. int. Med.*, 1968, *69*, 107). The exact etiology was not documented.

DR. OMMAYA: I have an aphorism which leads to a question. The aphorism is that the retrospectroscope tends to magnify usually what we like to see, and the prospectoscope magnifies what we do not like to see. Isn't it time that we consider prospective studies? I think the point has been made by Dr. Hardy that selective surgery with the transsphenoidal technique really opens up an avenue for treating these patients well before radiological criteria become significant. I would suggest that we now consider selection of patients using endocrinological criteria – and then as the prospective study dictates, medical management versus surgical management, using the transsphenoidal technique.

Summary

PETER O. KOHLER and GRIFF T. ROSS
NICHD, Bethesda, Md.

As pointed out in the preface, the Organizing Committee had three basic objectives when planning this symposium:

1. To summarize the present status of the art and science of diagnosing and treating human pituitary tumors.

2. To critically evaluate the results obtained among patients treated by experts using each of the several methods and to compare these results.

3. To define areas requiring further investigation. At the close of this last session, it seems appropriate to evaluate the extent to which the objectives of the committee have been attained.

As far as diagnosis is concerned, it is clear from the discussions that currently the evaluation of a patient with a suspected pituitary tumor should include a combination of 1) ophthalmologic, 2) endocrine, and 3) radiographic studies. Proponents of all these diagnostic modalities generally agree that visual field deficits with or without loss of visual acuity in a previously untreated patient represent a clear indication for further diagnostic studies. If neuroradiologic and endocrine tests confirm the presence of a pituitary tumor, some form of treatment is indicated. The definitive radiographic test is frequently the pneumoencephalogram with laminograms. An upward convexity of the diaphragm or pathological irregularities of the sella floor may indicate a tumor even in patients without enlargement of the sella.

A common problem in diagnosis in many medical centers concerns indications for advanced radiographic studies such as pneumoencephalograms and arteriograms in patients with no abnormalities of vision. These studies carry at least a small risk to the patient and may at times produce substantial discomfort. Both radiographic and endocrinologic evaluation provide data which may be helpful in deciding whether to pursue further studies or to temporize.

Considering radiographic studies first, Kaufmann has presented his criteria for making the diagnosis of non-tumorous enlargement of the sella turcica or 'empty sella'. These include tomograms which show the absence of erosion or changes above the diaphragm in a symmetrical sella with an intact, non-displaced, dorsum sella. DiChiro has cautioned that true volumetric enlargement of the sella always indicates some type of pathological change.

The use of cavernous sinograms to determine lateral extension of the tumor or magnification and subtraction arteriography to identify abnormal vasculature, tumor stain, or absence of the normal posterior pituitary blush appear to be promising methods for the early detection of pituitary tumors.

Endocrine studies have become increasingly sophisticated in the diagnosis of pituitary tumors and should be used in conjunction with the tomograms of the sella in making the decision to proceed to contrast X-ray studies and later to therapy. The combination of a definite anterior pituitary hormone deficit plus enlargement of the sella should suggest tumor until proven otherwise since the 'empty sella syndrome' is usually not associated with endocrine deficiencies. The basal serum prolactin appears to be valuable as a screening test for endocrine abnormalities. Many tumors which were previously thought to be non-functioning probably secrete prolactin even in patients without galactorrhea. The absolute basal level of prolactin and response to stimulation and suppression tests will help to differentiate tumor from other causes of hyperprolactinemia. Evaluation of other pituitary hormones for hypersecretion or deficiency is of obvious value in planning subsequent therapy.

Another more drastic diagnostic test which is emerging is the transsphenoidal pituitary biopsy prior to therapy. This has been recommended by many experts, and the procedure is now relatively safe. The diagnosis of an unsuspected intrasellar craniopharyngioma or a radioresistant cystic adenoma of the pituitary can be made by this technique.

Turning to treatment, there is little data concerning the clinical course of disease among patients receiving no treatment following definitive diagnosis of a pituitary tumor. While the numbers are small, 14 of 16 such patients in Sheline's series developed life threatening complications, suggesting that treatment should be undertaken once a diagnosis is established.

It seems clear that the objectives of therapy should be prevention or resolution of neurologic defects resulting from tumor growth while retaining or restoring normal anterior pituitary function among patients with chromophobe adenomas. In addition to these goals, elimination of the pathophysiologic effects of hormone excess is an objective of treatment in patients having hormone secreting tumors. In addition to functional objectives, prevention of recurrence of extrasellar disease is an indisputable goal since treatment of recurrent tumors seems to be associated with poor results irrespective of how the neoplasms are treated primarily. For large tumors where total ablation is impossible, conventional irradiation following maximal feasible surgical removal of tumor appears to be effective in preventing recurrences in the experience of Fager, Guiot and Sheline.

Some or all of these therapeutic goals have been achieved among patients treated with either surgery or irradiation or combinations of these procedures. However, the therapists have repetitively pointed out that it is difficult to be certain about the validity of comparisons when both the status of tumor at initiation of therapy and criteria of successful treatment were not uniformly defined. These deficiencies in the data minimize its usefulness for predicting response prior to treatment by the different methods available.

The use of heavy particle sources constitutes a significant addition to irradiation therapy for pituitary adenomas secreting hormones. Application is restricted to intrasellar tumors not previously irradiated, so that best results are achieved when the disease is recognized early. Similarly the best surgical results are obtained in transsphenoidal microsurgery as described by Hardy and Guiot when pituitary tumors are suspected and treatment initiated prior to enlargement of the sella. These exciting developments in therapy emphasize the importance of advancements in methodology for early diagnosis of pituitary neoplasms. However, some chromophobe tumors may become quite large while remaining asymptomatic so that delay in diagnosis with resultant large tumors requiring an intracranial surgical procedure probably can never be completely avoided.

It seems clear that experience with any therapeutic regimen is one determinant of the quality of results obtained. Since pituitary tumors are rare, accumulation of significant experience is unlikely outside of referral centers. Furthermore, as technology advances, requisite equipment for both diagnosis and treatment becomes more sophisticated, more expensive, and thus impractical for wide distribution. In the light of these considerations, restricting the treatment of patients suspected of having pituitary tumors to referral centers may be advantageous.

The final objective of the conference was to define areas for future research. Daughaday's hypothesis concerning a role for the hypothalamus in the pathogenesis of pituitary tumors merits additional study. Perhaps additional research directed toward understanding hypothalamic function will enable physicians to prevent neoplasms. As A. Lawrence points out, this hypothesis makes satisfactory medical therapeutic alternatives imaginable and stimulates the search for these. To secure adequate information on comparative efficacy of treatment requiring additional research is necessary. This will involve initial stratification of patients, random assignment to treatment protocols, and long term follow-up using well defined criteria for evaluating response.

Hardy has proposed a schema for the characterization of the extent of disease which is worthy of further evaluation, and Batzdorf has demonstrated the potential usefulness of computer science for storage, retrieval and analysis of these data.

Since pituitary tumors are uncommon, efficient accumulation of such data will require well organized collaborative studies, preferably at an international level. While the problems inherent in such an undertaking are formidable and unlikely to be surmonted quickly, the need for the information is sufficient to justify the effort.

Index of authors

Subject index

Prepared by W. van Westering, M. D., Amsterdam